ERRATUM

An error was introduced during the production of *Lilienfeld's Foundations of Epidemiology, Fourth Edition* (Schneider and Lilienfeld):

On p. 130, the equation for specificity should read:

$$Specificity = \frac{d}{b+d}$$

Lilienfeld's Foundations of Epidemiology

DONA SCHNEIDER, PH.D., M.P.H., F.A.C.E.

DAVID E. LILIENFELD, M.D., M.S. ENGIN., M.P.H., F.A.C.E.

Original Edition by ABRAHAM M. LILIENFELD, M.D., M.P.H., D.SC. (HON.), F.A.C.E.

OXFORD
UNIVERSITY PRESS

OXFORD
UNIVERSITY PRESS

Oxford University Press is a department of the University of
Oxford. It furthers the University's objective of excellence in research,
scholarship, and education by publishing worldwide.

Oxford   New York
Auckland   Cape Town   Dar es Salaam   Hong Kong   Karachi
Kuala Lumpur   Madrid   Melbourne   Mexico City   Nairobi
New Delhi   Shanghai   Taipei   Toronto

With offices in
Argentina   Austria   Brazil   Chile   Czech Republic   France   Greece
Guatemala   Hungary   Italy   Japan   Poland   Portugal   Singapore
South Korea   Switzerland   Thailand   Turkey   Ukraine   Vietnam

Published in the United States of America by
Oxford University Press
198 Madison Avenue, New York, NY 10016

Library of Congress Cataloging-in-Publication Data
Foundations of epidemiology.
Lilienfeld's foundations of epidemiology / Dona Schneider, David E. Lilienfeld; original
edition by Abraham M. Lilienfeld. — Fourth edition.
p. ; cm.
Preceded by Foundations of epidemiology / revised by David E. Lilienfeld,
Paul D. Stolley. 3rd ed. 1994.
Includes bibliographical references and index.
ISBN 978–0–19–537767–5
I. Schneider, Dona, 1946–.   II. Lilienfeld, David E. 1957–.   III. Title.
[DNLM: 1. Epidemiologic Methods.   2. Epidemiology. WA 950]
RA651
614.4—dc23
2015006834

9 8 7 6 5 4 3 2 1
Printed in the United States of America
on acid-free paper

Abraham Morris Lilienfeld (1920–1984), University Distinguished Service Professor at the Johns Hopkins University School of Hygiene and Public Health, wrote the first edition of this book in 1975/6. That edition reflected Lilienfeld's lifelong focus on teaching. One former student described him as having been born "with a piece of chalk in his hand," and with that chalk he would paint rainbows of epidemiology across the blackboard.

Students always had priority in scheduling meetings with Lilienfeld. When those meetings came at the end of the day, he would, at the last minute, regularly invite students home to continue the discussion over dinner. A blackboard hung in the family's kitchen to the side of the informal dining table for precisely this purpose. Doctoral students also sat at that table to review their thesis work with him, or, if more space was required, at the bigger table in the dining room.

Lilienfeld went to great lengths to teach and advocate for epidemiology in any and all venues. He was one of the founders of the University of Minnesota at Minneapolis Summer Program, where he taught epidemiology for three weeks each year. When Alexander Langmuir, his mentor, left Johns Hopkins to found the Epidemic Intelligence Service (EIS) at the Centers for Disease Control, he called upon Lilienfeld to teach introductory epidemiology to all EIS officers during the program's early years. When asked at the last minute to entertain a prominent Kenyan government economics official for the university president, Lilienfeld brought the guest home to "meet the family." During the evening, he regaled the visitor with tales about John Snow and the cholera outbreak investigations. He brought out and showed his guest a piece of the wooden water pipe involved in the outbreak that he husbanded that year as President of the American Epidemiological Society. A few years later, when the Kenyan official's son came to the United States after receiving his MD degree, he attended Johns Hopkins to study epidemiology.

Lilienfeld organized the Public Health Option in the pre-baccalaureate program at Johns Hopkins during the early 1970s, volunteering to teach an introductory epidemiology class for seniors. When the *American Journal of*

Epidemiology was struggling financially in the late 1960s, Lilienfeld suggested that the Society for Epidemiological Research (SER) might be interested in sponsoring the journal. The society subsequently did so. Lilienfeld took great pride in how many SER members learned about different aspects of epidemiology in the course of reading the journal. And, when the first edition of this text appeared, this consummate teacher insisted on keeping the price of the book as low as possible to facilitate access by all students, from undergraduates to post-doctoral fellows. The book appeared at a price of $19.95.

Abraham M. Lilienfeld embodied devotion to teaching about epidemiology to all who would listen. It is to his memory that we dedicate this book, in the spirit of introductory epidemiology as the cornerstone of public health and medicine.

CONTENTS

FOREWORD

The first edition of this text appeared in 1976, but, as explained to me on multiple occasions by the author (my father), its origins trace to more than two decades before. Abraham Morris Lilienfeld trained as an epidemiologist with a focus on infectious diseases. On completion of his training, he joined the epidemiology faculty at the Johns Hopkins School of Hygiene and Public Health (JHU), where he became interested in liver cirrhosis following his work on an infectious hepatitis outbreak in the early 1950s. The etiology of liver cirrhosis was not well understood at that time, but the prevalent hypothesis attributed the disease to alcoholism—not to an infectious agent. Lilienfeld examined the alcohol–liver cirrhosis relationship using the only epidemiologic methods he had available—those traditionally used to examine the etiology of infectious diseases. The utility of those methods for studying noninfectious diseases quickly became evident to him.

When Lilienfeld assumed leadership of the epidemiology program at Roswell Park Memorial Cancer Institute in Buffalo, New York, in 1953, he brought with him a plan to apply traditional epidemiologic methods to study the etiology of cancer. He conceptualized the issue of breast cancer mortality in a new way, with susceptibility to the disease varying with menopausal status, similar to the way susceptibility to an infectious agent varies based on immunization status. This change in framing the question allowed him to demonstrate the benefit of using traditional epidemiologic tools with the emerging diseases of the time—heart disease, cancer, and stroke.

Lilienfeld returned to JHU with a reputation as a methodological innovator. In 1965 the World Health Organization Cancer Unit asked him to collaborate on a book for health care professionals on epidemiologic methods for the study of cancer. *Cancer Epidemiology: Methods of Study* (1967) includes a discussion of John Snow and the mid-Victorian cholera outbreaks in the first five pages of the first chapter. Lilienfeld used this book in his courses on chronic disease epidemiology at JHU for several years. He noted that students found it helpful to have the material presented as a story, and he used the development of epidemiologic knowledge about cigarette smoking and lung cancer as his narrative.

In 1970, Lilienfeld became chair of epidemiology at JHU. With that appointment he took over responsibility for the department's introductory course. He taught the concepts and methods of epidemiology as foundational, truly believing the difference between chronic and infectious disease epidemiology to be an artificial one. By 1972, an entrepreneurial editor (Jeffrey House) at the Oxford University Press approached Lilienfeld about using his lecture notes as the basis for an introductory textbook in epidemiology. The professor declined, as he was lobbying Congress for the Surveillance, Epidemiology, and End Results (SEER) system as part of President Nixon's "War on Cancer," helping multiple doctoral students with their thesis research, developing a center for the epidemiology of gastrointestinal diseases, and continuing to teach his courses. He simply didn't have the time needed to write the book.

Two years later, in November 1974, Lilienfeld collapsed with a cardiac arrest during a lecture in the introductory course in epidemiology. After being resuscitated by the students, he found himself in a rehabilitation program and had to be out of the office for months. Needing a project to engage his considerable intellectual energy, Lilienfeld remembered the invitation to write an introductory textbook on epidemiology. An inquiry found the invitation still open. Within six months, the first draft was completed. Thus was born the **first edition** of *Foundations of Epidemiology* (1976). Students responded positively to the book, and it was adopted for many introductory epidemiology courses.

The **second edition** of the text appeared in 1980, a collaborative effort by father and son. The book was updated to reflect students' stated desires for a different narrative, as the smoking and lung cancer saga was becoming dated. As a result, the second edition shifted to narratives about oral contraceptives and cardiovascular diseases. The discussion of randomized controlled trials was also considerably expanded, reflecting epidemiologists' increasing use of them. The book was thoroughly updated, and the cover changed to show the point-contact spread of an infectious disease outbreak (although in production, the figure was mistakenly inverted).

The Lilienfelds were working on a **third edition** when the elder author died in 1984. Work on the revision was shelved until the early 1990s when a collaboration was struck with Paul Stolley. The didactic material in the third edition was broadened to accord with the expansion in epidemiologic activities during the 1980s. Demographic studies were discussed in a defined section, and the same was true of epidemiologic studies. A discussion of epidemiology in clinical practice was added.

For the **fourth edition**, the role of epidemiology within public health is the central theme. The chapter on inferences is moved forward, as many instructors now discuss causality early in their introductory epidemiology courses. The examples are updated, discussions about vital statistics are broadened to include birth as well as death, and recent concepts such as quality-adjusted life years (QALYs) and disability-adjusted life years (DALYs) have been added. To keep the book brief, it is purposely lean on figures and diagrams. To keep it affordable for students, it has no photos or color sidebars.

Those who have read previous editions of this text will find an old friend in this new edition, one you've known well for a long time, perhaps with some new attire and new stories to be shared. Hopefully, it succeeds in remaining true to the vision Lilienfeld had when creating the first edition describing an integrated field known as epidemiology. While today's world is different from that which he inhabited, and while the field itself has evolved, the core of the information remains as *Lilienfeld's Foundations of Epidemiology*.

DEL

PREFACE

This book is designed as a foundational text for introductory courses in epidemiology wherever they are offered—in schools of public health, medicine, dentistry, nursing, and the allied health professions, as well as undergraduate programs offered by two- and four-year liberal arts colleges and technical schools. The original 1976 edition of this text was written for precisely that purpose, and the fourth edition continues in the same tradition. We recognize, however, that pedagogical expectations for an introductory epidemiology text have changed over the years. Today, at the undergraduate level a successful text must address the set of expected discipline-specific learning outcomes developed from a national consensus of public health and liberal arts educators. At the graduate level such a text must help students develop the epidemiologic competencies that will aid them in their professional careers. We believe a foundational text can do both.

Because epidemiology is an inherently integrative discipline, it is not uncommon for texts to use different words to describe the same concept. For instance, some texts use the term *relative risk*, whereas others may use *rate ratio* or *risk ratio*. It can be confusing for students if their reading of the literature is not in line with the teachings in their introductory text. To address this dissonance, throughout this text complementary terms appear in parentheses and all definitions provided are synonymous with those from the *Dictionary of Epidemiology, 6th Edition*.

This text is divided into four parts. Part I (Introduction to Epidemiology) reviews the historical background and conceptual basis for epidemiology. Part II (Descriptive Studies) covers sources of epidemiologic data and the study designs that can be used to describe mortality and morbidity in human populations. The epidemiologic designs used to test hypotheses about health-related outcomes are discussed in detail in Part III (Analytic Studies), including the advantages and disadvantages of each. Finally, Part IV (Using Epidemiologic Information) includes chapters that show the reach of epidemiology into various disciplines—including field investigations, health care planning, and the clinical realms.

The reasoning processes used by epidemiologists to address health-related problems are illustrated throughout the book using both classic and contemporary examples. Problems sets are provided in some chapters to give students an opportunity to apply the epidemiologic methods and reasoning processes that constitute the field to contemporary health-related issues. Some of these issues are intentionally designed to evoke various viewpoints and should serve to spark classroom discussion. Thus, the text covers a broad reach of epidemiologic concepts and focuses on the interdisciplinary approach. We feel it important to describe not only how epidemiologic concepts developed over time, but also to demonstrate how the approach continues to be practical for understanding today's, and even tomorrow's, health-related outcomes.

I | Introduction to Epidemiology

The work of epidemiology is related to unanswered questions, but also to unquestioned answers.[1]

Patricia Buffler (2011)

PART I PROVIDES AN introduction to epidemiologic thinking and how it developed over time. The opening chapter explains how epidemiology uses a *comparative* approach, focusing on *disparities* (how health-related outcomes vary across time, in different places, and among different population subgroups). The epidemiologist's ultimate goal is to find, reduce, or eliminate those factors that cause disease and other adverse health outcomes. To achieve this goal, the epidemiologist must first determine who is at risk and why. The second step is for the epidemiologist to conduct carefully designed studies to test hypotheses about potential *etiological (causal) factors*.

Chapter 2 gives a brief account of the history of epidemiology, showing how epidemiology evolved into its present form. The major figures in the development of epidemiology are mentioned, and historical examples that demonstrate the uses of epidemiology are presented.

Chapter 3 covers the general principles and terminology used to classify diseases for the purposes of epidemiologic studies. The triad of agent–host–environment is discussed in detail, and the spectrum of disease, both infectious and noninfectious, with its associated terminology is introduced. Chapter 3 concludes with a discussion of herd immunity, the epidemiologic basis for national vaccination policies.

This introduction to epidemiology concludes with Chapter 4, which describes the way in which epidemiologists draw inferences from hypothesis-based studies. Of particular importance is how the epidemiologist determines whether the statistical results from these studies do or do not support a factor being causally-related to a particular health outcome.

Reference

1. Patricia Buffler, "Keynote address for the North American Congress of Epidemiology," Montreal, Canada, July 2011.

1 | Laying the Foundations

Epidemiology came to mean the study of disease, any disease, as
a mass phenomenon ... The physician's unit of study is a single
human being ... The epidemiologist's unit of study is ... an
aggregate of human beings.[1]

Major Greenwood (1932)

PIDEMIOLOGY IS "THE STUDY OF the occurrence and distribution of
health-related events, states, and processes in specified populations,
including the study of the determinants influencing such processes,
and the application of this knowledge to control relevant health problems."[2]
In other words, not only does epidemiology identify patterns of health-related
problems in populations, but it also investigates the underlying causes of
those problems and offers the results of well-designed studies as the basis
for implementing plans to improve the public's health. We must add that epidemiology is an integrative, eclectic science deriving concepts and methods
from other disciplines, especially anthropology, biology, geography, history,
sociology, and statistics. This interdisciplinary approach has led to epidemiology being taught not only in medical schools and schools of public health,
but also to undergraduates in both two-year and four-year liberal arts and
professional programs such as nursing and the allied health professions.

Epidemiologists are primarily interested in the way health outcomes differ according to *time, place,* and *persons.* They examine whether changes have
occurred in health-related states or events over days, months, or years (time);
whether one geographical area (place) differs from another in the frequency
of health-related outcomes; and whether the characteristics of individuals (persons) with a particular disease or condition distinguish them from
others.

Epidemiologists are concerned with the following characteristics of persons:

- Demographic factors such as age, gender, race, and ethnic group
- Biological factors such as circulating levels of antibodies, chemicals, and enzymes; blood constituents such as cells and platelets; and measurements of the physiological functions of organs and systems, such as blood glucose or hormone levels
- Social and economic factors such as socioeconomic status, educational background, occupation, and place of birth
- Behavioral factors such as tobacco and drug use, diet, and physical exercise
- Genetic factors such as blood groups or gene mutations

Understanding the confluence of these characteristics of persons in time and space, and being able to define each of them clearly and precisely at the outset of an epidemiologic inquiry, is the cornerstone to developing a good study design.

Purposes of Epidemiologic Inquiries

Epidemiologic studies are usually designed to yield information that can:

- Provide data that will help clarify the *etiology* or cause(s) of specific health outcomes
- Determine whether epidemiologic data are consistent with causal hypotheses developed clinically, experimentally, or from other studies
- Provide data that can help develop and evaluate preventive procedures, public health practices, and other types of health-related services

Etiological Studies

An example of how epidemiologists seek to determine *etiologic* (causal) *factors* comes from occupational epidemiology, where the frequency of disease may be observed to be higher among workers with particular exposures than among the general population. For instance, in 1955 the English epidemiologist Sir Richard Doll reported the occurrence of 18 cases of lung cancer among 105 asbestos factory workers. He concluded that asbestos was a cause of lung cancer, although the risk seemed confined to those with the greatest exposures.[3]

Selikoff and his colleagues examined the effects of asbestos on the end users of asbestos products by reviewing two decades of records from building insulation workers' unions in New York and New Jersey. Beginning on December 31, 1942, the deaths of members were followed to see what proportion died from lung cancer. The researchers found that of 255 union members, 45 died from cancers of the lung and pleura. They concurred with Doll that asbestos was a cause of lung cancer, even for workers who had lower exposures to asbestos than those experienced by the factory workers.[4]

Could cigarette smoking explain some of the relationship between asbestos and lung cancer? The investigators addressed this question by expanding their previous study to include all 17,800 asbestos insulation workers in the United States. Using data from a study conducted by the American Cancer Society to determine the rate of death from lung cancer in the general population, the researchers determined that asbestos insulation workers who smoked cigarettes were 53.2 times as likely to die from lung cancer compared with nonsmokers with no exposure to asbestos. For workers exposed to asbestos who did not smoke cigarettes, the elevation in risk was 5.2 times as high. Among the general population (those not exposed to asbestos in the workplace), cigarette smokers had a risk of lung cancer that was 10.8 times that of nonsmokers. The researchers concluded that asbestos was a cause of lung cancer, and that exposure to asbestos interacts with cigarette smoking to markedly increase that risk beyond that of either factor alone.[5]

It is not always true that exposure to chemicals increases the risk of adverse health outcomes. Indeed, occasionally an epidemiologic study finds that a chemical exposure provides a protective effect. A classic example of a protective effect is that of the presence of fluoride in drinking water reducing the risk of dental caries. Around 1915, a practicing dentist in Colorado formed the clinical impression that his patients with mottled teeth had fewer dental caries than his other patients.[6-8] By the late 1930s, dentists understood that patients presenting with mottled tooth enamel had been chronically exposed to high levels of fluoride in drinking water before their permanent teeth had erupted.[9-11] This combination of findings led the Public Health Service to conduct surveys of children aged 12–14 years in 21 cities in four states where the fluoride concentration in the water supply varied considerably.[12] The results showed that dental caries decreased with increasing fluoride content in drinking water, suggesting that adding fluoride to the water supply should decrease the frequency of dental caries (Figure 1.1).

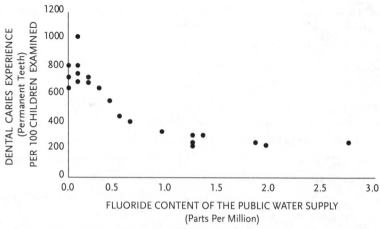

FIGURE 1.1 Relationship between the amount of dental caries (permanent teeth) observed in 7257 selected 12- to 14-year-old white school children of 21 cities of 4 states and the fluoride (F) content of public water supply.

SOURCE: Dean, Arnold, and Elvove (1942).[12]

The relationship between exposure to fluoride and reduced dental caries was then tested by experiment. The Public Health Service determined that fluoride would be added to the water supply of one community, and the water supply of a comparable community would remain naturally low. Over the course of several years, dentists could record the dental caries experience of school children in the communities and the rates could be compared. Several matched community studies were initiated, including one in 1945 comparing Newburgh and Kingston, New York.[13] After several years, school children in Newburgh (the town with fluoride added to the water supply) had 50 percent fewer decayed, missing, or filled teeth than school children in Kingston (the town without added fluoride). This example demonstrates how epidemiologic information is used to develop public health policy; namely, a practitioner's clinical impression led to an epidemiologic survey that then led to a well-designed epidemiologic experiment. The results of the experimental study eventually led to public health policy whereby fluoride was added to the drinking water supplies of many US communities.

Evaluating Consistency

It is fairly common for an epidemiologist to test an etiological hypothesis developed from clinical, experimental, or other studies to see whether it is consistent, i.e. whether the results will be the same if the study is repeated using various populations in other places or at different times. For example, oral contraceptives became widely available during the early 1960s. Case reports and the results of several epidemiologic studies showed relationships between oral contraceptive use and venous thromboembolism (blood clots), thrombotic stroke, and myocardial infarction.[14-16] Additional studies were undertaken to see if the findings held for women in different age groups.[17,18] Scores of epidemiologic studies followed and continue today comparing the risk of contraceptive use among women living in various countries, who have varying risk factors (smoking, family history of stroke), and who are taking different formulations of oral contraceptives, at different dosages, and for different lengths of time. The findings have been consistently demonstrated across multiple study populations over the years.

Basis for Preventive and Public Health Services

Epidemiologic data provide a means of evaluating the current health of populations, whether health-related outcomes vary over time, and whether prevention programs work. Examples of epidemiologic data include birth and death rates, as well as information gathered by disease registries and surveys of health risk behaviors. A complete discussion of these types of data appears in Part II of this text. Disease surveillance programs also add to the wealth of information on population health, as does the evaluation of the effectiveness of public health services. An in-depth discussion of the role of surveillance appears in Chapter 7, and new ways of obtaining surveillance data are covered in Chapter 14.

The study that determined the effectiveness of the Salk vaccine for preventing poliomyelitis is a classic example of how epidemiology contributes to preventive and public health services.[19] A more recent example is how epidemiologic data helped formulate recommendations for the human papilloma virus (HPV) vaccine program. Epidemiologic modeling suggested that vaccinating preadolescent females for HPV would reduce the number of cervical cancer cases in the vaccinated group by 62 percent. Vaccinating boys, however, would only reduce cervical cancer cases by 2 percent, a less cost-effective approach compared to a female-focused vaccination program.[20] Accordingly, HPV vaccination was originally recommended for girls alone. That recommendation was later amended to include boys when new epidemiologic data suggested that vaccinating boys would also reduce the occurrence of 7,000 penile, anal, and oropharyngeal cancers in the United States annually.[21] This example demonstrates how necessary it is to routinely review epidemiologic data in order to best design and implement successful public health prevention programs.

Epidemiologic information on how health status is distributed across time, place, and persons informs public health practice. It allows physicians and public health professionals to target populations where prevention, screening, and healthcare services should be focused in order to get the most out of public health resources. This holds true even if the underlying cause of a particular health state is not known. For example, diabetes mellitus was demonstrated to run in families by researchers at the Mayo Clinic as early as 1952.[22] The reason why this happens, whether there is a genetic etiology for diabetes, or whether environmental factors common to family members explain the development of diabetes, is not really important. All that a physician or public health practitioner needs to know is that there is an increased risk of developing diabetes among the family members of known diabetics. Thus, screening a diabetic patient's parents, siblings, and offspring will likely yield additional cases of the disease in this high-risk population.

Content of Epidemiologic Activities

Epidemiologists engage in two broad areas of study: observational and experimental epidemiology. Each area involves different methods.

Observational Epidemiology

The vast majority of epidemiologic studies fall into the observational category. For instance, the studies described above of employees exposed to certain chemical compounds, surveys of dental caries, and familial aggregation of diabetes, are all examples of observational investigations. Epidemiologists have developed appropriate methods for selecting populations and subgroups to observe, as well as various techniques for analyzing the information obtained from such studies. These topics are covered in Chapters 5 through 8 (Descriptive Studies) and in Chapters 9 and 10 (Observational Studies).

Occasionally, an investigator may observe the occurrence of a disease or other health-related outcome under existing conditions that closely approximate a controlled experiment. Inferences about causal factors derived from these *natural experiments* are considerably stronger than if they had been derived solely from observational studies. The studies in England by Doll, Hill, and Peto on the relationship between tobacco use and lung cancer illustrate this approach.[23-26] In 1951, the investigators ascertained the smoking habits of British male physicians aged 35 years and over and followed them

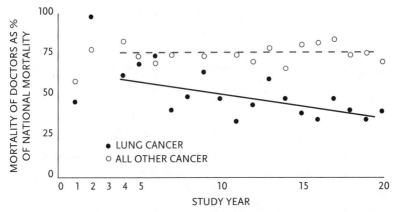

FIGURE 1.2 Trend in number of deaths certified in male doctors as percentage of number expected from experience of all men in England and Wales of same ages.

SOURCE: Doll and Peto (1976).[24] Copyright 1976, *British Medical Journal*. Reproduced with permission of BMJ Publishing Group, Ltd.

to determine their mortality from different causes, particularly lung cancer. Initial findings indicated that physicians who smoked cigarettes had a mortality rate from lung cancer that was about 10 times that of nonsmoking physicians.[23] Questionnaires were sent to the same physicians to determine their cigarette smoking habits in 1956, 1966, and 1971. Data from these surveys showed an approximately 50 percent decline in cigarette smoking among the physicians over the 20-year period.[24] The investigators then compared the cancer mortality experience for the physicians.[23] The mortality from lung cancer declined by about 40 percent with essentially no decline in other cancer deaths. In this case, the decline in cigarette smoking among male British physicians was a natural experiment that yielded a concomitant decline in lung cancer mortality for that group (Figure 1.2).[23]

Experimental Epidemiology

In controlled experiments, the investigator controls which population groups are exposed to specific *therapeutic* interventions (e.g., drugs to treat a disease, surgical procedures, and behavior modification) or *preventive* interventions (vitamin supplementation and smoking cessation programs). The Newburgh–Kingston dental caries study presented above was a controlled experiment. An important feature of experimental studies is that the investigator can randomly allocate subjects to the experimental and control groups, thereby minimizing the influence of factors other than the one being studied in the trial. The methods for assigning subjects in an experimental study are discussed in greater detail in Chapters 11 and 12.

Development and Evaluation of Study Methods

As new public health challenges emerged over time, epidemiologists developed new analytical methods to address them. Some of the methods were adapted from other disciplines, specifically those that utilized a *comparative* approach (comparing different time periods, places, and populations or subgroups). Epidemiologists use the comparative approach for various types of investigations, including those comparing infectious and noninfectious diseases, acute and chronic conditions effecting population health, public health prevention efforts, and medical interventions.[27]

The Sequence of Epidemiologic Reasoning

Epidemiologic reasoning is a two-stage process for clarifying the etiology of health-related states or outcomes. The sequence of reasoning is as follows:

1. Determine the statistical association between a characteristic and a health outcome
2. Derive causal inferences from the patterns of the statistical associations

The methods used to determine the statistical associations may be based on either group or individual factors. While there is a certain degree of overlap between these two categories, it is extremely useful to make the distinction between them. For example, *descriptive studies* (sometimes called *demographic studies*) allow the epidemiologist to compare the health status of different population groups in the expectation that any observed differences can be related to differences in the local environments, personal living habits, or even the genetic composition of these groups. Descriptive studies also provide information on trends in population health and may lead to hypotheses about why the observed patterns exist. The drawback of descriptive studies is that while data on the population being studied may be available, information on the individuals that make up that population may not. In those instances, the epidemiologist may rely on *ecological data* (also called *aggregate data, group data,* or *population data*) for making group comparisons. This lack of information on individuals presents a problem.

As an example, let us assume that Community A (with a high consumption of alcohol) has a higher mortality rate from lung cancer than

Community B (with no consumption of alcohol). This comparison suggests that drinking alcohol may be of etiological importance for developing lung cancer. However, the statistical relationship with alcohol only provides a clue for further investigation because of the problem of *ecological fallacy*, an erroneous conclusion that a statistical relationship existing at the group level also holds at the individual level.[28] While Communities A and B differ in their alcohol consumption, they may also differ in other factors not examined, such as cigarette smoking. One or more of these unexamined factors may be an underlying explanation for the observed lung cancer mortality experiences of the two communities, and not necessarily their alcohol consumption.[29–32]

After an association has been established from ecological data, clinical observations, or laboratory experiments, the epidemiologist attempts to determine whether the same association is present among individuals. Our ecological analysis suggested an association between alcohol consumption and developing lung cancer. Questions posed about individuals from both Communities A and B might include the following:

1. Do persons with the disease (lung cancer) have the characteristic (alcohol consumption) more frequently than those without the disease?
2. Do persons with the characteristic (alcohol consumption) develop the disease (lung cancer) more frequently than those who do not have the characteristic?

These questions can be addressed through cross-sectional, case-control, and cohort study designs, discussed in detail in Chapters 7, 9, and 10.

A Case Study Exemplifying the Epidemiologic Approach

One of the most common uses of the epidemiologic approach is the investigation of a foodborne outbreak. The term *outbreak* is often used to describe an excess of cases in a localized or time-limited situation, whereas the term *epidemic* is often preferred for describing a situation that is more widespread or that occurs over a longer period of time. While the primary goal of foodborne outbreak investigations is to identify the microbe or chemical contaminating the food and causing the illness, the secondary goal is to put safety measures into place (such as removing contaminated foodstuffs from stores, training food handlers to wash their hands, or repairing refrigeration units) to prevent a recurrence.

Foodborne outbreak investigations ascertain (1) whether there has been an outbreak and (2) whether there is a statistical association between the consumption of a specific food and a specific foodborne illness. Consider the classic example of an outbreak of gastroenteritis originally investigated by the New York State Department of Public Health. On an April day in 1940, the local health officer for Lycoming in Oswego County reported an apparent outbreak of acute gastrointestinal illness to the regional health office. An epidemiologist was assigned to investigate and learned that all persons known to be ill had attended a church supper the previous evening. As their family members who had not attended the event had not become ill, the epidemiologist focused on events related to the church supper. All attendees at the supper were interviewed to determine whether or not they developed symptoms of gastroenteritis. If so, they were asked when (day and hour) the symptoms first appeared. Everyone was asked which food(s) they consumed at the supper. Of the 80 attendees, 46 persons were found to have had symptoms of gastroenteritis.[33]

The first step in assessing whether an outbreak has occurred requires calculating the *crude attack rate*.

$$Crude\,attack\,rate = \frac{Number\,of\,persons\,ill\,with\,disease}{Number\,of\,persons\,attending\,the\,event}$$

In this case, the crude attack rate was almost 58 percent (46/80), far beyond what might be expected in the general population (the *endemic* or background rate of disease) or what might occur from seasonal or random variation. This finding led the epidemiologist to conclude that he was dealing with a probable foodborne outbreak.

The second step in an outbreak investigation is to develop a *case definition* that includes time, place, and person variables, as well as diagnosis or symptomatology. In our example, the case definition was as follows: All persons who developed acute gastrointestinal *symptoms* within 72 hours after eating supper on April 18, 1940 (*time*), and who were among attendees (*persons*) of the Oswego Church supper in Lycoming, New York (*place*). Every individual who attended the event was interviewed (whether they became ill or not) to determine what foods (including water and condiments) they did or did not consume. If they became ill, it was important to determine the time when their symptoms first appeared. The information was then entered into a *line listing* (spreadsheet) and used to develop two epidemiologic tools: a table of food-specific attack rates and an *epidemic curve*.

The attack rates for each food served at the church supper were calculated using the following formula:

$$Food\text{-}specific\ attack\ rate = \frac{Number\ of\ persons\ who\ ate\ the\ food\ and\ became\ ill}{Total\ number\ of\ persons\ who\ ate\ the\ food}$$

To identify the contaminated food, the epidemiologist then calculated the ratio of food-specific attack rates (*rate ratio*) for each menu item and compared the results to identify which food(s) were the likely cause of the illness.

$$Rate\ ratio = \frac{Food\text{-}specific\ attack\ rate\ for\ those\ who\ become\ ill}{Food\text{-}specific\ attack\ rate\ for\ those\ who\ remained\ well}$$

Table 1.1 shows that persons who ate the vanilla ice cream at the church supper were 5.7 times more likely to become ill than those who did not eat it, representing the greatest discrepancy between the attack rates of those consuming and not consuming each specific foodstuff. The epidemiologist was able to conclude that the vanilla ice cream was the likely source of the contamination that caused the illness.

Laboratory investigations may be undertaken to identify the chemical or microorganism that contaminated the food and was responsible for the outbreak. Samples from remaining food items may further inform the investigation, as well as biological samples (stool and/or blood) from individuals who became ill and from those who prepared or served the food. It may be impossible to sample the food identified as the source of the outbreak if it was completely consumed or discarded. In these instances, the investigator may make efforts to track food items back into the food supply or use an additional tool—the epidemic curve—to aid in the identification of the most likely agent. A full discussion of the epidemic curve is presented in Chapter 3.

Foodborne and other types of outbreaks may be difficult to investigate because the world has become a complex place. Interstate and international travel, trade agreements, and the rapid transport of goods and foodstuffs can make it difficult to work through foodborne outbreaks. When the outbreak described above occurred in 1940, surveillance systems with real-time reporting did not exist. In 1996, the United States Centers for Disease Control and Prevention (CDC) put into place *FoodNet*, an active surveillance network covering 10 areas of the United States (Connecticut, Georgia, Maryland, Minnesota, New Mexico, Oregon, Tennessee, and selected counties in California, Colorado, and New York).[34] FoodNet requires reporting

TABLE 1.1 Food-Specific Attack Rates

FOOD	ATE THE FOOD				DID NOT EAT THE FOOD				RATE RATIO*
	ILL	WELL	TOTAL	ATTACK RATE (%)	ILL	WELL	TOTAL	ATTACK RATE (%)	
Baked ham	29	17	46	63	17	12	29	59	1.1
Spinach	26	17	43	60	20	12	32	63	1.0
Mashed potato	23	14	37	62	23	14	37	62	1.0
Cabbage salad	18	10	28	64	28	19	47	60	1.1
Jello	16	7	23	70	30	22	52	58	1.2
Rolls	21	16	37	57	25	13	38	66	0.9
Brown bread	18	9	27	67	28	20	48	58	1.2
Milk	2	2	4	50	44	27	71	62	0.8
Coffee	19	12	31	61	27	17	44	61	1.0
Water	13	11	24	54	33	18	51	65	0.8
Cakes	27	13	40	68	19	16	35	54	1.3
Ice cream (van)	43	11	54	80	3	18	21	14	5.7
Ice cream (choc)	25	22	47	53	20	7	27	74	0.7
Fruit salad	4	2	6	67	42	27	69	61	1.1

* RATE RATIO IS CALCULATED AS RATIO OF CALCULATED ATTACK RATES. FOR INSTANCE, FOR BAKED HAM, THE RATE RATIO IS 0.63/0.59, OR 1.1.
SOURCE: Centers for Disease Control and Prevention (1981). [33]

of all laboratory-confirmed cases of infections caused by *Campylobacter,* *Cryptosporidium, Cyclospora, Listeria, Salmonella,* Shiga toxin-producing *Escherichia coli* (STEC 0157 and non-0157), *Shigella, Vibrio,* and *Yersinia,* as well as hospitalized cases of hemolytic uremic syndrome (a complication of STEC). FoodNet does not, however, serve the purpose of national outbreak surveillance in real time. To that end, the CDC maintains the *National Outbreak Reporting System* (NORS)[35] to track all foodborne, waterborne, and other types of enteric outbreaks in all US states and territories. NORS became Web-based as of 2009, allowing faster responses to outbreaks by state and local public health agencies. The data generated from NORS should allow epidemiologists and health policymakers to design and implement more effective measures to reduce the burden of foodborne and waterborne outbreaks on the population. Similar national foodborne disease surveillance systems have been developed in the United Kingdom (by the Health Protection Agency), France (a network of 14 National Reference Centers), and other European countries, under the aegis of the World Health Organization.

The interested reader can find information on the historical use of the Lycoming outbreak in Gross's description of the outbreak investigation 35 years after it occurred.[36] The techniques used in the Lycoming outbreak investigation have now been used by epidemiologists for more than a century, although the statistical analyses used have evolved since the first known effort to investigate a foodborne outbreak in England in 1902.[37]

Summary

Epidemiology is a comparative science in which the investigator examines the relationship of health-related outcomes with the presence or absence of various factors in populations. Descriptive studies are used to formulate etiological hypotheses about the patterns of these outcomes based on time, place, and person factors. Analytic studies (observational and experimental) are used to test hypotheses and to provide insights into the potential causes of the outcomes being evaluated. Epidemiologic activities include (1) descriptive and observational studies, where the investigator does not control exposure to subjects in the study, (2) experimental studies, where the investigator does control subjects' exposure, as well as (3) the development and evaluation of new study methods.

Epidemiologic reasoning is a two-stage process for clarifying the etiology of health-related states or outcomes. The first stage is deriving a statistical association between a characteristic and a health outcome, a task that may be achieved through the use of descriptive studies. Conclusions based on statistical relationships derived from descriptive studies must be formulated carefully, however, as they are based on population data and are prone to ecological fallacy.

The second stage of epidemiologic reasoning requires testing causal hypotheses (generated from the first stage) using analytic methods. An example of the second stage was offered in the investigation of a foodborne outbreak. The source of an outbreak could be found by comparing the attack rates among persons who consumed a given food with those for persons who did not consume that food. The food item with the greatest disparity in attack rates (rate ratio) was the likely source of the outbreak.

References

1. Major Greenwood, *Epidemiology: Historical and Experimental.* Baltimore: Johns Hopkins Press, 1932.
2. Miquel Porta, ed., *A Dictionary of Epidemiology, 6th Edition.* New York: Oxford University Press, 2014.
3. Richard Doll, "Mortality from Lung Cancer in Asbestos Workers," *British Journal of Industrial Medicine* 12 (1955): 81–86.
4. Irving J. Selikoff, Jacob Churg, and E. Cuyler Hammond, "Asbestos Exposure and Neoplasia." *JAMA* 188 (1964): 22–26.
5. Irving J. Selikoff, E. Cuyler Hammond, and Herbert Seidman, "Mortality Experience of Insulation Workers in the United States and Canada, 1943–1976," *Annals of the New York Academy of Medicine* 330 (1979): 91–116.
6. F. S. McKay and G. V. Black, "Mottled Teeth: An Endemic Developmental Imperfection of the Enamel of the Teeth Heretofore Unknown in the Literature of Dentistry," *Dental Cosmos* 58, no. 5 (1916): 477–484.
7. F. S. McKay and G. V. Black, "An Investigation of Mottled Teeth," *Dental Cosmos* 58 (1916): 627–644; 781–792; 894–904.
8. F. S. McKay, "Mottled Enamel: A Fundamental Problem in Dentistry," *Dental Cosmos* 67, no. 9 (1925): 847–860.
9. H. Trendley Dean and Elias Elvove, "Some Epidemiological Aspects of Chronic Endemic Dental Fluorosis," *American Journal of Public Health and the Nation's Health* 26, no. 6 (1936): 567–575.
10. H. Trendley Dean, "Endemic Fluorosis and Its Relation to Dental Caries," *Public Health Reports* 53, no. 33 (1938): 1443–1498.
11. H. Trendley Dean, Phillip Jay, Francis A. Arnold, Jr., Frank J. McClure, and Elias Elvove, "Domestic Water and Dental Caries, Including Certain Epidemiological Aspects of Oral *L. acidophilus,*" *Public Health Reports* 54, no. 21 (1939): 862–888.
12. H. Trendley Dean, Francis A. Arnold, and Elias Elvove, "Domestic Water and Dental Caries," *Public Health Reports* 57, no. 32 (1942): 1155–1179.
13. David B. Ast and Edward R. Schlesinger, "The Conclusion of a Ten-Year Study of Water Fluoridation," *American Journal of Public Health and the Nation's Health* 46, no 3 (1956): 265–271.

14. J. Boyce, J. W. Fawcett, and E. W. Noall, "Coronary Thrombosis and Conovide," *Lancet* 1, no. 7272 (1963): 111.
15. Collaborative Group for the Study of Stroke in Young Women. "Oral Contraception and Increased Risk of Cerebral Ischemia or Thrombosis," *New England Journal of Medicine* 288, no. 17 (1973): 871–878.
16. M. P. Vessey and J. I. Mann, "Female Sex Hormones and Thrombosis. Epidemiological Aspects," *British Medical Bulletin* 2, no. 34 (1978): 157–162.
17. J. I. Mann, Richard Doll, Margaret Thorogood, M. P. Vessey, and W. E. Waters, "Risk Factors for Myocardial Infarction in Young Women," *British Journal of Preventive & Social Medicine* 30, no. 2 (1976): 94–100.
18. J. I. Mann, M. H. W. Inman, and Margaret Thorogood, "Oral Contraceptive Use in Older Women and Fatal Myocardial Infarction," *British Medical Journal* 2, no 6033 (1976): 445–447.
19. Francis T Jr, Korns RF, Voight RB, et al. An Evaluation of the 1954 Poliomyelitis Vaccine Trials. *American Journal of Public Health and the Nation's Health* 45, Part 2 (1955): 1–63.
20. A. V. Taira, C. P. Neukermans, and G. D. Sanders, "Evaluating Human Papillomavirus Vaccination Programs," *Emerging Infectious Diseases* 10, no. 11 (2004): 1915–1923.
21. Centers for Disease Control and Prevention. "Vaccines: HPV Vaccine FAQS." Available at http://www.cdc.gov/vaccines/vpd-vac/hpv/vac-faqs.htm.
22. Arthur G. Steinberg and Russell M. Wilder, "A Study of the Genetics of Diabetes Mellitus," *American Journal of Human Genetics* 4, no. 2 (1952): 113–135.
23. Richard Doll and A. Bradford Hill, "Smoking and Carcinoma of the Lung," *British Medical Journal* 2, no. 4682 (1950): 739–748.
24. Richard Doll and Richard Peto, "Mortality in Relation to Smoking: 20 Years' Observations on Male British Doctors," *British Medical Journal* 2, no. 6051 (1976): 1525–1536.
25. Richard Doll, Richard Gray, Barbara Hafner, and Richard Peto, "Mortality in Relation to Smoking: 22 Years' Observations on Female British Doctors," *British Medical Journal* 280, no. 6219 (1980): 967–971.
26. Royal College of Physicians. *Smoking and Health Now: A new report and summary on smoking and its effects on health.* London: Royal College of Physicians of London, Pitman Medical and Scientific Publishing Company, 1971.
27. Abraham M. Lilienfeld, "Epidemiology of Infectious and Non-Infectious Disease: Some Comparisons," *American Journal of Epidemiology* 97, no. 3 (1973): 135–147.
28. Hal Morgenstern, "Uses of Ecologic Analysis in Epidemiologic Research," *American Journal of Public Health* 72, no. 12 (1982): 1336–1344.
29. Leo A. Goodman, "Ecological Regressions and Behavior of Individuals," *American Sociological Review* 18 (1953): 663–664.
30. Steven Piantadosi, David P. Byar, and Sylvan B. Green, "The Ecological Fallacy," *American Journal of Epidemiology* 127, no. 5 (1988): 893–904.
31. William S. Robinson, "Ecological Correlations and the Behavior of Individuals," *International Journal of Epidemiology* 38, no. 2 (2009): 337–341.
32. H. C. Selvin, "Durkheim's Suicide and Problems of Empirical Research," *American Journal of Sociology* 63, no. 6 (1958): 607–619.

33. Centers for Disease Control and Prevention Epidemiology Program Office. "An Outbreak of Gastrointestinal Illness Following a Church Supper, Lycoming, Oswego County, New York, June 19, 1940." Atlanta, GA: US Department of Health and Human Services, Public Health Service, 1981.

34. Centers for Disease Control and Prevention. "Foodborne Diseases Active Surveillance Network (FoodNet)." Available at http://www.cdc.gov/foodnet/.

35. Centers for Disease Control and Prevention, "National Outbreak Reporting System (NORS, Food)." Available at http://www.cdc.gov/nors/.

36. Michael Gross, "Oswego County Revisited," *Public Health Reports* 91 (1976): 168–170.

37. Alfredo Morabia and Anne Hardy, "The Pioneering Use of a Questionnaire to Investigate a Food Borne Disease Outbreak in Early 20th Century Britain," *Journal of Epidemiology and Community Health* 59 (2005): 94–99.

Problem Set: Chapter 1

1. A large Coast Guard training center served a special breakfast for 535 recruits who were landlocked over a major holiday weekend. The clinic physician at the training center, Dr. Treadwater, began seeing recruits with the same symptoms (nausea, vomiting, and diarrhea) throughout the morning and into the afternoon. In total, 58 recruits were being treated for what appeared to be the same illness before the end of the day. Dr. Treadwater felt strongly that the clinic was dealing with a foodborne outbreak. Help Dr. Treadwater by calculating the crude attack rate for the suspected foodborne outbreak following the special breakfast.

2. Dr. Treadwater was concerned that additional recruits may have been ill but not ill enough to come to the clinic for treatment. The physician assistant at the clinic, PA Ondeck, was charged with surveying all of the recruits about which food items they ate at the special breakfast and whether or not they experienced similar symptoms. PA Ondeck found a few additional cases, and he created a line listing of the recruits' responses to his questions. The line listing appears below.

FOOD	CONSUMED FOOD		DID NOT CONSUME FOOD	
	NUMBER WELL	NUMBER ILL	NUMBER WELL	NUMBER ILL
Tomato juice	204	47	263	21
Cantaloupe	290	53	177	15
Creamed chipped beef	147	60	320	8
Potatoes	161	44	306	24
Eggs	169	39	298	29
Pastry	204	34	263	34
Toast	238	46	229	22
Milk	301	50	166	18

Help PA Ondeck by creating a table that includes the food-specific attack rates following the special breakfast that morning.

3. Dr. Treadwater asks PA Ondeck for the rate ratios to narrow down which food item might have been contaminated with the causative agent of the outbreak. Help PA Ondeck by calculating the rate ratios for each item to one decimal point and enter them into your table.

4. Dr. Treadwater asks you which food item you believe is the likely cause of this "common source" outbreak. Explain your choice.

5. Why might so many of the recruits who ate the creamed chipped beef not have become ill? Why might some who did not eat it still become ill?

6. What additional investigations could be done to determine the source of the likely causative agent?

7. How can such foodborne outbreaks be prevented at the Coast Guard training center in the future?

2 | Threads of Epidemiologic History

Don't you (forget about me)[1] . . .

Keith Forsey and Steve Schiff (1984)

PIDEMIOLOGY IS AN ECLECTIC DISCIPLINE, so its history is generally interwoven with that of other academic disciplines. In the nineteenth century, however, epidemiology began developing its own philosophy, concepts, and methods. This chapter focuses on two major components that helped the discipline develop its unique framework: theories of disease etiology and the development of epidemiologic methods.

Theories of Disease Etiology

The idea that the environment can influence the occurrence of disease had its origins in antiquity. For instance, circa 400 BCE, Hippocrates' *On Airs, Waters, and Places* stressed:

> Whoever wishes to investigate medicine properly, should proceed thus: in the first place to consider the seasons of the year . . . Then the winds . . . We must also consider the qualities of the waters . . . And the mode in which the inhabitants live, and what are their pursuits, whether they are fond of drinking and eating to excess, and given to indolence, or are fond of exercise and labor, not given to excess in eating and drinking.[2]

The Greek physician was not alone in his concerns. In the first century BCE, the Roman architect for Caesar Augustus, Vitruvius, wrote about the dangers of locating a city near fetid swamplands:

> For when the morning breezes blow toward the town at sunrise, if they bring with them mist from marshes and, mingled with the mist, the poisonous

breath of creatures of the marshes to be wafted into the bodies of the inhabitants, they will make the site unhealthy.[3]

In the same time period, Pliny the Elder noted the deleterious effect of occupational exposures to asbestos and mercury,[4] and the Roman poet Lucretius wrote:

> ... when men are following up the veins of gold and silver, probing with the pick deep into the hidden parts of earth, what stenches Scaptensula [a town in Thrace] breathes out underground? And what poison gold mines may exhale! How strange they make men's faces, how they change their colour! Have you not seen or heard how they are wont to die in a short time and how the powers of life fail those, whom the strong force of necessity imprisons in such work?[5]

Though some diseases were linked with environmental and occupational exposures in early history, they did not seem to cause significant concern. In contrast, contagions seemed to arise without warning and often caused panic among the populace. Early attempts to control contagions are demonstrated by the Biblical edict that the leper must "live outside the camp,"[6] as well as the Byzantine emperor Justinian's proclamation of the first effective quarantine laws in 549 CE, requiring that travelers from territories struck by plague be isolated and avoided.[7]

Why did contagions arise? Italian physician and scholar Girolamo Fracastoro (1478–1553) is usually credited with being the first to suggest that "seeds of contagions" caused specific diseases.[8] One of his contemporaries, Girolamo Cardano, expanded on this concept in 1557, noting that "seeds of disease were minute animals, capable of reproducing their kind."[9] That contagions could be caused by a *contagium vivum* (living organism) was a bold idea that spurred the imaginations of inquiring minds. In 1658, for example, the German Jesuit scholar Athanasius Kircher published *Scrutinium Pestis* in which Kircher referred to "true latent germs" and claimed to have seen living microorganisms in the blood of those struck by the bubonic plague.[10] As this was 25 years before Anton von Leeuwenhoek is credited with discovering microorganisms through a microscope, it is possible that what Kircher saw were red blood cells. His ideas, however, gained support among many prominent physicians.

Contagium vivum was not the only theory advanced as the cause of epidemics. Ancient China and India had long held that polluted air (dust, fog, haze, or poison gases) could cause disease. The idea that "bad air" (malaria) caused epidemics also took hold in the West during the 1700s. This *miasma theory* asserted that air containing decaying organic matter (*miasmata*) could make individuals ill. Thus it was the environment (which could be identified by the bad smell in the air) that was assumed to cause individuals to become ill, not the transfer of a contagion between individuals.

The two theories of the causes of epidemics challenged each other for supremacy for two centuries. A leading exponent of the *contagium vivum* theory was New England clergyman Cotton Mather. Mather's knowledge of the work of Kircher, Leeuwenhoek, and others led him to infer the concept of a germ theory of disease. He became an early advocate of smallpox inoculation, proposing that "animalcula" caused the disease.[11] In contrast, Benjamin Rush, one of the eighteenth century's leading physicians, felt compelled to adopt the miasma theory when the *contagium vivum* hypothesis failed to explain the yellow fever epidemics that then plagued North America.[12] The idea that a *vector* (mosquito) could be involved in transmitting a germ from person to person could not yet be imagined.

After 1800, three individuals—an Italian lawyer, a French physician, and a German anatomist—made valuable contributions to the *contagium vivum* theory. The first, Agosino Bassi, showed that small organisms within a host could produce disease. Over 25 years of careful experiments on muscardine, a fatal disease of silkworms, Bassi traced what he called the "fatal thing" from its entry into the silkworm until it caused the silkworm's death. He identified a fungus as the culprit, and recommended the use of disinfectants and other techniques to reduce the contagion. Bassi was subsequently honored for saving the Italian silk industry.[13]

The second contributor, French physician Pierre-Fidèle Bretonneau, showed communicable diseases to be "specific." In 1826 Brettoneau distinguished between scarlet fever and diphtheria and documented that the lesions on the mucous membranes of diphtheria patients go through cyclical changes in appearance as the disease progresses. His careful observations clarified that the different presentations of diphtheria were the same disease, simply in different stages.[14]

In 1840, the third contributor, German anatomist Jacob Henle, wrote *Von den Miasmen und Kontagien*, summarizing for the first time all of the scientific evidence for and against the doctrine of *contagium vivum*. While Henle was not able to identify a specific microbe as the cause of a specific disease, he is widely considered the cofounder of the theory of microorganisms as the cause of infective diseases. His student, Robert Koch, later discovered the tubercle bacillus as the cause of tuberculosis and, in 1905, received the Nobel

Prize in Physiology and Medicine for his efforts linking microbes to specific diseases.

The *contagium vivum* theory appeared in the English literature in the nineteenth century. In 1851, the *Lancet* published excerpts from "On the Nature of Epidemics," a paper presented to the London Epidemiological Society by John Grove. Grove explained that whether an epidemic afflicts plants or man, the cause must be something that has the power to reproduce itself, something no purely chemical process can do. Two years later the author submitted another paper to the Society that stated, "Wherever the agents of communicable diseases have been demonstrated, they have uniformly been shown to depend upon some form of cell-life."[15]

By the mid-1800s the *contagium vivum* theory was widely espoused by European physicians and scientists. The theory began to merge with the evolving concept that better data and statistical methods could bring about a better understanding of disease. Thus began the development of epidemiology as a distinct discipline.

Development of Epidemiologic Methods

The essence of the epidemiologic study is the comparison of groups of people with regard to a characteristic of interest. The earliest recorded account of such a comparison appears in the Old Testament in the first chapter of the Book of Daniel, when Nebuchadnezzar (king of Babylon) commanded his chief officer to feed some Jerusalem children a daily portion of the king's food and wine for a period of three years. Daniel declined the offer. The chief office challenged Daniel that his health would not be as good as that of those who ate the king's food. Daniel posed a test—some servants would eat the king's food, and the Jerusalem children would eat only legumes and water for 10 days. At the end of the 10 days, the chief officer found the Jerusalem children "appeared fairer, and they were fatter in the flesh, than all the youths that did eat of the king's food."[16]

While Daniel's challenge allowed for a comparison, it wasn't until the scientific revolution of the 1600s that the modern course of epidemiology began to evolve. During this period, scientists reasoned that if mathematical relationships could be found to describe, analyze, and understand the physical universe, then similar relationships must exist in the biological world. *Laws of mortality* referred to generalized statements about the relationships between disease (measured by death rates) and man. For specific aspects of disease, attempts were made to formulate *laws of epidemics*.

Initial Efforts

One of the first individuals to work within the context of such laws was the London tradesman, John Graunt. An intellectually curious man, Graunt collected the *Bills of Mortality*, which had been initiated in 1603 by the parish clerks of both London and a town in Hampshire. In 1662, Graunt published his *Natural and Political Observations mentioned in a following index and made upon the Bills of Mortality.*[17] This work was groundbreaking in that Graunt was the first to search for patterns of mortality and fertility using population-based records and, additionally, that he explicitly listed the errors and ambiguities in the data he used.

Graunt observed three distinct patterns in the bills: an annual excess of male births, high infant mortality, and a seasonal variation in mortality. He distinguished two broad causes of death—the acute and the "chronical" diseases—as well as noting an urban–rural difference in mortality. From the collected data, Graunt constructed the first known *life table*, which summarized the mortality experience of a population by providing the number of deaths, percent, or probability of living or dying over a lifetime—a truly outstanding achievement (Table 2.1). He also proposed that each country prepare similar tables to be compared and used to construct a general *law of mortality* akin to Newton's laws of motion in the physical world.

TABLE 2.1 Life Table of Deaths in London

BY AGE	DEATHS	SURVIVORS
0	---	100
6	36	64
16	24	40
26	15	25
36	9	16
46	6	10
56	4	6
66	3	3
76	2	1
80	1	0

"Where as [sic] we have found, that of 100 quick Conceptions about 36 of them die before they be six years old, and that perhaps but one surviveth 76, we, having seven Decads between six and 76, we sought six mean proportional numbers between 64, the remainer, living at six years, and the one, which survives 76, and finde, that the numbers following are practically near enough to the truth; for men do not die in exact Proportions, nor in Fractions . . ."
SOURCE: Graunt's *Observations*[17]

The Comparative Framework

At its core, epidemiology is about comparing groups, as exemplified by two eighteenth-century papers. The first was a 1747 report of an experiment by James Lind, an English naval physician interested in the etiology and treatment of scurvy. Lind took to sea onboard the *Salisbury* 12 patients with fulminant scurvy. All the seamen had "putrid gums, spots, and lassitude, with weakness of their knees . . ." Of the 12, two were given a quart of cider each day; two gargled with elixir of vitriol (a mixture of sulfuric acid, alcohol, and aromatics such as ginger and cinnamon) three times a day; two were given two spoonsful[s] of vinegar three times a day; two of the worst patients were "put under a course of sea water"; two were given two oranges and one lemon each day; and the two remaining patients took "the bigness of a nutmeg three times a day." The seamen all drank barley water and "were gently purged three or four times during the course."[18]

The consequence of Lind's experiment was that the men who ate the oranges and lemons recovered quickly, one being fit for duty by the end of day six. The other recovered sufficiently to nurse the rest of the sick. Lind inferred that eating citric acid fruits cured scurvy and that it would also prevent the disease. The British Navy accepted his analysis only decades later, requiring that limes or lime juice be incorporated into onboard diets beginning in 1785; hence, the British nickname for seamen, "Limeys."

Daniel Bernoulli published the second noteworthy paper on epidemiology in 1760. After evaluating the available evidence, Bernoulli concluded that persons inoculated with smallpox were conferred with lifelong immunity against the disease. Using a life table, he determined that inoculation at birth would increase life expectancy.[19] Although smallpox has now been eradicated, Bernoulli's model remains important for considering other devastating infections that confer lifetime immunity to survivors, such as measles.

Several years later, at the end of the eighteenth century, the French Revolution had a even further-reaching influence on epidemiology. It allowed individuals from the lower classes to assume positions of leadership in medicine, exemplified by Pierre Charles-Alexandre Louis. Louis was very much aware of the need for discovering laws of nature in medicine and pioneered the use of statistical methods, his *"méthode numerique."* Perhaps his most famous study is the one where he demonstrated that bloodletting was not efficacious for treating disease, thus helping halt its use in medical practice.[20]

One of the builders of the "Paris Hospital" during the first part of the nineteenth century, Louis was a renowned teacher. Students from both Europe and the Americas sought him out for training (Figure 2.1). Two of

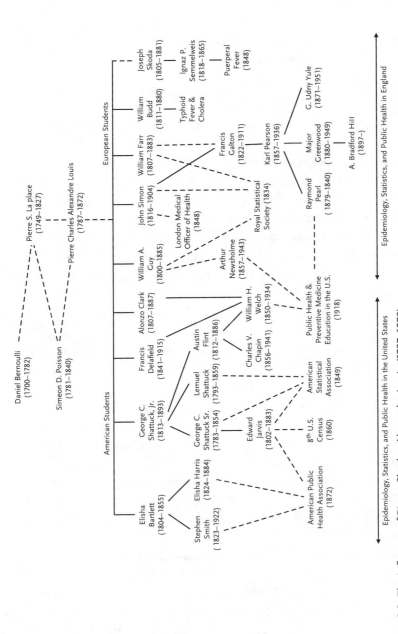

FIGURE 2.1 The influence of Pierre Charles-Alexandre Louis (1787–1872).

his students, William Augustus Guy and William Farr, were instrumental in the development of epidemiology in Victorian England, becoming intimately associated with the Statistical Society of London (later the Royal Statistical Society). Guy became a pioneer in the public health movement in England, and Farr, as the first Compiler of Abstracts of the Registrar General's Office, organized the world's first modern vital statistics system. Farr also conducted his own statistical analyses and provided significant insights into the development of epidemiologic methods (Table 2.2).[21]

The London Epidemiological Society

The London Epidemiological Society was organized in 1850, spurred by concerns over another cholera outbreak in the city. Benjamin G. Babington served as the Society's first president. Founding members included John Simon (Medical Officer of Health for London), Thomas Addison (Addison's disease), Richard Bright (Bright's disease), John Snow (then known for administering chloroform as an anesthetic), and Thomas Watson, all prominent London physicians. The Society quickly expanded its scope to include all epidemics, not just cholera. Its report on smallpox vaccination, for example, was the major reason for the passage of the Vaccination Act of 1853, mandating vaccination on a nationwide basis.[22]

Cholera

John Snow conducted a series of classical studies of cholera in London showing that *V. cholerae* was transmitted by water. As a vegan and teetotaler who joined the Temperance Movement in 1830, the Victorian physician considered the mouth to be the portal for all pathogens. During the 1849 London cholera outbreak, Snow first formulated his theory that cholera was transmitted by water. When the 1854 epidemic began, he plotted cholera deaths on a map of London. Finding the greatest concentration of deaths around Golden Square in Soho, Snow lobbied the local politicians to shut down the community water pump on Broad Street (now Broadwick Street). The epidemic abated, but it is unclear whether removal of the pump handle aided in the epidemic's decline.

At the same time, Snow noted that the Lambeth Company and the Southwark and Vauxhall Company supplied water to most homes located south of the Thames. He also noted that the companies' water mains were interspersed, so houses on the same street received water from different sources. Snow knew that while both companies had proximate water sources on the Thames during the 1849 epidemic, the Lambeth Company had moved

TABLE 2.2 Examples of William Farr's Understanding of Epidemiologic Concepts

EPIDEMIOLOGIC CONCEPT	FARR'S STATEMENT
Scope of epidemiology	"The causes that make the rates of mortality vary may be considered under 2 heads— 1. Causes inherent in the population itself, such, for example, as sex and age. 2. Causes outside the population, such as air, water, food, clothing, dwellings, or such groups of causes as are involved in residence, and relation of the several parts to each other in time and space."
Person-years	"The year of life is the lifetime unit. It is represented by one person living through a year; or by two persons living through half a year."
Relationship of death rate and probability of dying (or living)	"The rate of mortality serves to give the probability of living a year."
Standardized mortality rate	"[If] the number of boys under 5 years of age was 147,390, the annual rate of mortality in the healthy districts [the standard population] was .04348; . . . 6,347 deaths which would have happened in London . . . continuing the process . . . the mortality in London should [be] 15 in 1,000."
Dose-response effect	"The effects are in some regulated proportion to the intensity of the causes."
Need for large numbers of population and biological inferences	"When the number of cases is considerable the relative mortality is most correctly expressed and . . . slight differences deserve little attention."
Herd immunity	"The small-pox would be . . . sometimes arrested, by vaccination which protected a part of the population."
Prevalence = incidence × duration	"In estimating the prevalence of disease, two things must be distinctly considered; the relative frequency of their attacks, and the relative proportion of sick-time they produce. The first may be determined at once, a comparison of the number of attacks with the numbers living; the second by enumerating several times the living and the actually sick of the disease, and thence deducing the mean proportion suffering constantly. Time is here taken into account: and the sick-time, if the attacks of two diseases be equal, will vary as their duration varies, and whatever the number of attacks may be, multiplying them by the mean duration of each disease will give the sick-time."
Case-control and cohort studies	"Is your inquiry to be retrospective or prospective? If the former the replies will be general, vague, and I fear of little value."

SOURCE: Lilienfeld and Lilienfeld.[21]

TABLE 2.3 Deaths from Cholera per 10,000 Houses by Source of Water Supply, London, 1854

WATER SUPPLY	NUMBER OF HOUSES	DEATHS FROM CHOLERA	DEATHS IN EACH 10,000 HOMES
Southwark and Vauxhall Company	40,046	1,263	315
Lambeth Company	26,107	98	37
Rest of London	256,423	1,422	59

DATA SOURCE: *Snow On Cholera* (1936).[23]

its source upriver, where the Thames was less polluted. During the 1854 epidemic, Snow (1) ascertained the total number of houses supplied by each water company, (2) calculated cholera death rates per 10,000 houses for the first seven weeks of the epidemic, and (3) compared them with those for the rest of London (Table 2.3). His findings demonstrated that the cholera mortality rates in homes supplied by the Southwark and Vauxhall Company were eight or nine times as great as those supplied by the Lambeth Company.[23]

John Snow's achievement was based on the logical organization of observations, his recognition of a natural experiment in the 1854 outbreak, and the quantitative approach in analyzing the occurrence of disease. Snow's report led to legislation mandating that all London water companies filter their water by 1857,[24] and he was celebrated by being elected President of the Medical Society of London. Later, however, he was discredited for advocating against clean air legislation.

Typhoid Fever

A different epidemiologic approach to disease is embodied in William Budd's 1857–1873 studies of typhoid fever. Budd, an active member of the London Epidemiological Society and a student of Louis, practiced medicine in his native English village of North Tawton. Budd's observations of the village's environmental conditions led him to argue against the miasmatic origin of typhoid fever:

> Much there was, as I can myself testify, offensive to the nose, but [typhoid] fever there was none. It could not be said that the atmospheric conditions necessary to [typhoid] fever was wanting [sic], because while this village remained exempt, many neighboring villages suffered severely from the pest . . . Meanwhile privies, pigstyes, and dungheaps continued, year after year, to exhale ill odours, without any specific effect on the public health . . . I ascertained by an inquiry conducted with the most scrupulous care that for fifteen years there had been

no severe outbreak of this disorder, and that for nearly ten years there had been but a single case. For the development of this fever a more specific element was needed than either the swine, the dungheaps, or the privies . . .[25]

After observing more than 80 patients with typhoid fever, Budd hypothesized that the disease was spread by contagion. He inferred this by observing instances of three or four successive cases in the same household, and also by documenting that three individuals who had left the village during the epidemic spread the disease to some of their new contacts. Budd traced instances of person-to-person contact resulting in typhoid fever in villages previously free of the disease, despite village environmental conditions similar to those of North Tawton. He concluded that typhoid is a "contagious or self-propagating fever" that manifests as an intestinal disturbance, and that it was passed between individuals via contact with infected feces. In 1880, the typhoid fever bacillus was finally described.

Other European Efforts

Louis's teachings also influenced physicians across Europe outside the United Kingdom, notably Austria and Denmark. Many of his students were encouraged to collect and analyze data on medical outcomes in order to demonstrate the effectiveness of treatments and determine the causes of epidemics. Two specific examples serve to demonstrate how gathering such data led to an improved understanding of disease: puerperal fever and measles.

Puerperal Fever

Joseph Skoda, a leading internist at the Vienna Medical School, used and taught Louis's numerical method. His student, Ignaz Semmelweis, noted changing trends of maternal mortality from puerperal (childbed) fever in two maternity wards of the *Allgemeines Krankenhaus*, a large Viennese maternity hospital. Between 1833 and 1840, midwifery students, medical students, and physicians were equally distributed between these two wards, which did not differ in maternal mortality. In 1840 the training system was changed, with one ward training midwives and the other training medical students and physicians. A difference in the maternal mortality rates of the two wards then appeared and continued from 1841 to 1846 (9.9 percent in the ward used by medical students and physicians, 3.9 percent in the ward used by midwifery students).

Semmelweis observed that the medical students and physicians performed autopsies prior to their attendance in the maternity wards, whereas the midwifery students did not. This led him to hypothesize that the high maternal mortality rate resulted from the transmission of infectious material from the autopsy room to the maternity clinic. In 1847 Semmelweis instituted the practice of having physicians and medical students wash their hands with chlorinated solutions before performing deliveries. The death rate fell to 1.3 percent in 1848, equaling that in the ward used by the midwifery students.[26] Despite these findings, the idea that doctors spread disease with dirty hands was soundly rejected by the medical community. Semmelweis was totally discredited and committed to an asylum at age 47, where he died from being beaten by the guards. Two years later, in 1867, British physician Joseph Lister began championing the use of carbolic acid as an antiseptic in the surgical theater.

Measles

A cabinetmaker from Copenhagen arrived at the Faroe Islands (population 7,864) on March 28, 1846 and developed symptoms of measles early in April. Though cases of measles had historically occurred in the Faroes, there had been no such cases since 1781. Within the next six months, 6,100 Faroe Islanders came down with measles and 170 died of the disease. The Danish government sent a 26-year-old physician, Peter Ludwig Panum, to deal with the situation.

Visiting 52 villages across the Faroes, Panum personally treated 1,000 cases of measles. His observations on several thousand cases yielded information on the circumstances and dates of their exposure to the infection, as well as the dates on which the *exanthem* (rash) appeared. From these observations, Panum discovered that measles had a 13- to 14-day incubation period. He also determined that the patient is likely to be infectious for a few days prior to the eruption of the exanthem, and is not infectious while the scabs are being shed. Panum's observations led him to conclude that measles is transmitted by direct contact between an infected and susceptible individual, and that it does not arise spontaneously by miasma. He also suggested that one attack of measles conferred lifelong immunity (validated when the Faroes had another measles epidemic in 1875 and only persons under 30 years of age became ill).[27]

Much of what we know about the epidemiology of measles today derives from Panum's observations. We have since learned, however, that the measles virus is transmitted by droplets that are sprayed out when infected people sneeze or cough. *Susceptible* individuals become infected when they breathe in the droplets or touch *fomites* (inanimate objects) contaminated with the virus and then touch their noses or mouths.

American Beginnings

Pierre Charles-Alexandre Louis's influence was not restricted to Europe, as many Americans went to Paris to study under his tutelage. For example, Henry I. Bowditch, Oliver Wendell Holmes Sr., and George C. Shattuck Jr. all studied under Louis for several years prior to becoming professors of medicine at Harvard University (see Figure 2.1). Lemuel Shattuck, cousin to George who had studied under Louis, prepared the 1850 landmark report outlining the basis for public health organization at the state and local levels.[28] Lemuel Shattuck was a founding member of the American Statistical Association and was active in offering detailed recommendations for creating a vital statistics system, a census, disease nomenclature for causes of death, and the collection of data by age, race, sex, occupation, and more. One of George C. Shattuck Sr.'s students, Edward Jarvis, was the third president of the Association and responsible for the reorganization of the 1860 US census, thus facilitating its use by epidemiologists and biometricians.

In New York, another group of Louis's students influenced the development of epidemiology and public health in the United States. Elisha Bartlett (the first individual to provide a rationale for a control group in an epidemiologic study), Alonzo Clark, and Francis Delafield taught at either the Columbia University College of Physicians and Surgeons or the Bellevue Hospital Medical College. Their positions in these prestigious institutions placed them all in prominent positions to effect change. Among their students were Elisha Harris (first vital registrar in New York City) and Stephen Smith (first president of the American Public Health Association, founded in 1872). Louis's teachings continued to flow through the medical and public health communities in the United States throughout the late nineteenth and well into the early twentieth century.

New Diseases Demand New Methods

Louis's *méthode numerique* set the stage for statisticians interested in health to develop new methods to analyze their data and share the results. For instance, Francis Galton (developer of the normal distribution and the correlation coefficient) became a close colleague of Karl Pearson (discover of the chi-square distribution) and the two were among the founders of the journal *Biometrika*. In Britain, the Ministry of Health created the position of medical statistician in 1919, hiring Major Greenwood (later a professor of epidemiology and vital statistics at the London School of Hygiene and Tropical

Medicine). Greenwood recruited Austin Bradford Hill, a pioneer in study methods (see below). In the United States, the US Public Health Service and its Hygienic Laboratory (later to become the National Institutes of Health) were founded in 1897. These agencies attracted several epidemiologic pioneers who developed experimental and field methods to address the emerging diseases of the time, one of which was cancer.

Cancer

The American Association for Cancer Research, founded in 1907, served the same role in the development of cancer epidemiology that the London Epidemiological Society had served in Victorian epidemiology, providing a forum to discuss scientific papers on cancer. Its publication, the *Journal of Cancer Research/American Journal of Cancer,* contained a comprehensive set of global cancer research publication abstracts that proved to be a significant scientific resource. The principal scientific question of the day was whether cancer was increasing. Unfortunately, the only available data—mortality statistics—had deficiencies that made it difficult to discern trends in cancer occurrence. It became clear that a population-based surveillance system that listed all persons with cancer (a *cancer registry*) was needed in order to provide an answer.

Within a year of its founding in 1937, the United States National Cancer Institute (NCI) launched the First National Cancer Survey (FNCS) to assess the burden of cancer in the United States. The FNCS surveyed ten metropolitan areas/states, finding stomach cancer the most common of all cancers. In 1940, the NCI convened a meeting of the nation's public health and medical leaders to discuss the stomach cancer data. At that meeting, human genetics pioneer Madge Macklin outlined how to conduct an epidemiologic cohort study—an approach still in use today.

Modern Epidemiology

By the time of World War II, most of the study methods now used by epidemiologists had been developed. After the war, there was an immediate need for trained epidemiologists to serve in public health and biomedical research agencies, such as the Centers for Disease Control and Prevention and the *Institut National de la Santé et de la Recherche Médicale.* Two areas in particular generated significant a strong demand for epidemiologic training: the *randomized controlled (clinical) trial,* and the relationship between cigarette smoking and lung cancer.

Randomized Controlled Trials

Assessing the efficacy of disease treatment and prevention efforts had been an ongoing challenge for centuries. The current approach, however, began its development around the turn of the twentieth century. In 1904, Karl Pearson, a founder of modern biostatistics, was asked by the British War Office to evaluate a new approach to preventing bacterial infections. Pearson began developing measures of association between exposure and health outcomes (e.g., correlation coefficients), a process of evaluation that continues through the present. When asked to examine a new and potentially revolutionary treatment for infections, Pearson's protégé, Major Greenwood, conducted the assessment, finding it not as effective as was hoped.

The importance of using an epidemiologic approach to clinical data was sealed in 1937 when the *Lancet* asked Major Greenwood's then protégé, (Austin) Bradford Hill, to write a series of articles describing mathematical statistics used in a clinical context. The well-received series and subsequent book established Hill as an emerging expert in epidemiology. One comment in the book is of particular note: "By the allocation of the patients to the two groups we want to ensure that these two groups are alike except in treatment ... [and] this might be done ... by a random division of the patients ..."[29] Hill's understanding of randomization went beyond that of English statistician Ronald A. Fisher (who developed the concept for statistical significance tests). Hill used randomization as a means to prevent bias from being introduced into the experimental trial.

After World War II, new therapeutics and preventive agents rapidly moved forward in development. One such agent was streptomycin, an experimental treatment for tuberculosis; another was a vaccine against pertussis (whooping cough). Both treatments were tested using Hill's randomization approach. Although the pertussis vaccine trial starter earlier, the streptomycin trial published its results first.[30] Both randomized controlled trials were considered successes, and the epidemiologic study design became incorporated as a standard in the field.

Smoking

In 1947, in response to rising lung cancer mortality, the British government asked Bradford Hill to investigate the role of the increasing rate of cigarette smoking as the possible cause. Hill and his protégé, Richard Doll, used a case-control design to address the issue. Their study, conducted in the late

1940s, used hospitalized patients in the United Kingdom who had lung cancer as the cases and those with other diseases as controls. The team found a clear association between cigarette smoking and lung cancer. Their findings were opposed by R. A. Fisher, who (as a pipe smoker himself) strongly noted that correlation does not imply causation.

Concurrent with Hill and Doll's efforts in Britain, two American groups simultaneously published their results on the relationship of cigarette smoking to lung cancer (Morton L. Levin and colleagues at the Roswell Park Memorial Institute formed one team, and a Washington University medical student, Ernst Wynder, with his mentor/collaborator, American pulmonary surgeon Evarts Graham, the other). The Levin paper was originally rejected by the *Journal of the American Medical Association*, but when the journal received a second paper with similar results from the Washington University team, the editor was faced with a dilemma. How could the journal reject one paper but publish the other co-authored by the prominent pulmonary surgeon that had similar results? The answer was to publish both papers at the same time.

The three case-control studies with similar findings were all published in 1950, stimulating discussion about the relationship between cigarette smoking and lung cancer. Shortly thereafter, three large cohort studies were launched to confirm the findings. The United States Veteran's Administration Life Insurance study, the American Cancer Society Hammond-Horn study, and the British Doctors Study provided such strong epidemiological data that by 1962 in Britain and 1964 in the United States, the Royal Society of Medicine and the United States Surgeon General, respectively, deemed cigarette smoking to be a cause of lung cancer.

Summary

Diverse threads of history combined to create the fabric of epidemiology. It took the development of numerical methods beginning in the eighteenth century, the development of a vital statistics system and standardized data collection during the nineteenth and twentieth centuries, and the development of various comparative study designs thereafter to create the cloth. It took changes in disease patterns, large data sets, and the need for an expanding community of epidemiologists to add texture, to make the cloth stronger and able to endure the inevitable challenges faced by an emerging discipline. Perhaps Sir Isaac Newton summarized the situation well when he observed, "If I have seen further it is by standing on ye sholders [*sic*] of Giants."[31]

References

1. Keith Forsey and Steve Schiff. "Don't You (Forget About Me)" by Simple Minds. New York: Virgin Records, Ltd., 1984.
2. Hippocrates. "On Airs, Waters, and Places" (circa 400 BCE) in *The Genuine Works of Hippocrates, Volume 1.* Translated by F Adams. New York: William Wood & Company, 1939, 19–41.
3. Vitruvius. *De Architectura. Volume I* (circa 15 BCE). Translated by Morris Hicky Morgan. Cambridge, MA: Harvard University Press, 1914.
4. Pliny. *Naturalis Historia. Gaius Plinius Secundus, Volume IX* (Pliny the Elder, circa 77–79 CE). Translated by D. E. Eichholz. Cambridge, MA: Harvard University Press, 1942.
5. Lucretius. *On the Nature of Things* (Titus Lucretius Carus, circa 50 BCE). Translated by C. Bailey. Oxford: Clarendon Press, 1910.
6. Leviticus 13: 46. *The Holy Bible*, King James Edition. New York: Oxford Edition, 1769.
7. Pablo F. Gomez, "Quarantine," in *Encyclopedia of Pestilence, Pandemics, and Plagues, Vol I*, ed. J. P. Byrne. Westport, CT: Greenwood Press, 2008, 584–86.
8. Girolamo Frascatoro, *De Contagione et Contagiosis Morbis.* (1546). Translated by W. C. F. Wright. New York: G. P. Putnam's Sons, 1930.
9. George Rosen, *A History of Public Health*, p. 84. Baltimore: Johns Hopkins University Press, 1938.
10. Paula Findlen, *Athanasius Kircher: The Last Man Who Knew Everything.* New York: Routledge, 2004.
11. Cotton Mather, *The Angel of Bethesda: An Essay upon the Common Maladies of Mankind* (First Edition, 1724). Worcester, MA: American Antiquarian Society, 1972.
12. Benjamin Rush, *An account of the bilious remitting yellow fever, as it appeared in the city of Philadelphia, in the year 1793.* Edinburgh: John Moir, 1796.
13. Giovanni P. Arcieri, *Agostino Bassi in the History of Medical Thought.* New York: The Vigo Press, 1938.
14. Paul Triaire, *Bretonneau et ses correspondants.* Paris: Felix Algan, Libraire Editeur, 1892.
15. John Grove, "On Contagion and Infection in Relation to Epidemic Diseases" (Read before the Epidemiological Society, August 1853). *The Monthly Journal of Medical Science*, 73, no. 3 (1853): 396–413.
16. Daniel 1: 16, The Holy Bible, King James Edition. New York: Oxford Edition, 1769.
17. John Graunt, *Natural and Political Observations mentioned in a following index and made upon the Bills of Mortality.* London, 1662. Reprinted Baltimore: Johns Hopkins University Press, 1939.
18. James Lind, *A Treatise on the Scurvy. In Three Parts. Containing an Inquiry into the Nature, Causes, and Cure of that Disease. Together with a Critical and Chronological View of what has been published on the subject.* Edinburgh: Sands, Murray and Cochran, 1752.

19. Daniel Bernoulli, *An attempt at a new analysis of the mortality caused by smallpox and of the advantages of inoculation to prevent it* (1790) in *History of Actuarial Science, Vol VIII*, eds. S. Haberman and T. A. Sibbett. London: William Pickering, 1995.

20. P. C. A. Louis, *Researches on the Effects of Bloodletting in Some Inflammatory Diseases: Together With, Researches on Phthisis* (Paris, 1936). Reprinted Birmingham, AL: Classics of Medicine Library, 1986.

21. David E. Lilienfeld and Abraham M. Lilienfeld, "Epidemiology: A Retrospective Study," *American Journal of Epidemiology* 106 (1977): 445–459.

22. *Transactions of the Epidemiological Society of London, Vol I, 1963*. London: Forgotten Books, 2012.

23. John Snow, *On the Mode of Communication of Cholera* (London, 1854).Available at http://www.deltaomega.org/documents/snowfin.pdf.,

24. G. Tellnes, "Public Health and the Way Forward," in *Public Health in Europe: 10 Years European Public Health Association*, ed. W. I. Kirch. Berlin, Heidelberg, New York: Springer-Verlag; 2003, 41–46.

25. William Budd, *Typhoid Fever: Its Nature, Mode of Spreading and Prevention* (1873). Reprinted New York: American Public Health Association, 1931.

26. Ignaz Semmelweiss, *The Etiology, Concept, and Prophylaxis of Childbed Fever* (Vienna, 1863). Reprinted in Birmingham, AL: Classics of Medicine Library, 1941.

27. Peter Ludvig Panum, *Observations Made During the Epidemic of Measles on the Faroe Islands in the Year 1846* (Copenhagen, 1847). Translated by A. Sommerville. New York: F. H. Newton, 1940.

28. Lemuel Shattuck, *Report of the Sanitary Commission of Massachusetts*. Boston: Dutton and Westworth, 1850.

29. Austin Bradford Hill, *Principles of Medical Statistics*. London: Lancet, 1937.

30. Medical Research Council. "Streptomycin Treatment of Pulmonary Tuberculosis," *British Medical Journal* 2, no. 4582 (1948): 769–782.

31. *The Correspondence of Isaac Newton*, ed. H. W. Turnbull. Chicago, IL: Royal Society at the University Press, 1958.

3 | Selected Epidemiologic Concepts

The classification of facts, the recognition of their sequence and
relative significance is the function of science, and the habit
of forming a judgment upon these facts unbiased by personal
feeling is characteristic of what may be termed the scientific frame
of mind.[1]

Karl Pearson (1892)

M ANY OF THE FUNDAMENTAL CONCEPTS of epidemiology evolved from
studies of infectious diseases. However, many are equally applicable to noninfectious diseases and conditions. For instance, both
infectious and noninfectious diseases can be acquired from either *exogenous*
(*extrinsic* or *external*), or *endogenous* (*intrinsic* or *internal*) sources. Influenza
virus (infectious) and lead poisoning (noninfectious) are examples of exogenous sources of disease. Examples of endogenous sources of diseases
include cystitis (infectious, from a subject's own normal flora) and familial hypercholesterolemia (noninfectious, an inherited genetic defect in the
receptor for low-density lipoprotein). There are other ways to conceptualize
diseases, as well. This chapter reviews those concepts of greatest value to the
epidemiologist.

Agent, Host, and Environment

Patterns of infectious disease depend upon factors that influence the probability of contact between an etiologic *agent* and a susceptible person, or
host, facilitated by the *environment* in which they coexist. This interaction of factors is sometimes called the *epidemiologic triad*. Over the years,

epidemiologists have expanded the definition of etiologic agent to cover all causes of adverse health outcomes, not only infectious diseases. Table 3.1 presents a classification scheme covering both endogenous and exogenous factors as etiologic agents of human disease. Note that nutritive agents are endogenous, whereas chemical and physical agents in the environment are exogenous.

Table 3.1 also lists host and environmental factors that make individuals more or less likely to be either susceptible or exposed to the agents of

TABLE 3.1 Agent, Host, and Environmental Factors that Interact to Produce Human Disease

AGENTS OF DISEASE	EXAMPLES
Nutritive elements	
Excess	Cholesterol, obesity
Deficiency	Vitamins, proteins
Chemical agents	
Poisons	Carbon monoxide, drugs
Allergens	Ragweed, poison ivy
Physical agents	Ionizing radiation, mechanical
Infectious agents	
Parasites	Hookworm, malaria
Bacteria	Tuberculosis, strep throat
Fungi	Pneumocystis pneumonia, athlete's foot
Rickettsia	Lyme disease, typhus
Viruses	Measles, rabies
Prions	Creutzfeldt-Jakob Disease, Kuru

HOST FACTORS	EXAMPLES
Genetic/Ethnic	Cystic fibrosis, Tay-Sachs disease
Age	Alzheimer's disease
Sex	Breast cancer, prostate cancer
Physiologic state	Pregnancy, puberty
Immunologic state	Immunization, prior infection
Human behavior	Personal hygiene, tobacco use

ENVIRONMENTAL FACTORS	EXAMPLES
Physical environment	Climate change, natural or man-made disaster
Biologic environment	Population density, arthropod vectors
Socioeconomic environment	
Occupation	Exposure to dangerous conditions
Economic status	Stress, crowding, nutritional status
Disruption	War, migration

disease. Host factors can be personal characteristics such as an individual's age, gender, or genetic factors. They can also be related to an individual's immunologic experience or personal behaviors.

The environment that allows the host and agent to come into contact may exist for a very brief or extended period of time. Environmental conditions also pose limitations on the ability of a disease agent to survive. For example, arid conditions or cold temperatures may reduce the ability of viruses to survive for long periods outside the human body, rain may wash dust or other allergens out of the air, or a dam may create a pool of water that promotes the survival and spread of a parasite. The environment may also alter population mobility and restrict interpersonal contact among susceptible hosts. For instance, bad weather may cause school closings and reduce the spread of viral illnesses among children; civil strife may cause refugees to band together in temporary camps and become more susceptible to outbreaks of disease; or friends may grow apart with changed behaviors, such as smoking cigarettes or changing their diets.

Scientific disciplines are usually concerned with one category of potential etiologic factors and their relationship with specific health outcomes. For instance, the geneticist concentrates on genetic factors for disease, the microbiologist on infectious agents, and the sociologist on human behavior, ethnic groups, and socioeconomic environments. The epidemiologist, however, integrates information about health-related states and events across disciplines. It is this focus on the interaction of time, place, and person factors that makes the disease classification framework in Table 3.1 an epidemiologic concept.

The Natural History of Disease

The *natural history of disease* refers to the progression of a given disease from the time of its biological onset until its resolution, either through recovery, disability, or death. The concept can be applied to both infectious and noninfectious diseases, reflecting the course of a disease if there is no intervention. Figure 3.1 shows that the disease process begins when a *susceptible* individual has an exposure to a disease-causing agent. The disease progresses along a *spectrum of disease* ranging from a *subclinical phase* where the host has no symptoms, into a *clinical phase* where symptoms are apparent, and then to disease resolution.

Consider the example of cerebrovascular disease, a chronic, noninfectious disease to which everyone is susceptible. Atherosclerotic changes may begin

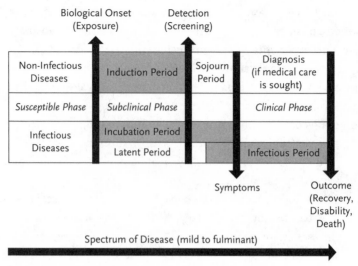

FIGURE 3.1 The spectrum of disease.

in the carotid arteries during childhood, although no symptoms will likely be apparent. The time required for a chronic disease to become symptomatic is called the *induction period*. At some point during the induction period it may be possible for the disease to be detected through screening (*sojourn period*). Unfortunately, cerebrovascular disease is not usually diagnosed until significant symptoms, such as a transient ischemic attack (TIA) or stroke, occur. The disease then moves into the *clinical phase*, and the outcome will likely depend upon the medical care sought.

In infectious diseases the spectrum of disease is sometimes called the *gradient of infection*, and the way it progresses has a great deal to do with the characteristics of the infectious agent, the dose of the agent received, and the immune response of the host. Infectious agents also have characteristics that help us understand how dangerous they can be. The first of these is *infectivity*, or the ability of an agent to enter a susceptible host. Infectivity of an agent is statistically expressed as the proportion of exposures that result in infection:

$$Infectivity = \frac{Number\ of\ hosts\ infected}{Number\ of\ susceptibles\ exposed} \times 100$$

Examples of agents with high infectivity are the measles and smallpox viruses. Low infectivity is exemplified by both *Mycobacterim tuberculosis* (the causal agent for tuberculosis) and *Mycobacterim leprae* (the causal agent for leprosy).

The second characteristic of agents is *pathogenicity*, or the ability of the agent to survive and multiply in sufficient numbers to produce clinical disease among those infected. It is statistically expressed as:

$$Pathogenicity = \frac{Number\ of\ clinical\ cases}{Number\ of\ hosts\ infected} \times 100$$

The Human Immunodeficiency Virus (the causal agent for Acquired Immunodeficiency Syndrome, or AIDS) and common cold viruses have high pathogenicity, while the poliovirus and *Chlamydia trachomatis* have low pathogenicity.

The final characteristic of agents is *virulence*, the ability of the agent to cause death or permanent disability among those that develop clinical disease. The statistical formula for calculating virulence is:

$$Virulence = \frac{Number\ of\ deaths\ or\ permanent\ disability}{Number\ of\ clinical\ cases} \times 100$$

High virulence is characterized by the rabies and Ebola viruses. Examples of low virulence include the common cold and rubella (the causal agent for German measles) viruses.

Knowing the infectivity, pathogenicity, and virulence of an agent enables the epidemiologist to predict what will happen if susceptible individuals are exposed and there are no available treatments for the resulting infections. It is entirely possible for an etiologic agent to be highly infective but not very pathogenic, or for an infection to progress to mild clinical disease among certain populations but be very deadly to others. For example, Epstein-Barr virus infects most people at some time during their lives. Infants are susceptible as soon as maternal antibodies to the virus disappear. While it is common for young children to be infected with the virus, many display no symptoms or only a brief, mild illness. When infection occurs during early adulthood, however, clinical cases of infectious mononucleosis may persist with serious symptoms for several months, often requiring hospitalization.[2]

Consider the spectrum of an infectious disease as shown in the lower half of Figure 3.1. After exposure, the infected host enters the incubation period, where the agent begins to multiply. At the beginning of the incubation period is the *latent period*, a time when the agent is not yet being shed. Once the agent has reached numbers sufficient to be passed on to another susceptible host, the *infectious period* begins. Note that it is quite possible for persons to be infectious before they develop symptoms of their disease. This means that individuals with *inapparent infections* may become *carriers* of the agent, not knowing they are ill. A well-known example of this situation is that of Mary Mallon ("Typhoid Mary"), the first person in the United States to be identified as an inapparent carrier of the infectious agent *Salmonella typhi*. Over the course of her work as a cook in New York between 1900 and 1907, Mary Mallon infected more than 50 people, at least three of whom died. Mallon never developed symptoms of her disease, refused to believe she was infected, and continued to spread typhoid throughout the city until being permanently quarantined on North Brother Island in the East River.[3]

As epidemiology is not an exact science, it should not be surprising for the reader to learn that not all textbooks agree on the terminology that should be used to describe the natural history of disease as described in Figure 3.1. Some texts eliminate the sojourn period, instead describing chronic diseases as having only *induction* (the time between exposure and the beginning of the disease process) and *latency* (the time between the beginning of the disease process and manifestation of symptoms) periods before diagnosis. They may also describe infectious diseases as having *incubation* (the time of infection and the appearance of symptoms), *latency* (the period between the time of infection and the start of the infectious period) and *infectious* (the time when the disease is able to be transmitted to others) periods. Which terminology is used often depends upon the target audience for the text.

It is important for epidemiologists to understand the full spectrum of disease for several reasons. First, inapparent cases play a significant role in the spread of infectious agents. Consider, for instance, a susceptible individual exposed to the measles (rubeola) virus. The incubation period for measles ranges from 7 to 18 days from exposure until symptoms appear.[4] The infectious period for shedding the virus is up to four days before the rash develops and up to five days afterward. It then follows that the latent period, where the virus has not yet multiplied in sufficient numbers to be shed, can be as short as three days (7 days from exposure minus 4 days before the rash develops) or as long as 14 days (18 days from exposure minus 4 days before the rash develops), depending upon the infective dose received and the host's own immune response. The infectious period would therefore last up to nine days (4 days before the rash develops plus 5 days afterward). While clinical disease (fever, runny nose, and a rash) develops in more than 90 percent of measles cases, some infected persons develop no symptoms. The disease will not become apparent in these individuals, but they will infect others for the entire infectious period.[4]

A second reason for the importance of knowing the natural history of disease is for designing epidemiologic studies, for example in identifying the relevant period of exposure when cases should develop. The spectrum of disease is often exemplified by describing the *iceberg phenomenon*, where the tip of the iceberg (above the water) represents the proportion of diagnosed disease and the submerged portion represents all cases of the disease remaining undiagnosed, misdiagnosed, or unreported.[5] The iceberg phenomenon has been variously called "ears of the hippopotamus" and "crocodile's nose" in parts of the world where icebergs are unknown.[6] Regardless of the term used, the phenomenon reflects the need for both clinical medicine and public health to learn as much about a disease as possible in order to minimize the burden of that disease on a population.

A third reason for the epidemiologist to understand the full spectrum of disease relates to the importance of screening for diseases. Many of these diseases, if caught early, might be prevented from progressing, or they might be cured. Putting effective screening programs into place that can identify individuals who are in a subclinical phase of a noninfectious disease, then, has the potential for reducing the burden of these diseases on populations. A discussion of population-based screening can be found in Chapter 7; individual screening is discussed in Chapter 13.

Modes of Transmission

Infectious disease outbreaks are often classified by the ways in which they spread through populations, or their *modes of transmission*. Table 3.2 begins with a categorization of the modes by their *dynamics of spread*, or the way in which the infectious agent moves through a population. Outbreaks may be linked to a *common vehicle* such as a contaminated food, air, or water supply that can infect many individuals so exposed. Outbreaks might also be *propagated*, passed from host to host by serial transfer (such as respiratory infections or sexually transmitted diseases). Other modes of transmission in a propagated epidemic include passing on the disease through *vectors* (insects or animals) or *fomites* (inanimate objects). Some infectious diseases spread through a population in more than one way, depending upon the characteristics of the agent and its ability to survive in a variety of environments. Consider malaria, for example. The disease is primarily propagated via an insect vector (the *Anopheles gambii* mosquito), but it can also be transmitted through a common vehicle (blood transfusion infected with the *Plasmodium* parasite).[7,8] Depending on its dynamic of spread, malaria can be either a propagated or common-vehicle epidemic.

Table 3.2 contains additional classification systems for the modes of transmission of propagated epidemics. These classification systems are important, as they provide a basis for developing public health measures that can help prevent or stop the spread of epidemics in the community. One example of public health prevention measures linked to the *portal of entry and exit* classification is the "cough into your sleeve" health education campaign, designed for everyone from preschoolers in the classroom to commuters on public transit. Coughing into your sleeve rather than contaminating the air of those close to you reduces droplet spread of the infectious agent, the pathway needed to spread the agent via the respiratory route. Similarly, an aggressive handwashing campaign for food handlers and the cleaning of food preparation surfaces with a solution of bleach and water can reduce the risk of transmitting *Salmonella*, an infectious agent transmitted through the gastrointestinal tract (oral–anal route, sometimes referred to as "fingers-feces-mouth").

The epidemiologist must determine the *principal reservoir* of an infectious agent to provide the knowledge necessary to stop outbreaks, and even to help formulate programs to eradicate infectious diseases. For instance, it has long been known that the only reservoir for the smallpox virus is man. That knowledge made the disease a potential target for a global eradication campaign, promulgated through a rigorous program that included rapid case identification, isolation of cases, and the creation of a *cordon sanitaire* (barrier to disease). The *cordon sanitaire* is a buffer zone of nonsusceptibles that stops the spread of disease, achieved by implementing a ring-vaccination program around the case to prevent further transmission. In 1980, the World Health Organization officially declared smallpox to be globally eradicated, the first human disease to achieve that status (although the United States and Russia retain laboratory stocks of the virus). If smallpox had more than one principal reservoir of infection, or if it *cycled through nature* in a complex way, eradication of naturally occurring smallpox might have been impossible. Indeed, earlier efforts to globally eradicate malaria, yellow fever, and yaws were unsuccessful, although the incidence of these diseases has been dramatically reduced. Infectious diseases that are now close to being globally eradicated are those where man is the only reservoir (such as polio) and/or where the cycle of the agent through nature is understood and the pathway can be disrupted (such as guinea-worm disease).[10]

Although originally developed for infectious diseases, the framework for transmission has been applied to diseases and disorders associated with

TABLE 3.2 Classification of Infectious Diseases by Their Modes of Transmission, with Examples*

DYNAMICS OF SPREAD	
COMMON SOURCE	PROPAGATED (HOST-TO-HOST)
Ingestion	Gastrointestinal route
cholera	Shigella
E. coli 0157:H7	pinworms
Inhalation	Respiratory route
Legionella	measles virus
Hanta virus	influenza virus
Inoculation	Genitourinary/mucosal
hepatitis B	gonorrhea
HIV	HIV
PROPAGATED (VECTOR)	PROPAGATED (FOMITE)
Animal	Combs, brushes, towels, drinking glasses
rabies	pediculosis (head lice)
Insect	herpes
malaria	
PORTAL OF ENTRY AND EXIT	
Upper respiratory tract	Lower respiratory tract
diphtheria	tuberculosis
strep throat	pneumonia
Gastrointestinal tract	Genitourinary tract
Salmonella (typhoid)	chlamydia
rotavirus	HIV
Conjunctiva	Percutaneous
trachoma	Yellow fever
viral conjunctivitis	malaria
PRINCIPLE RESERVOIR	CYCLE OF INFECTION IN NATURE
Man	Man–man
hepatitis A	influenza
poliomyelitis	Man–arthropod–man
Other vertebrates (zoonoses)	malaria
tularemia	Vertebrate–vertebrate–man
rabies	psittacosis
Free-living agent	Vertebrate–arthropod–vertebrate–man
tetanus	viral encephalitis
	Complex cycles
	helminthic infections

* Diseases may be classified in more than one category.

noninfectious agents, specifically behaviors. These agents have been termed *social contagions*. Social contagions are usually spread within a network of persons, but they may also be spread outside of the immediate network to the larger population. Examples of social contagions include cigarette smoking and obesity. Influencing the network may provide one means by which transmission of a social contagion can be halted.

Herd Immunity

Individuals who develop immunity to an infectious disease, either through immunization or recovery, serve as bodyguards against the spread of that disease within their community. We have already described how the ring-vaccination technique helped in the global eradication of smallpox. The technique, however, was applied only after a case of smallpox became apparent to public health officials. When dealing with inapparent infections, preventing an outbreak becomes a more complex task.

Consider an immune individual coming into contact with an inapparent carrier of the measles virus. The immune individual will not become infected and pass measles on to others, but rather serves as a barrier to disease spread. The proportion of immune individuals required to prevent a disease from becoming epidemic in a community is the level of *herd immunity*. The level of herd immunity required to prevent the spread of an outbreak varies with the specific disease agent. It also depends upon the degree to which infected individuals are capable of transmitting the infection (host immunity), the length of time during which they are infectious (infectious period), and the size and social behavior of the community.

In 1840, William Farr observed, "the smallpox would be disturbed, and sometimes arrested, by vaccination, which protected a part of the population . . ." By the 1920s, the concept of herd immunity was used to study how outbreaks moved through populations. Mathematical models of the spread of infectious agents showed that the smaller the community, the lower the probability of contact between a susceptible person and an infectious one.[11] While the models are theoretically true, the reality is that individuals with inapparent infections may travel well beyond their immediate communities. Their movements can rapidly spread an epidemic, creating a series of outbreak "hot spots." That is exactly what happened during the severe acute respiratory syndrome (SARS) epidemic of 2002, when an outbreak in southern China spread to more than two dozen countries in North and South America, Europe, and Asia before it was contained.

A very practical aspect of herd immunity is that an entire population (100 percent) does not have to be immunized to prevent the spread of an epidemic.[12] This knowledge is useful in the formulation of national vaccination policies. In the United States, for instance, children are vaccinated for measles, mumps, and rubella (MMR vaccine) with two doses, the first administered between 12 and 18 months of age and the second, at least 1 month after the first dose and before 4 years of age (before entering school).[13] This policy works to control transmission of the rubella virus and successfully prevents congenital rubella syndrome as long as 80 to 85 percent of the population is immunized.[14]

Over time, the risks to populations from vaccine-preventable diseases may change because of falling immunization rates, a rise in the proportion of immune-compromised individuals, and an increase in population mobility, especially from global travel. In response to these and other factors, in 2012 the Advisory Committee on Immunization Practices (AICP) recommended that students at all post–high school educational institutions and international travelers provide proof of immunity to measles, mumps, and rubella (laboratory confirmation of immunity or immunization record) and that persons with HIV be vaccinated if they do not have evidence of current severe immunosuppression. This is a clear expansion of the recommendations that preschool children be the focus of the MMR vaccine program, an expansion designed to increase herd immunity across the United States.[15]

In some countries, outbreaks of vaccine-preventable childhood diseases have followed the trend of parents not vaccinating their children out of safety concerns. In Japan, for example, a national vaccination program against measles began in 1978. In 1994, some children had an allergic reaction to the gelatin in the MMR vaccine and the policy was modified from mass obligatory immunization to voluntary individual immunization. Outbreaks of measles immediately occurred in Japan, and a revised immunization program was introduced. Such programs should be effective in controlling the disease as long as a 90 percent vaccine level can be maintained.[16] In contrast, Finland introduced a mandatory two-dose MMR vaccine program in 1982, covering more than 95 percent of the population. While there have been a few cases of measles that were imported from travelers arriving in Finland, the country has had no outbreaks of measles, mumps, or rubella since 1995.[17]

Resistance to vaccine programs continues in many parts of the world, and those preparing to work in medicine, nursing, and public health should be prepared to address this issue with the populations they serve. The resistance to vaccines is often fueled by individuals and groups seeking to instill fear of vaccine programs among the general public for a variety of reasons. These may include well-educated individuals who believe that a natural lifestyle is preferable to vaccines, civil libertarians who believe that mandatory vaccine programs threaten the independence of the individual, parents who mistakenly fear that vaccines cause cancers and autism, tribal leaders who spread rumors that vaccines are secret plots by Westerners to sterilize the population, and extremist organizations that equate vaccine programs with Western incursions that pollute their culture. Those working in vaccine programs must understand the reasons for resistance to vaccine programs if they are to develop successful strategies to overcome it.

The Epidemic Curve

Chapter 1 included the example of an outbreak traced to a single food item, vanilla ice cream. Figure 3.2 shows the *epidemic curve* from that outbreak, indicating the rate at which the cases manifested symptoms.[9] As might be typical of a foodborne epidemic, there was a rapid onset of cases of the disease, but the outbreak was limited in terms of time, place, and persons.

The incubation period for various infectious agents has been a subject of interest in epidemiology dating back to the middle 1800s. At that time, a leading physician at the Smallpox and Vaccination Hospital in London, George Gregory, observed that while each disease had a characteristic incubation period, it could vary somewhat from person to person. Epidemiologists later determined that this variation in incubation periods depended upon the *dosage* of the infectious agent, its *portal of entry*, and the *rate and degree of immune response* by the host. The epidemic curve for all cases in a common source outbreak, then, would likely be *skewed to the right*, reflecting cases with a longer incubation period. Sartwell observed that the typical epidemic curve for a common source outbreak has a lognormal distribution, in other words, a normal distribution in which the x-axis is the logarithm of time rather than time itself.[18] To demonstrate this, an epidemic curve representing a lognormal distribution with a right skew (reflecting cases with a longer incubation period) is shown in Figure 3.3.

It is possible for an epidemic curve from a common source outbreak to have different shapes. For example, if the exposure was prolonged or sporadic, the epidemic curve could be flattened or even demonstrate multiple peaks. The epidemiologist uses the epidemic curve as an essential graphic

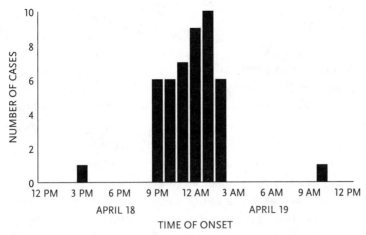

FIGURE 3.2 Cases of gastrointestinal illness by time of onset of symptoms (hour categories) Oswego County, New York, April 19, 1940.

SOURCE: Centers for Disease Control and Prevention (1981).[9]

tool because it allows a common source epidemic to be described using only three factors:

1. The distribution of times and onset of illness of the cases.
2. The incubation period of the disease.
3. The time of exposure.

If only two of these factors are known, it is possible to deduce the third.

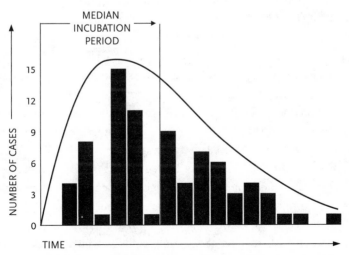

FIGURE 3.3 Example of an epidemiologic curve from a common source outbreak.

To illustrate, assume that physicians in a community begin to see multiple cases of *Salmonella* over a period of a two weeks. The epidemiologist starts to investigate the outbreak by identifying all the cases and creating an epidemic curve. Because the incubation period for *Salmonella* is known, the epidemiologist can estimate the time of exposure by identifying the median point on the epidemic curve (the preferred measure of central tendency because of the skewness in incubation periods) and then work backward to estimate the likely time of exposure. The location and activities of the cases at the likely time of exposure should lead to the common source of the outbreak. Likewise, if sufficient information is available to construct the epidemic curve, and the time of a common exposure is known, the epidemiologist can determine the probable type of infectious disease from the incubation period.

Consider another example. A water fountain in a public park is contaminated with *Salmonella*. Rather than cases of the disease becoming apparent in a short period of time, new cases could continue to occur for an extended period (a season or perhaps a full year) unless the source of the contamination is located and remediated. Since the agent of disease is known (the cases of *Salmonella* having been diagnosed), and because each infectious disease agent has its own characteristic incubation period,[4] the epidemiologist can again gain insight into the outbreak from observing the epidemic curve. If the epidemic curve has multiple peaks, the whereabouts and activities of the cases that occurred at the time of the beginning of the incubation period for each peak should suggest the water fountain as the source of infection. If the epidemic curve is flat, then the epidemiologist will have to estimate the time of exposure for each case rather than for the cases as a whole. Once the common exposure for each case is identified, the role of the drinking fountain will come to light, and the work of remediating the source of the outbreak can commence.

Epidemiologic reasoning using the epidemic curve is widely used to investigate infectious disease outbreaks, but the curves are also applicable to veterinary and botanical settings as well as to noninfectious conditions. For instance, exposure to radiation was recognized as a possible etiological factor for leukemia in the 1930s.[19] Investigators interested in understanding the induction period for the disease approached it in two ways.[20] First they analyzed the cases of leukemia that occurred after the 1945 atomic bomb explosion in Hiroshima, which can be regarded as a single exposure. The investigators compared the annual incidence of leukemia following explosion of the bomb among those who were located less than 1,000 meters from the *hypocenter* (the location of the bomb at the time of the explosion, or *ground zero*) with the incidence among those who were 2,000 meters or more from the center, generally considered an unexposed group. As expected, the annual leukemia incidence rate was higher among those closer to the hypocenter. The epidemic curve, however, showed that the incidence of leukemia peaked in the period 1951 to 1952, about six years after initial exposure to radiation in Hiroshima.

Next, the researchers evaluated reports of ankylosing spondylitis patients who developed leukemia following radiation treatment by either a single exposure or multiple exposures over a number of years.[20] This time, they determined that the epidemic curve peaked at about four years after exposure to radiation and that 90 percent of the cases occurred within nine years. From these two findings, they concluded that the search for etiological factors for leukemia among adults should focus on the 10-year period before the onset of the disease.

Another example of reasoning about etiologic factors for noninfectious diseases using the epidemic curve is that which examined the changing pattern of mortality from leukemia among English and Welsh children less than five years of age between 1931 and 1953.[21] Hewitt created a series of curves for childhood leukemia mortality and noted that not only did the curves change over time, they showed a remarkable similarity to epidemic curves reflecting the incubation periods for various infectious diseases. Could the difference in the mortality curves be due to changes in exposure to etiologic agents? As the mortality from childhood leukemia peaked at three to four years of age, could the modal point on the curve be used to estimate the induction period and perhaps identify etiologic factors for the disease?

As the Hiroshima data confirmed the link between radiation exposure and leukemia, Hewitt wondered if exposure to X-rays offered a potential explanation for the rise in childhood leukemia. This possibility stimulated investigations into the relationship between prenatal and postnatal X-rays and other procedures, and the occurrence of childhood leukemia. A connection was found between intrauterine radiation (mainly X-rays of the pelvis) and childhood leukemia,[22] but subsequent studies suggested that only part of the increase in childhood leukemia death rates could be explained by such exposures.[23-25] More than half a century and hundreds of publications after Hewitt's original observation, concerns remain about the risks of exposing the fetus and/or child to various types and levels of X-rays (diagnostic, CT scan, therapeutic) and the consequent development of adverse birth outcomes and childhood malignancies.[26,27]

In infectious diseases, the incubation period reflects the multiplication of an organism and its interaction with host defenses. This knowledge led multiple investigators to speculate on whether the infectious model could be applied to noninfectious diseases such as cancer. In the laboratory setting, the distribution of time from exposure until the manifestation of cancers among irradiated mice has been found to have a lognormal distribution, similar to an epidemic curve reflecting a common-vehicle outbreak. Lognormal distributions have also been found in a range of occupational exposures resulting in cancer; exposures to drugs and vaccines leading to adverse health events (e.g., chloramphenicol and the development of aplastic anemia); genetic disorders; and serum cholesterol, blood pressure, and mortality from coronary heart disease.

Summary

The occurrence of disease requires the interaction of an agent with a host in a given environment, otherwise known as the *epidemiologic triad*. The interaction may reflect a population's single exposure to an infectious or noninfectious agent resulting in a common-vehicle outbreak. Another possibility is that an infectious agent is spread via serial transfer from an infected individual to a susceptible host. Once the agent has been introduced to a susceptible host, a series of biological events takes place leading to subclinical followed by clinically apparent disease. The time period from exposure to disease resolution is the spectrum of disease.

The terminology used to describe the natural history of diseases varies by textbook and audience. Chronic diseases have induction and latency periods before the disease becomes symptomatic. Infectious diseases have incubation (the time of infection and the appearance of symptoms), latency (the period between the time of infection and the start of the infectious period), and infectious (the time when the disease is able to be transmitted to others) periods. The sojourn period is the time before symptoms appear, but when the disease may be detected through screening.

The concept of herd immunity provides a basis for population-based vaccination programs. As the proportion of the population immunized (either by previous exposure to the agent or by vaccination) increases (i.e., is no longer susceptible), the opportunity for transmission of the agent within that population declines. For most infectious agents, the level of herd immunity required to cease disease transmission is less than 100 percent. How a population achieves that level may differ depending upon how policies surrounding vaccine programs are implemented.

Each disease has a characteristic incubation period, and the distribution of the time periods when cases become symptomatic is displayed in an epidemic curve. The distribution of the epidemic curve tends to skew to the right for common source outbreaks or epidemics, reflecting the variation in host response that may yield differences in incubation or induction periods. For propagated outbreaks that spread serially, the epidemic curve may be flattened. Whether the curve is skewed, has multiple peaks, or is flat, the epidemic curve is an essential tool for the epidemiologist. It takes into account three factors: (1) the distribution of times and onset of illness of the cases, (2) the incubation period of the disease, and (3) the time of exposure. If only two of the three are known, the third can be deduced.

References

1. Karl Pearson, *The Grammar of Science*. London: Walter Scott, 1892.
2. I. Grotto et al., "Clinical and Laboratory Presentation of EBV Positive Infectious Mononucleosis in Young Adults," *Epidemiology & Infection* 131, no. 1 (2003): 683–689.
3. Anthony Bourdain, *Typhoid Mary: An Urban Historical*. New York: Bloomsbury, 2001.
4. David L. Heymann, *Control of Communicable Diseases Manual*. Washington, DC: American Public Health Association, 2015.
5. J. M. Last, "The Iceberg: 'Completing the Clinical Picture' in General Practice," *Lancet* 282, no. 7297 (1963): 28–31.
6. Miquel Porta, ed., *A Dictionary of Epidemiology, 6th Edition*. New York: Oxford University Press, 2014.
7. Mary Mungai, Gary Tegtmeier, Mary Chamberland, and Monica Parise, "Transfusion-Transmitted Malaria in the United States from 1963 through 1999," *New England Journal of Medicine* 344, no. 26 (2001): 1973–1978.
8. A. K. Owusu-Ofori, C. Parry, and I. Bates, "Transfusion-Transmitted Malaria in Countries Where Malaria Is Endemic: A Review of the Literature From Sub-Sahara Africa," *Clinical Infectious Diseases* 51, no. 10 (2010): 1192–1198.
9. Centers for Disease Control and Prevention Epidemiology Program Office, "An Outbreak of Gastrointestinal Illness Following a Church Supper, Lycoming, Oswego County, New York, June 19, 1940," Atlanta, GA: US Department of Health and Human Services, Public Health Service, 1981.
10. Walter R. Dowdle, "The Principles of Disease Elimination and Eradication," *MMWR Supplements* 48, S1 (1999): 23–27.
11. M. S. Bartlett, "Measles Periodicity and Community Size," *Journal of the Royal Statistical Society* 120, no. 1 (1957): 48–70.
12. John P. Fox et al., "Herd Immunity: Basic Concept and Relevance to Public Health Immunization Practices," *American Journal of Epidemiology* 94 (1971): 179–118.
13. American Academy of Pediatrics. "2015 Immunization Schedules." Accessed March 24, 2015. http://www2.aap.org/immunization/IZSchedule.html.

14. R. M. Anderson and D. J. Nokes, "Mathematical Models of Transmission and Control," in *Oxford Textbook of Public Health, 2nd Edition*, eds. W. W. Holland and R. Detels. Oxford: Oxford University Press, 1991.

15. Advisory Committee for Immunization Practices, "ACIP Provisional Recommendations: Prevention of Measles, Rubella, Congenital Rubella Syndrome (CRS), and Mumps." December 2012. Available at http://www.acphd. org/media/284696/mmr-oct-2012.pdf.

16. Yusike Maitani and Hirofumi Ishikawa, "Effectiveness Assessment of Vaccination Policy Against Measles Epidemic in Japan Using an Age–Time 2-Dimensional Mathematical Model," *Environmental Health and Preventive Medicine* 17, no. 1 (2012): 34–43.

17. I. Davidkin et al., "MMR Vaccination and Disease Elimination: The Finnish Experience." *Expert Review of Vaccines* 9, no. 9, (2010): 1005–1053.

18. Phillip E. Sartwell, "The Distribution of Incubation Periods of Infectious Disease," *American Journal of Epidemiology* 51 (1950): 310–318.

19. Richard Doll, "Hazards of Ionising Radiation: 100 Years of Observations on Man." *British Journal of Cancer* 72, no. 6 (1995): 1339–1349.

20. S. Cobb, N. Miller, and N. Wald, "On the Estimation of the Incubation Period in Malignant Disease," *Journal of Chronic Diseases* 9, no. 4 (1959): 385–393.

21. David Hewitt. "Some Features of Leukemia Mortality," *British Journal of Preventive & Social Medicine* 9, no. 2 (1955): 81–88.

22. Alice Stewart, Josephine Webb, and David Hewitt, "A Survey of Childhood Malignancies," *British Medical Journal* 1, no. 5086 (1958): 1945–1508.

23. Brian MacMahon, "Prenatal X-ray Exposure and Childhood Cancer," *Journal of the National Cancer Institute* 28, no. 5 (1962): 1173–1191.

24. S. Graham, M. L. Levin, A. M. Lilienfeld, et al. "Preconception, Intrauterine, and Postnatal Irradiation as Related to Leukemia," in *Epidemiological Approaches to the Study of Cancer and Other Chronic Diseases*, ed. W. Haenszel. Washington, DC: US Government Printing Office; 1966, 347–71.

25. E. L. Diamond, H. Schmerler, and A. M. Lilienfeld, "The Relationship of Intra-Uterine Radiation to Subsequent Mortality and Development of Leukemia in Children: A Prospective Study," *American Journal of Epidemiology* 97, no. 5 (1973): 283–313.

26. International Commission on Radiological Protection, "Pregnancy and Medical Irradiation," *Annals of the ICRP* 30, no. 1 (2000): iii–viii, 1–43. Available at http://www.icrp.org/publication.asp?id = ICRP%20Publication%2084.

27. H. B. Kal and H. Struikmans, "Pregnancy and Medical Irradiation: Summary and Conclusions from the International Commission on Radiological Protection," Publication 84 (Dutch), *Nederlands Tijdschrift voor Geneeskunde* 146, no. 7 (2002): 299–303.

Problem Set: Chapter 3

1. The local health officer for the town of Casserole, Falleen Soufflé, received reports from three physicians that they were taking care of local residents who

had diarrhea, abdominal cramps, vomiting, chills, and fever. The physicians each sent a stool sample from one of their patients for culture. The same strain of salmonella was isolated in all three samples. In all, 119 patients were identified, and the times of onset of the disease were tabulated as follows:

JANUARY 7		JANUARY 8		JANUARY 9	
TIME	CASES	TIME	CASES	TIME	CASES
6–7:59 am	2	12–1:59 am	5	12–1:59 am	3
8–9:59 am	5	2–3:59 am	3	2–3:59 am	2
10–11:59 am	11	4–5:59 am	3	4–5:59 am	0
12–1:59 pm	18	6–7:59 am	3	6–7:59 am	1
2–3:59 pm	10	8–9:59 am	4	8–9:59 am	0
4–5:59 pm	7	10–11:59 am	6	10–11:59 am	1
6–7:59 pm	5	12–1:59 pm	8	12–1:59 pm	0
8–9:59 pm	4	2–3:59 pm	4	2–3:59 pm	0
10–11:59 pm	4	4–5:59 pm	3	4–5:59 pm	0
		6–7:59 pm	3	6–7:59 pm	0
		8–9:59 pm	2	8–9:59 pm	0
		10–11:59 pm	2	10–11:59 pm	0

    a. Make a graph of the epidemic curve.

    b. What type of outbreak does this curve suggest? Why?

    c. What are the possible reasons for the bimodality of this type of epidemic curve?

    d. Three factors are necessary to describe an epidemic, but if only two are known it is possible to deduce the third. Which two factors does Health Officer Soufflé know? Which factor will she be able to deduce?

    e. Having deduced the third factor, what might be the next step in the investigation?

2. Sunnyside Up is a town of 5,000 persons that experienced a serious outbreak of pertussis (whooping cough) last year. Shortly after that outbreak, the state health department conducted a survey of the town's residents to determine how many persons were susceptible to *B. pertussis*, the causal agent for the disease. The survey included blood samples that showed that 1,000 town residents had developed antibodies to *B. pertussis*; that is, they were immune to reinfection.

    During the first two weeks of this year, many patients again presented to the local hospital with pertussis and Dr. Egghead (the physician-in-chief) contacted the state health department for assistance. Over the next two months, local physicians diagnosed some 300 cases of pertussis among Sunnyside Up residents; 60 of these cases died from the disease. Once the outbreak had concluded, the state health department again surveyed town residents, collecting blood samples from each to see how many had been exposed to the agent. Of the 4,000 residents susceptible to infection, 600 had developed infections with *B. pertussis*. Dr. Egghead is trying to characterize the outbreak for the local medical society and has asked for your help as the local epidemiologist.

    Help Dr. Egghead by calculating the infectivity, pathogenicity, and virulence of the causative agent for the recent outbreak of pertussis in Sunnyside Up.

3. Down the road from Sunnyside Up is the sleepy town of Scrambled, with a population of 2,000. When the state health department conducted its pertussis survey in Sunnyside Up last year, it conducted one in Scrambled, as well. As it turned out, 1,000 Scrambled residents were immune to *B. pertussis*. When 20 residents of Scrambled developed pertussis over a 4-week period in late spring (5 died), Dr. Over-Easy (Dr. Egghead's counterpart in Scrambled) began a survey of all town residents, obtaining blood from each to see if they had been infected. The results of the blood tests showed that 40 Scrambled residents had been infected since the state's survey last year. Scrambled's mayor, I. M. Poached, insisted that the culprit came from Sunnyside. Dr. Over-Easy isn't so sure.

   Help Dr. Over-Easy determine the infectivity, pathogenicity, and virulence of *B. pertussis* in this outbreak.

4. Create a table to compare the characteristics of the causative agent in Sunnyside Up with those of the causative agent in Scrambled. Using this information, what can Dr. Over-Easy tell Mayor Poached about the outbreak?

5. Pancake Row is a college town of 100,000 persons directly across Brunch Lake from Sunnyside Up. Over a weekend round of golf with Nurse Sugar Molasses, the head of student health at Pancake Row College, Mayor Maple Syrup said, "Those 2,500 students make your college the biggest population group in Pancake Row. Is there any chance of any health problems cropping up your way?"

   "No, Mayor, I heard about the pertussis outbreak, but I think we're good. I thought that we might have a problem with measles, but it turns out that 40 percent of the students have already been vaccinated against it. My one concern is a sophomore who came into the clinic with what looks like measles."."

   "Measles?" the mayor responded. "I thought that vaccinations had eliminated that disease years ago."

   "Only if people get vaccinated," Nurse Molasses said.

   As soon as they finished the round of golf, Nurse Molasses returned to campus and was told by the on-call physician, Dr. Milk N. Oatmeal, that the sophomore had a confirmed case of measles. "The measles virus is highly contagious," the doctor said. "It can be spread by serial transfer through coughing and sneezing, close personal contact, or direct contact with infected surfaces for up to two hours. An infected person can transmit the virus from four days prior to the onset of the rash to four days after the rash erupts. To halt any potential outbreak, the student body has to reach a 90 percent level of herd immunity within days. Therefore, anyone lacking proof of vaccination will be given a measles vaccine immediately. There's a shortage of measles vaccines in the state, so we need to know how many doses of the vaccine it will take to stem the outbreak."

   Help Dr. Oatmeal and Nurse Molasses by estimating the minimum number of vaccine doses that need to be administered to students not previously immunized to ensure there will be no measles epidemic at Pancake Row College.

4 | Inferring Causal Relationships

> Epidemiology at any given time is something more than the total
> of its established facts. It includes their orderly arrangement into
> chains of inference which extends more or less beyond the bounds
> of direct observation.[1]
>
> *Wade Hampton Frost (1936)*

C HAPTERS 1, 2, AND 3 INTRODUCED the epidemiologic approach to
studying the health of populations using information from the triads "time, place, and person" and "agent, host, and environment."
Once a pattern of health outcomes is observed, the epidemiologist begins
the process of trying to determine why it exists—the underlying cause(s).
The framework used by the epidemiologist to test whether a relationship
between a potential cause and effect does or does not exist is called *causal
inference*.[2] The conceptual aspects of the framework are introduced in this
chapter to help the reader understand how statistical methods and study
designs help the epidemiologist build a case for cause. The clinical applications of the framework will be further considered in Chapter 13, and the field
applications in Chapter 14.

Showing Cause

Finding a statistical association between two or more variables in an epidemiologic study does not necessarily indicate a causal relationship. The epidemiologist must consider the possibility that the statistical association occurred
by *chance* alone. It is also possible that the association may be *artifactual*
(*spurious*), the result of biased methods of data collection, nonrepresentative

sampling methods, misclassification of exposure or disease, or other study errors. Most of these problems can be avoided by well-designed epidemiologic studies.

Sometimes an analysis will yield results that identify a true statistical association, yet it may still be *noncausal*. This is because many variables can occur together without necessarily being a part of a causal chain. For example, left-handed individuals suffer more unintentional injuries compared to those who are right-handed. The association is a true one, but is it causal?

Establishing a *causal association* requires using a framework that withstands scientific scrutiny. One of the earliest frameworks of *causal criteria* can be traced to the German pathologist Jakob Henle in 1840, prior to the discovery of bacteria as agents of disease. One of Henle's students, Robert Koch, revised the criteria during the late 1880s; the result is now termed the *Henle-Koch postulates* (*Koch's postulates*).[3]

The Henle-Koch postulates are threefold:

1. The organism must be found in all cases of the disease.
2. The organism can be isolated from patients with the disease and grown in pure culture.
3. When the pure culture of the organism is inoculated into susceptible animals or humans, it must reproduce the disease.

By the beginning of the twentieth century, advances in sanitation, nutrition, and water supply led to changes in patterns of mortality. Deaths from infectious diseases declined, and noninfectious diseases became more prominent. As useful as the Henle-Koch postulates may have been, they did not lend themselves to identifying causal factors for noninfectious diseases, especially those with long incubation periods.

In 1959, Yerushalmy and Palmer proposed an updated framework to address the problem of showing cause with noninfectious diseases.[4] Their work was subsequently revised and extended by Lilienfeld,[5] and Stallones advanced this discussion into the formulation used in the landmark 1964 Surgeon General's report linking cigarette smoking and lung cancer.[6] The resultant framework became known as the *Surgeon General's criteria* and included the following:

1. *Consistency*—When the same results are found by different investigators in different places and among different groups using different methods, the likelihood of a causal effect is increased.

2. *Strength of association*—The stronger the statistical association, especially in the absence of other potentially causative or confounding factors, the more likely the relationship is to be causal.
3. *Specificity*—If a specific outcome among a specific population at a specific place and time has no other likely explanation, the likelihood of a causal effect is increased.
4. *Temporality*—The cause must precede the effect, and it must take into account anticipated time delays required for the effect to occur.
5. *Coherence*—The association should not conflict with existing knowledge of the disease gained through biological, clinical, epidemiological or sociological research.

In the year following the Surgeon General's report, British epidemiologist A. Bradford Hill gave the President's address at the Royal Society of Medicine, where he listed "considerations of causal inference."[7] Hill included the Surgeon General's criteria his considerations, but he also added three more:

1. *Dose-response relationship*—A change in the amount of exposure should generally lead to a respective change in the incidence of the effect.
2. *Plausibility*—A plausible biological mechanism between the exposure and the outcome is helpful for showing cause, but it may not be known or even partially known in some instances.
3. *Experiment*—An experimental study (human or animal) that demonstrates that the outcome can be altered is helpful but not always possible.

Taken together, the eight considerations became known as the *Bradford Hill criteria* (*Hill's postulates*). Hill reinforced the fact that as an *inductive* science, epidemiology is unable to *prove* cause. Rather, the epidemiologist *infers* causality to identify *etiological factors* (*causal factors, causal associations,* or *risk factors*).[8] He noted that this is a pragmatic approach, as:

All scientific work is incomplete—whether it be observational or experimental . . .
"Who knows," asked Robert Browning, "but the world may end tonight?" True, but on available evidence, most of us make ready to commute on 8:30 the next day.[9]

Since Hill's address, epidemiologists have struggled with various sets of postulates and causal models, probing for ways to infer causation that can hold up to epidemiologic, legal, and scientific challenges. In 1976, Evans synthesized a framework applicable to both infectious and noninfectious diseases—the *Unified Concept of Causation*.[10] Epidemiologists did not, however, adopt this conceptualization, and the discussion shifted to whether causes were *necessary* (the outcome cannot occur without the causal factor being present) or *sufficient* (the presence of the causal factor must cause the outcome) to cause a particular outcome. For example, an individual cannot develop acquired immunodeficiency syndrome (AIDS) without first being infected with human immunodeficiency virus (HIV). Thus, infection with HIV is a necessary cause for an individual to develop AIDS. On the other hand, not all individuals infected with HIV develop AIDS. This means that HIV is not a sufficient cause of AIDS, and other factors must also be at work. Table 4.1 gives additional examples.

Though the concept of necessary and sufficient causes may help the epidemiologist in assessing causation, there are complex diseases with important risk factors that are neither necessary nor sufficient to cause disease, as exemplified by smoking and lung cancer. Cigarette smoking is strongly associated with the development of lung cancer (fulfilling the Surgeon General's criteria), yet some nonsmokers develop the disease; therefore, smoking is not a necessary cause. Many persons who smoke cigarettes do not develop lung cancer; therefore, smoking is not a sufficient cause. Rothman suggested that sufficient causes were actually made up of components, none of which caused the outcome on its own but would do so in conjunction with other components. Hence, the concept of *sufficient components* was presented in a model using *causal pies*. If sufficient components occurred together, they would trigger the effect.[11]

TABLE 4.1 Examples of Necessary and Sufficient Causes for Select Diagnostic (Dx) Conditions

		NECESSARY FACTOR	
		YES	NO
SUFFICIENT FACTOR	YES	Measles virus (Dx: measles)	Radiation (Dx: lung cancer)
		Maternal consumption of alcohol (Dx: fetal alcohol syndrome)	Postmenopausal estrogens (endometrial cancer)
	NO	Presence of *Streptococcus mutans* (Dx: dental caries)	Hypertension (Dx: acute coronary syndrome)
		Chickenpox virus infection (Dx: shingles)	Exposure to sunlight (Dx: skin cancer)

The sufficient components model has been criticized as *deterministic* in that it either triggered an effect or it did not (yes/no). The model was also criticized as not being flexible enough to account for a dose-response relationship. A reformulation of the sufficient components model was offered by Parascandola and Weed,[12] suggesting that each component adds to the probability of an outcome rather than joining together to trigger an effect. This approach allowed for the consideration of dose-response effects.

In 2005, Greenland offered a *counterfactual model of causation* for decisions related to health policy.[13] This approach utilizes statistical modeling to ask the question, "What if?" For instance, how would the outcome change if a patient with a chronic disease were treated immediately instead of in a week, a month, or a year? Using statistical modeling, the epidemiologist can evaluate the effect of removing an etiological factor or changing conditions on various outcomes. Susser and Schwartz extended the counterfactual model to uses beyond those of health policy. They identified causal factors in social epidemiology by using an unexposed group as a proxy for the counterfactual.[14] At this time, the counterfactual model is rapidly becoming the standard for showing cause in both epidemiological and medical research.[15] The reader interested in using counterfactual modeling techniques should seek guidance from more advanced epidemiology texts.

Confounding and Effect Modification

When the association between an etiologic factor and an outcome is influenced by a third variable that leads to an inaccurate comparison, the association is *confounded*. The third variable is called a *confounding factor* or *confounder*. Consider the association between consuming alcohol, smoking cigarettes, and lung cancer. Cigarette smoking is a risk factor for lung cancer. Persons who smoke cigarettes also tend to drink more alcohol than those who do not smoke. Those who smoke more cigarettes tend to drink more than those who smoke fewer cigarettes. Thus, if we were examining the association between alcohol consumption and lung cancer, cigarette smoking would be a confounding factor. While this illustration uses only one risk factor and one confounding factor, the concept can be extended to multivariate situations where the statistical associations among variables may be complex. It is important for the epidemiologist searching for causal relationships to remain aware of the possibility of confounding and to use epidemiologic tools and reasoning to minimize the likelihood of drawing inaccurate conclusions.

Three tools are often used to address the issue of confounding in the design phase of an epidemiologic study:

1. *Restriction*: The study can be restricted to a specific population group or to subjects that meet various selection criteria in order to control for the effect of known confounders. For example, Colaco and colleagues investigated whether toilet training strategies (child-centered or parent-centered) were associated with dysfunctional voiding in childhood.[16] The investigators evaluated two groups of children aged 4–12 years, one group presenting with urge incontinence and the other serving as normal controls. Participation was restricted, in that children with anatomical malformations of the urinary tract, diabetes mellitus, proteinuria, or history of neurological conditions were excluded from the study. These conditions are known to cause dysfunctional voiding and, if included, could cause the results to be confounded. The study found that the method of toilet training was not associated with dysfunctional voiding.

2. *Matching*: Study participants can be matched for the potential confounding variable. For instance, twin studies examined the relationship of cigarette smoking and early death, finding excess mortality among the twins that smoked compared to those who did not smoke or who smoked less. Identical (monozygotic) twins were matched to control for genetics, and both identical and fraternal (dizygotic) twins were matched to control for the potential confounding of early life experiences and exposures (especially diet).[17]

3. *Adjustment*: The effect of confounding may be mitigated by statistical adjustment, methods that take the confounder into account. In brief, the epidemiologist measures the crude association between an exposure and an outcome of interest, repeats the analysis after adjusting for each potential confounder, and then compares the results of the crude and adjusted measures (Chapter 5 covers this technique in depth). An analysis in 1990 by Hirayama exemplifies this approach.[18] The researcher found that the risk for lung cancer in women who consume alcohol increased with ascending consumption (Figure 4.1). This result suggests that drinking alcohol is associated with the risk of developing lung cancer. When the data were adjusted for differences in cigarette smoking patterns, the association disappeared (Figure 4.2). In this instance, cigarette smoking was a confounding variable. Its presence misled the investigators about the role of alcohol in the development of lung cancer until they unraveled the confounding.

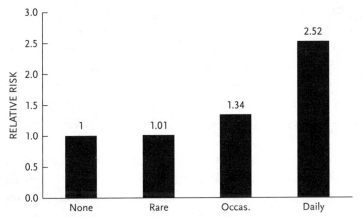

FIGURE 4.1 Relative risks for lung cancer in women by frequency of alcohol
consumption.

SOURCE: Adapted from Hirayama (1990).[18]

Adjusting for confounders may be accomplished by using a *stratified analysis,* where variables are broken into levels (*strata*) and then reanalyzed. A commonly used approach is the *Cochran-Mantel-Haenszel* statistical technique, where each stratum is assigned an appropriate weight, and the weights are used to calculate an adjusted relative risk[19] (see Chapter 10). Alternatively, multivariate techniques (multiple and logistic regression and log-linear models) may be used. Regardless of the multivariate approach employed, the epidemiologist mathematically models the occurrence of disease based upon the presence or absence of possible risk factors and confounders.

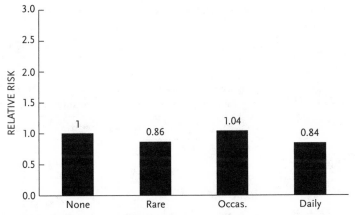

FIGURE 4.2 Relative risks for lung cancer in women by frequency of alcohol
consumption, adjusted for cigarette smoking.

SOURCE: Adapted from Hirayama (1990).[18]

These statistical techniques allow for several *independent variables* (*potential confounders*) to be considered in the model simultaneously. If the study does not adequately control for the presence of confounding variables, the inferences drawn from the results may not be well founded.

It is possible that risk factors may interact to create a *synergistic* (*enhanced*) or *antagonistic* (*diminished*) causal effect, sometimes referred to as *effect modification* or *interaction*. The epidemiologist uses these terms to describe two or more factors that together can prevent, cause, or change effects. For example, exposure to asbestos fibers and cigarette smoking interact to cause lung cancer at a greater rate than would either individually. While the two risk factors may each be causally related with lung cancer, together they work synergistically. The *relative risks* (relationship of the individual risks) for developing lung cancer among smoking and nonsmoking asbestos insulation workers are shown in Table 4.2 to illustrate such enhancement.

The terminology used by epidemiologists to describe effect modification and interaction continues to evolve.[21] For instance, Vanderweele defined the terms as separate concepts, with interaction being "the effects of two interventions," and effect modification being "the effect of one intervention varying across strata of a second variable."[22] Thus, there is still much debate in the epidemiologic literature about the appropriate way to assess and analyze a data set for confounding, effect modification, and interactions. When such relationships are found, they must be fully described when the results of the study are presented. The epidemiologist may point out, for example, that men and women showed different responses to varying dosages of a treatment, or that children in a particular age group were especially prone to particular types of unintentional injuries. Such information becomes the bedrock for inferring cause.

TABLE 4.2 Age-Adjusted Lung Cancer Mortality Rates per 100,000 Man-Years with Rate Ratios* by Cigarette Smoking and Occupational Exposure to Asbestos Dust

	NONSMOKERS	CIGARETTE SMOKERS
NOT EXPOSED TO ASBESTOS DUST	11.3 (1.0)	122.6 (10.9)
EXPOSED TO ASBESTOS DUST	58.4 (5.2)	601.6 (53.2)

* Rate ratios in parentheses are based on nonsmokers not exposed to asbestos dust as the referent group.
DATA SOURCE: Hammond et al. (1979).[20]

Legal and Policy Implications

All of the postulates and models discussed above provide guidelines for *inferring* (not proving) *causal relationships*. As the conclusions drawn from epidemiologic studies may impact public health, public policy, and clinical decisions, the epidemiologist must be clear on this point when reporting study results.

The epidemiologist may also serve as a resource to the courts when environmental or occupational exposures, or the use of a product (pharmaceutical, medical device, or consumer product such as tobacco) is associated with injury. Two questions arise when determining liability:

1. Is the alleged exposure a cause of the disease in question?

When testifying on such matters, it is important for the epidemiologist to carefully explain the process of drawing a causal inference. By educating both the courts and those who craft legislation, the epidemiologist may prevent erroneous rulings and the supposition that all causal criteria must be met to assert that an exposure causes an outcome.

For example, exposure to asbestos has long been recognized as an occupational health problem linked to mesothelioma, lung cancer, and other respiratory diseases. The World Health Organization, the World Bank, and other national and global organizations have called for a ban on its use. As with the tobacco industry in earlier decades, the asbestos industry hired consultants to testify against causal claims, both in occupational injury cases and to national legislative bodies considering bans on asbestos use. The industry hired consultants to challenge select evidence, generating doubt in the minds of jurors and policymakers about cause. The epidemiologist, however, examines the totality of the evidence before rendering a conclusion about the question of cause, and bears the burden of educating the public about the process. In 2012, the Joint Policy Committee of the Societies of Epidemiology (JCP-SE, representing at least 10 epidemiologic organizations from around the globe) called for an international ban on asbestos use. Using wide media coverage, the JCP-SE educated policymakers about how epidemiologists draw conclusions about cause. Shortly after the statement was issued, the Canadian government recognized chrysotile asbestos as a hazardous substance and promised aid to mining communities to shift their economic activities. The JCP-SE's efforts clearly made inroads into bringing legitimacy to ending asbestos mining and use, a global public health issue.[23]

2. Is it more likely than not that the injury resulted from that exposure?

Once causation is inferred, the epidemiologist must assess whether the exposure caused the injury in a particular plaintiff. One common model used by courts in the United States is to ask whether it is "more likely than not" that the individual's injury resulted from the exposure. To address this question, the epidemiologist calculates the probability that a given case of disease resulted from exposure to the etiologic factor. If the probability is greater than 50 percent, the epidemiologist may conclude that the factor is more likely than not the cause of the litigant's case of disease (see also Chapters 9 and 10 for discussions of population-attributable fraction). In cases involving occupational exposures where the probability of exposure is high, additional epidemiologic calculations may be needed to demonstrate the risk.

Again, consider the relationship between asbestos and lung cancer demonstrated in Table 4.2. The lung cancer mortality rates for those exposed to asbestos dust were increased more than four-fold regardless of whether the study subjects smoked cigarettes (a known cause of lung cancer) or not. Based on these data and additional epidemiologic analyses, the epidemiologist would conclude that an individual who had been exposed to asbestos dust and who died from lung cancer *more likely than not* developed that cancer as a result of their exposure to asbestos. Epidemiologic studies such as these have led many courts around the world to award compensation for injuries incurred by workers exposed to asbestos.

Summary

Epidemiologic inferences may lead to a public health action; to changes in clinical practice, health education, legislation, or public policy; or to new research directions. An example of the role of epidemiologic data influencing public policy is that of US legislation regulating smoking in public places. The restrictions are designed to protect the general population, including children and the most vulnerable, from exposure to environmental tobacco smoke. Other examples of health education efforts include emphasizing the use of condoms to aid in the prevention of HIV infection, the need to reduce alcohol intake during pregnancy to prevent fetal alcohol syndrome, the use of seat belts to reduce auto accident injuries, and the role of dietary change in reducing heart disease.

Experimentation and the determination of biological mechanisms that initiate and promote the disease process provide the most direct evidence of a causal relationship between a risk factor and a disease outcome. Causation in infectious disease is still demonstrated by the Henle-Koch postulates. In fact, Fredricks and Relman updated these postulates in 1996 by incorporating the DNA typing of microorganisms.[24]

For noninfectious health outcomes, epidemiologic studies can provide very strong support for hypotheses describing both direct and indirect associations. Inferences from such studies must not be made in isolation, and they must comport, when the knowledge exists, with human biology. In the absence of that knowledge, epidemiologic and other evidence can accumulate to the point where a causal hypothesis becomes highly probable. Although an element of subjectivity will always remain, a causal hypothesis developed under accepted postulates or using appropriate causal models can be sufficiently probable to provide a reasonable basis for successful preventive and public health actions.

References

1. Wade Hampton Frost, "Introduction," in *Snow on Cholera*, p. ix. New York: The Commonwealth Fund, 1936. Available at http://www.ncbi.nlm.nih.gov/pmc/articles/PMC2601508/?page = 1
2. Miquel Porta, ed., *A Dictionary of Epidemiology, 6th Edition*. New York: Oxford University Press, 2014.
3. R. Koch R, "Über den augenblicklichen Stand der bakteriologischen Choleradiagnose," *Zeitschrift für Hygiene und Infectionskrankheiten* 14 (1893): 319–333.
4. J. Yerushalmy and Carroll E. Palmer, "On the Methodology of Investigations of Etiology Factors in Chronic Diseases," *Journal of Chronic Diseases* 10, no. 1 (1959): 27–40.
5. Abraham M. Lilienfeld, "On the Methodology of Investigations of Etiologic Factors in Chronic Diseases: Some Comments," *Journal of Chronic Diseases* 10, no. 1 (1959): 41–46.
6. Richard Kluger, *Ashes to Ashes*. New York: Vintage, 1997.
7. Henry Blackburn and Dawin Labarthe, "Stories from the Evolution of Guidelines for Causal Inference in Epidemiologic Associations: 1953–1965," *American Journal of Epidemiology* 17, no. 12 (2012): 1071–1077.
8. Austin Bradford Hill, "Statistical Evidence and Inference" in *Principles of Medical Statistics* (pp. 309–323). New York: Oxford University Press, 1971.
9. Austin Bradford Hill, "President's Address: The Environment and Disease: Association or Causation?" *Proceedings of the Royal Society of Medicine* 58 (May 1965): 295–300.
10. Alfred S. Evans, "Causation and Disease: The Henle-Koch Postulates Revisited," *Yale Journal of Biology and Medicine* 49 (1976): 175–195.

11. Kenneth J. Rothman, "Causes," *American Journal of Epidemiology.* 104, no. 6 (1976): 587–592.
12. M. Parascandola and D. L. Weed, "Causation in Epidemiology," *Journal of Epidemiology & Community Health* 55, no 12 (2001): 905–912.
13. Sander Greenland, "Epidemiologic measures and policy formulation: lessons from potential outcomes," *Emerging Themes in Epidemiology* 2 (2005): 5, doi:10.1186/1742-7622-2-5.
14. Ezra Susser and Sharon Schwartz, "Are social causes so different from all other causes? A comment on Sander Greenland," *Emerging Themes in Epidemiology* 2 (2005): 4, doi:10.1186/1742-7622-2-4.
15. M. Hofler, "Causal Inference Based on Counterfactuals," *BMC Medical Research Methodology* 5 (2005): 28, doi:10.1186/1471-2288-5-28.
16. Marc Colaco, Kelly Johnson, Dona Schneider, and Joseph Barone, "Toilet Training Method Is Not Related to Dysfunctional Voiding," *Clinical Pediatrics* 52, no. 1 (2013): 49–53.
17. J. Kaprio and M. Koskenvuo, "Twins, Smoking and Mortality: A 12-year Prospective Study of Smoking Discordant Twin Pairs," *Social Science & Medicine* 29, no. 9 (1989): 1083–1089.
18. Takeshi Hirayama, *Life-Style and Mortality: A Large-Scale Census-Based Cohort Study in Japan.* Basel: S. Karger, 1990.
19. Nathan Mantel and William Haenszel, "Statistical Aspects of the Analysis of Data from Retrospective Studies of Disease," *Journal of the National Cancer Institute* 22 (1959): 719–748.
20. E. Cuyler Hammond, Irving J. Selikoff, and Herbert Seidman, "Asbestos Exposure, Cigarette Smoking, and Death Rates," *Annals of the New York Academy of Sciences* 330 (1979): 473–490.
21. Anders Ahlbom and Lars Alfredsson, "Interaction: A Word with Two Meanings Creates Confusion," *European Journal of Epidemiology* 20, no. 7 (2005): 563–564.
22. Tyler J. VanderWeele, "On the Distinction between Interaction and Effect Modification," *Epidemiology* 20, no. 6 (2009): 863–871.
23. Wael K. Al-Delaimy, "The JPC-SE Position Statement on Asbestos: A long-overdue appeal by epidemiologists to ban asbestos worldwide and end related global environmental injustice," *Environmental Health Perspectives* 121, no. 5 (2013): a144–a145.
24. David N. Fredricks and David A. Relman, "Sequence-based Identification of Microbial Pathogens: A reconsideration of Koch's postulates. *Clinical Microbiology Reviews* 9, no. 1 (1996): 18–33.

II | Descriptive Studies

As our world continues to generate unimaginable amounts of
data, more data lead to more correlations, and more correlations
can lead to more discoveries.[1]

Hans Rosling (2011)

CHAPTERS 5 THROUGH 8 deal with the conduct and interpretation
of descriptive studies. Such studies are used to track the health of
populations and to search for associations between patterns of particular health outcomes and possible etiologic factors that explain
those patterns. While descriptive studies can help the epidemiologist generate hypotheses about the etiologies of population health
outcomes, they cannot assess the risk for those outcomes among
individuals. Individual risk must be evaluated through the use of
analytic studies. These will be covered in Part III.

Descriptive studies focus on the use of vital statistics (birth and
death information) as well as morbidity data to assess population
health. Since these data are often readily available and inexpensive to obtain, the epidemiologist can track population health over
time and generate hypotheses about particular patterns seen in
the data. Chapter 5 demonstrates how vital statistics are assembled and describes the advantages and problems of working with
information about birth and death in the population as a whole.
Chapter 6 provides examples of how birth and death are used to
examine population health, including following patterns over time
(secular trends), comparing places, and examining differences
among groups of persons.

The ways in which morbidity data are gathered, including the
role of surveillance, are covered in Chapter 7. Particular emphasis

is placed on the cross-sectional survey and the use of screening populations for disease. Measures of screening test performance are covered, along with a discussion of the role of these tests for public health. Examples of how epidemiologists use morbidity data are provided in Chapter 8, including the identification of clusters in time and/or space. The epidemiologist always remembers that when clusters are identified, descriptive studies may only suggest a hypothesis regarding the cause or provide an initial test of a hypothesis. To test an etiologic hypothesis about a cluster, an epidemiologic study that can assess individual risk must be conducted.

Reference

1. Hans Rosling, "Pumphandle Lecture for the John Snow Society," London, September 2011.

5 | Vital Statistics

> Vital statistics forms perhaps the most important branch of
> Statistics, as it deals with mankind in the aggregate.[1]
>
> *Sir Arthur Newsholme (1924)*

THE USE OF A POPULATION census can be traced to ancient civilizations such as Egypt, Greece, and Rome. A census could be used to record households, persons, or specific types of property in order to tax the population or to impose a military draft. The recording of vital events (births, deaths, marriages and divorce) was not of interest to civil authorities, so that task was left to religious institutions. Beginning in the fifteenth century, all Spanish churches began maintaining registers of births, baptisms, marriages, and deaths. Parishes across northern Europe followed suit during the sixteenth century, and Buddhist temples started to track births, deaths, and marriages in the seventeenth century.[2]

The first civil registration of vital events is credited to the Incas, who used a system of colored strings and knots to record the number of births and deaths each month, as well as the number of men who went to war and died in service. In colonial America, civil authorities in Virginia and Massachusetts absorbed the responsibility of keeping track of vital events. In Europe, the Napoleonic Code (1804) spurred civil authorities to assume the role of keeping vital records so that the state could confer citizenship and guarantee the rights of its citizens.[2] Public records on vital events are now maintained by civil units (tribes, municipalities, states/provinces, and nations) in many parts of the world to document citizenship, validate marital status, ensure inheritance rights, help settle legal claims, and more. In total, the individual records are reported as *vital statistics*.

England and Wales created the General Register Office in 1836 to guarantee property rights among the landed gentry and to provide key information on births and deaths needed by the British life insurance industry. William Farr was hired as "Examiner and Compiler of Abstracts," a junior-level position which he elevated and expanded over the course of 40 years. Farr not only gathered and compiled vital registrations, he also pioneered their use in monitoring the health of populations (see Chapter 2). His regular reporting and efforts at standardizing the coding of outcomes was unsurpassed during his lifetime.[3] The United States did not produce a comparable set of vital statistics for the entire nation until 1933, almost a century later.[4] Currently, the US National Vital Statistics System (NVSS) receives vital statistics data from each of the fifty states, New York City, the District of Columbia, and the US territories (American Samoa, the Commonwealth of the Northern Marianas, Guam, Puerto Rico, and the US Virgin Islands). The NVSS is administered by the National Center for Health Statistics (NCHS), a division of the Centers for Disease Control and Prevention (CDC).

Not all geographic areas of the world have civil registration systems that include the births and deaths of all their inhabitants. Because of cost, civil strife, lack of infrastructure, and other limitations, some regions have only partial information and others have none. Nations with stable governments and significant infrastructures are the ones most likely to have complete coverage of all vital events in their jurisdictions. The United Nations issued recommendations for the establishment of vital statistics systems in 2010, providing suggested forms for registering live births, deaths, fetal deaths, marriages, and divorces.[5] Among the types of data provided by a vital statistics system, the epidemiologist is primarily concerned with *mortality* (deaths) and *natality* (births).

Mortality

Mortality statistics provide information helpful in the formulation of public policies that can prevent early and perhaps needless deaths. What are the leading causes of death? How do they differ geographically, and what are the likely reasons for any disparities? The epidemiologist asks these types of questions in an effort to identify health issues in the community and to generate hypotheses about the etiologic factors that are important contributors to adverse health outcomes and premature death.

Mortality Data

In the United States, local units submit their death certificate data electronically to their states, and the states, in turn, report it to the NCHS using standard variables such as name, gender, birth date, Social Security number, place of residence, place of death, and the cause(s) of death.[6] The immediate cause of death is entered first, then any intermediate conditions contributing to the death, and finally the underlying cause. Mortality data sets for public use are available for researchers to query online by using the CDC WONDER website.[7] US mortality data sets are also available for download from the NCHS website.

Sometimes the epidemiologist wants to link records from various databases to obtain information about occupational history, outpatient pharmaceutical use, parental background, or hospital treatment before death. For example, the National Death Index (NDI) is a computer file of all deaths in the United States that can be linked to other databases through combinations of Social Security numbers, names, and dates of birth. To obtain data sets that include any form of personal identification, the epidemiologist must submit a research protocol to an institutional review board (IRB) outlining how the information on individuals will be handled such that their privacy is maintained.

The World Health Organization (WHO) collects and disseminates global mortality data. Gathering such data is difficult; in 2005, only 23 of 192 countries had reliable information on death registration, and 75 countries had no cause-specific mortality information available.[8] To improve the quality of these data, the WHO provides a simple death data collection form with instructions for individuals charged with completing the information.[5] Figure 5.1 provides an example of a completed WHO death certificate. Note that the form asks for *antecedent causes of death*, similar to the death certificate used in the United States.

Classification of Cause of Death

The *International Classification of Diseases* (ICD) is the global standard for coding causes of death on death certificates. The ICD system is revised about once a decade, with the 11th revision expected to be released in 2017. Not all nations adopt new ICD revisions at the same time, and not all those completing death certificates necessarily fill them out completely or accurately. For instance, the United States lagged significantly behind other nations in adopting ICD-10, primarily because many computing systems were programmed to use ICD-9 and the costs to upgrade to ICD-10 were high.

Because the individual completing a death certificate may not be familiar with the deceased's medical history, the reliability of the information relating causes of death may be less than optimal. Many studies have evaluated

Cause of death		Approximate interval between onset and death
I Disease or condition directly leading to death *	(a) Cerebral hemorrhage due to (or as a consequence of)	4 hours
	(b) Metastasis of the brain due to (or as a consequence of)	4 months
Antecedent causes Morbid conditions, if any, giving rise to hte above cause, stating the underlying condition last	(c) Breast cancer due to (or as a consequence of)	5 years
	(d)	
II Other significant conditions contributing to death, but not related to the disease or conditions causing it	Arterial hypertension Diabetes mellitus	3 years 10 years
* This does not mean the mode of dying, e.g. heart failure, respiratory failure. It means hte disease, injury, or complication that caused death.		

FIGURE 5.1 Example of a completed World Health Organization cause of death certificate.

SOURCE: Copyright 2010, World Health Organization. Reproduced with permission of the World Health Organization.

the accuracy of the cause-of-death statements on the death certificate.[9–13] AIDS/HIV infection, for example, was underreported as an underlying cause of death during the early years of the epidemic.[14] Similarly, in Japan, mortality from multiple sclerosis was underreported, as many deaths were attributed to "cerebral sclerosis" (stroke).[15] In contrast, stroke may be over-reported as an underlying cause of death. As an example, a Framingham, Massachusetts study reported that for about 40 percent of deaths attributed to stroke, no evidence of stroke could be found.[16] Other studies have shown that even when physicians evaluate the same case histories, they often differ in the way they report the underlying cause on the death certificate.[17–19] Changes in coding practices may also lead to perceived changes in mortality, even when there has been no change in the actual mortality experience of a population.

Autopsy data, hospital records, and other sources of mortality data may provide accurate information about details omitted from the death certificate, but hospitalized cases or a series selected from coroner's inquests are neither representative of that population nor of the population as a whole.[20–22] The decline in the autopsy rate, especially in the United States, is an additional problem. Before 1970, accreditation standards required teaching hospitals to have a 25 percent autopsy rate; nonteaching hospitals needed 20 percent. That requirement no longer exists, and because the cost of an autopsy is not covered by insurance plans, the US hospital autopsy rate fell to less than 5 percent in 2010.[23]

While the use of the medical autopsy has declined, the *verbal autopsy* has gained as a technique for estimating the cause of death, especially in large areas of India, China, and 36 other places around the world.[24] The verbal autopsy is a technique whereby questions are asked of next of kin about the signs, symptoms, medical history, and circumstances preceding their loved one's death. The WHO issued standards for the verbal autopsy in 2012, including a questionnaire.[25] While the information obtained from a verbal autopsy may not be as accurate as that obtained by the civil registration of deaths, it helps describe the causes of death at the population level.

Mortality Measures

The most frequently used measure of mortality is the *mortality rate* or *death rate*, which has three essential elements:

1. A defined *population at risk*.
2. A time period.
3. The number of deaths occurring in that population during the time period.

Rates are usually calculated on an annual basis and expressed per a given population size, such as 1,000 persons, 100,000 persons, or 1,000,000 persons. The former is used for common causes of death; the latter two are used when the epidemiologist is reporting on selected outcomes (such as deaths from motor vehicle accidents) or rare events (such as deaths from venomous snake bites).

Crude death rates measure the risk of dying for an individual who might be selected randomly from the total population at risk in a given time period. While crude death rates can be expressed for any given population size, global data are often reported as per 1,000 per year. In contrast, US vital statistics report crude death rates per 100,000 per year. The following equation can be adjusted for any population size.

$$Crude\,death\,rate\,per\,1,000\,per\,year = \frac{Number\,of\,deaths\,in\,a\,given\,year}{Population\,at\,risk\,during\,that\,year} \times 1,000$$

Because populations often grow or shrink over the time interval being investigated, the epidemiologist typically uses the midpoint population of the time period for rate calculations. For example, suppose the population at risk was 10,000 persons on January 1 of a study year, but by December 31 of that year there had been mass inmigration, and the population was now 15,000 persons. It is appropriate to use the midpoint population estimate of 12,500 persons as the denominator for rate calculations.

Death rates can also be *specific*, reflecting the risk of dying for an individual that belongs to a particular subgroup of the population at risk. Specific rates can be calculated for selected person characteristics such as age, gender, marital status, or ethnicity. For instance, *age-specific death rates* can be calculated for 0- to 9-year-olds, 10- to 19-year-olds, 20- to 29-year-olds, and so on. It is not uncommon for the epidemiologist to calculate specific rates for multiple person-characteristics at the same time. For example, *age-gender specific death rates* can be calculated to allow for the comparison of 15- to 24-year-old males with that for 15- to 24-year-old females. As with crude death rates, cause-specific death rates are often reported as per 1,000 per year for global data, whereas those based on US vital statistics are usually reported as per 100,000 per year.

$$Specific\ death\ rate\ per\ 1{,}000\ per\ year = \frac{\begin{array}{c} Number\ of\ deaths \\ in\ a\ subgroup \\ in\ a\ given\ year \end{array}}{\begin{array}{c} Population \\ of\ that\ subgroup \\ during\ that\ year \end{array}} \times 1{,}000$$

The epidemiologist uses *cause-specific death rates* to compare the burden of various diseases on the population, either for the total population or for subgroups of that population. For instance, the epidemiologist may be interested in mortality from motor vehicle accidents for a specific population. The cause-specific rate for motor vehicle accidents would be calculated as:

$$Cause\text{-}specific\ death\ rate\ per\ 1{,}000\ per\ year = \frac{\begin{array}{c} Number\ of\ deaths\ from \\ motor\ vehicle\ accidents \\ in\ a\ given\ year \end{array}}{\begin{array}{c} Population\ at\ risk \\ during\ that\ year \end{array}} \times 1{,}000$$

The calculation could be even more specific, addressing only drivers less than 25 years of age.

$$\text{Cause-age-specific death rate per } 1,000 \text{ per year} = \frac{\begin{array}{c}\textit{Deaths from motor}\\ \textit{vehicle accidents for}\\ \textit{drivers} < 25 \textit{ years old}\\ \textit{in a given year}\end{array}}{\begin{array}{c}\textit{Population} < 25 \textit{ years}\\ \textit{old during that year}\end{array}} \times 1,000$$

The *case-fatality rate* is similar to the cause-specific mortality rate, but instead of the denominator being the total population at risk, it is only those persons who develop a given disease or other adverse health outcome during a given period of time. By convention, the case-fatality rate is considered a proportion and calculated as a percentage. It is used to estimate the risk of dying during a given time period for only those individuals with the condition. If the disease is an infectious agent, the case-fatality rate reflects the infectious agent's virulence, although virulence includes cases in the numerator who recover but may be left with a significant disability, such as a crippled limb from polio or deafness from rubella (see Chapter 3). Case-fatality rates may be specifically calculated for age, gender, and any other factor of epidemiologic importance.

$$\text{Case-fatality rate (\%)} = \frac{\begin{array}{c}\textit{Deaths from a given disease}\\ \textit{during a time interval}\end{array}}{\begin{array}{c}\textit{Number of cases of that disease}\\ \textit{during the same time interval}\end{array}} \times 100$$

It is important to draw the distinction between cause-specific death and case-fatality rates because imprecision in using the terms may result in misunderstanding. For instance, assume a population has 10,000 people, and in a given year half of them develop disease Q (5,000). Of those that develop disease Q, 100 die from the disease. The epidemiologist wishes to know the cause-specific annual mortality rate per 100,000 for disease Q in this population. That rate would be 1,000 per 100,000 persons per year ((100/10,000) × 100,000), reflecting the entire population. The case-fatality rate, however, would be 2 percent ((100/5,000) × 100), indicating that one out of every 50 persons who developed disease Q died from the disease. The risk of death from disease Q was not to the entire population but only to those contracting it.

Standardizing Mortality Rates

The risk of dying generally increases with age. Thus, populations having large proportions of older members are likely have higher crude death rates compared to those with primarily younger ones. The epidemiologist uses a statistical adjustment technique called *standardization* to remove the effect of population differences, such as age, in data sets. The two most widely used methods of standardization are the *direct* method that uses a weighted average to yield an *age-standardized rate* or *age-adjusted rate* (AAR) and the *indirect* method that yields a *standardized mortality ratio* (SMR). Standardization techniques can also be applied to other types of rates such as morbidity or injury rates, especially to deal with structural differences in populations (i.e., age, gender, social class, or family size). In studies of infant mortality, for instance, the epidemiologist often adjusts for birth weight because it is a strong predictor of infant death. Studies of pregnancy outcomes often use adjustment for the age of the mother since maternal age is a predictor of some adverse birth outcomes.

Consider the mortality experience of two populations: Florida, with an aging population, and Alaska, with a relatively young one. Beginning in the 1930s, large numbers of retirees moved to Florida from the less temperate Northeast and Midwest regions of the United States. In contrast, Alaska was the least populous territory (becoming a state in 1959), and those who moved there were primarily young workers seeking adventure and employment in the expanding fishing, mining, and oil extraction industries. The difference in the population distributions was quickly reflected in the crude death rates for the states, with Florida's crude mortality rate more than double that for Alaska by 1970. Table 5.1 shows the crude mortality rates for both states in 1988.

Now assume the epidemiologist wants to compare the mortality experience of the two states in 2010, but is still concerned about the differences in the age structures of the states' populations. To control for these potential differences, the epidemiologist will age-adjust the rates, either using the direct or indirect method of standardization.

TABLE 5.1 Crude Mortality Rates for Florida and Alaska, 1988

VARIABLE	FLORIDA	ALASKA
Number of deaths*	131,044	2,064
Total population**	12,335,000	524,000
Crude mortality rate	1,062.2 per 100,000	393.9 per 100,000

DATA SOURCES: *VITAL STATISTICS OF THE UNITED STATES (1991).
**US Bureau of the Census (1988 est.).

Direct Method

Epidemiologists have used direct standardization of death rates for more than 150 years. They adjust the data by first constructing a table that contains the age-specific death rates for the populations to be compared. The age-specific rates are calculated directly from the numbers of deaths in each age category (the numerator, from vital statistics) and their respective populations at risk (the denominator, from the census). Age-specific rates can also be obtained directly from tables calculated through readily available online programs such as CDC WONDER (See Table 5.2).

The next step is to select a *standard population*. The choice of a standard depends upon the type of comparisons to be made. For instance, if the epidemiologist wants to compare current standardized rates with historically reported ones, they might select the standard used for the historical calculations, recalculate the historical rates using a more current standard, or both. In nineteenth century Britain, vital statistics reports changed the standard population each time there was a new national census (the first year of each decade). The practice changed when the 1901 census of England and Wales was adopted as the general standard for age-adjustment in both Britain and the United States. The 1901 standard remained in force until the United States accepted the 1940 US Census as its standard.[26] That standard remained in

TABLE 5.2 Age-Specific Mortality Rate Calculations per 100,000 for Florida and Alaska, 2010

AGE (YEARS)	NUMBER OF DEATHS*		POPULATION *		AGE-SPECIFIC RATES PER 100,000	
	FLORIDA	ALASKA	FLORIDA	ALASKA	FLORIDA	ALASKA
<1	1,403	43	208,724	10,828	672.2	397.1
1–4	282	19	864,782	43,168	32.6	44.0
5–9	125	7	1,080,255	50,890	11.6	13.8
10–14	157	15	1,130,847	50,816	13.9	29.5
15–19	602	43	1,228,382	52,141	49.0	82.5
20–24	1,207	84	1,228,758	54,416	98.2	154.4
25–34	2,835	130	2,289,545	103,125	123.8	126.1
35–44	4,494	196	2,431,254	92,974	184.8	210.8
45–54	12,001	466	2,741,493	111,026	437.8	419.7
55–64	20,528	633	2,337,668	85,909	878.1	736.8
65–74	28,600	684	1,727,940	35,350	1,655.2	1,934.9
75–84	45,525	706	1,097,537	14,877	4,147.9	4,745.6
85+	56,025	702	434,125	4,711	12,905.3	14,901.3

DATA SOURCE: CDC WONDER. http://wonder.cdc.gov/

effect until 1998, when all US health statistics were required to be adjusted to the 2000 US Census. The significance of picking one standard population versus another has been investigated, and while there are changes in the magnitude of the adjusted rates, the relative differences between the rates being compared are not much affected.[27] Thus, the population standard or standards selected should be appropriate for comparative and reporting purposes. In the Florida and Alaska example, the epidemiologist decides to use the 2000 US standard million population as the standard.

The final step in direct standardization is to multiply the age-specific death rates by their respective population standards to get the number of deaths *expected* in each age category. The expected numbers of deaths are then tallied and the sums divided by the total number in the population standard. The result is the *age-adjusted (age-standardized)* rate for each state. Table 5.3 shows that when the rates were directly standardized for age, Florida's mortality rate fell to 700.9 per 100,000 population and Alaska's rose to 771.2 per 100,000.

If the epidemiologist had chosen the 1940 or 1970 US population as the standard, would it have mattered in the calculations? Table 5.4 shows those

TABLE 5.3 Calculating Age-Adjusted Mortality Rates per 100,000 for Florida and Alaska, 2010, Using the 2000 US Standard Million Population

AGE (YEARS)	AGE-SPECIFIC RATES PER 100,000		2000 US STANDARD MILLION	EXPECTED NUMBER OF DEATHS	
	FLORIDA	ALASKA		FLORIDA	ALASKA
< 1	672.2	397.1	13,818	9,288,459.6	5,487,127.8
1–4	32.6	44.0	55,317	1,803,334.2	2,433,948.0
5–9	11.6	13.8	72,533	841,382.8	1,000,955.4
10–14	13.9	29.5	73,032	1,015,144.8	2,154,444.0
15–19	49.0	82.5	72,169	3,536,281.0	5,953,942.5
20–24	98.2	154.4	66,478	6,528,139.6	10,264,203.2
25–34	123.8	126.1	135,573	16,783,937.4	17,095,755.3
35–44	184.8	210.8	162,613	30,050,882.4	34,278,820.4
45–54	437.8	419.7	134,834	59,030,325.2	56,589,829.8
55–64	878.1	736.8	87,247	76,611,590.7	64,283,589.6
65–74	1,655.2	1,934.9	66,037	109,304,442.4	127,774,991.3
75–84	4,147.9	4,745.6	44,841	185,995,983.9	212,797,449.6
85+	12,905.3	14,901.3	15,508	200,135,392.4	231,089,360.4
Total			1,000,000	700,925,296.4	771,204,417.3
Age-adjusted rate per 100,000				700.9	771.2

DATA SOURCE: CDC WONDER. http://wonder.cdc.gov/

TABLE 5.4 Age-Adjusted Mortality Rates for Florida and Alaska in 2010 Using Various US Population Standards, with Crude Mortality Rates and Rate Ratio Comparisons

STANDARD	AGE-STANDARDIZED MORTALITY RATES PER 100,000, 2010		RATE RATIO
	FLORIDA	ALASKA	
1940 US standard million	413.7	428.8	0.96
1970 US standard million	557.2	583.6	0.95
2000 US standard million	700.9	771.2	0.91
Crude rate	924.4	524.9	1.76

DATA SOURCE: CDC WONDER. http://wonder.cdc.gov/

results, along with the crude mortality rates and *rate ratios* (RRs) for making comparisons. Florida's crude mortality rate was 76 percent higher than that for Alaska in 2010 (RR = 1.76), but the state's mortality experience was actually a bit lower than Alaska's when the epidemiologist weighted the data to control for differences in the age structures of the populations (RR = 0.94 to 0.96). Note that the choice of the population standard differed in terms of the magnitude of the calculated rates, as the 1940 US standard million reflects a much younger national population structure whereas the 2000 standard reflects an aging US population. The RRs, however, were not much changed.

Indirect Method

When the available information is insufficient to calculate age-specific rates, the epidemiologist needs to use the indirect method of adjustment. For example, in an occupational cohort, the number of workers in each age group may be known, and the total number of deaths may be known, but the ages of those who died may not be available. In indirect adjustment, the epidemiologist uses the mortality experience of a standard population to estimate the number of deaths that would occur in a study population (the *expected*). The estimate is then compared with the actual number of deaths (the *observed*) and multiplied by 100 to yield the SMR.

$$SMR\,(\%) = \frac{Observed\ number\ of\ deaths\ during\ an\ interval}{Expected\ number\ of\ deaths\ during\ that\ same\ interval} \times 100$$

If the observed mortality is the same as the expected mortality, the SMR will be 100 (percent). An SMR greater than 100 indicates that mortality is higher in the observed group than would be expected in the standard population; an SMR less than 100 indicates it is lower than expected.

TABLE 5.5 Calculating Standardized Mortality Ratios (SMRs) for Florida and Alaska, 2010

AGE GROUP (YEARS)	2010 US DEATH RATE PER 100,000	POPULATION (MILLIONS)		EXPECTED DEATHS	
		FLORIDA	ALASKA	FLORIDA	ALASKA
<1	623.4	208,724	10,828	1301.2	67.5
1–4	26.5	864,782	43,168	229.2	11.4
5–9	11.5	1,080,255	50,890	124.2	5.9
10–14	14.3	1,130,847	50,816	161.7	7.3
15–19	49.4	1,228,382	52,141	606.8	25.8
20–24	86.5	1,228,758	54,416	1062.9	47.1
25–34	102.9	2,289,545	103,125	2355.9	106.1
35–44	170.5	2,431,254	92,974	4145.3	158.5
45–54	407.1	2,741,493	111,026	11160.6	452.0
55–64	851.9	2,337,668	85,909	19914.6	731.9
65–74	1,875.1	1,727,940	35,350	32400.6	662.8
75–84	4,790.2	1,097,537	14,877	52574.2	712.6
85+	13,934.3	434,125	4,711	60492.3	656.4
Total		18,801,310	710,231	186,529.5	3,645.3
Number of deaths observed in 2010				173,791	3,728
SMR				93.2	102.3

DATA SOURCE: CDC WONDER. http://wonder.cdc.gov/

To calculate indirectly adjusted rates, the epidemiologist constructs a table containing the number of persons in each age group of the study populations to be compared. Table 5.5 shows the 2010 US census estimates for the Florida and Alaska populations. The *age-specific death rates* for a standard population are then selected and entered into the table. Again, the choice of a standard should make sense relative to the comparisons being made. The Florida–Alaska example uses age-specific death rates from US vital statistics for the nation in 2010.

The third step in indirect adjustment is to multiply the numbers in each age stratum of the study populations by the respective age-specific death rates from the standard. This calculation estimates the number of deaths that would be observed in each age category if the study populations had the same age-specific death rates as the standard population. The expected numbers of deaths are then totaled for each of the places being compared.

The final step is to divide the total number of deaths in the study population (the observed) by the total number of expected deaths, and multiply that result by 100 to produce a percentage. In the example, Florida had an SMR of 93.2 and Alaska had an SMR of 102.3. The SMR indicates the relationship of each state's mortality experience relative to that of the United States as a whole (SMR = 100). In other words, the population of Florida is dying at a rate 6.8 percent lower than the mortality rate for the nation; that for Alaska is dying at a rate 2.3 percent greater than that for the nation.

The crude rates, the directly standardized (AARs), and the indirectly standardized (SMRs) rates present different ways of examining mortality data. Each method of adjustment has advantages and disadvantages; the epidemiologist chooses the method of adjustment based upon the research question and the available information. Crude rates are the simplest to calculate and reflect the actual number of events in a population. Clearly, Florida had more deaths per 100,000 population (the crude rate) in 2010 than did Alaska. This does not mean, however, that Alaska was a healthier place to live or that an individual's risk of dying in Florida was greater than if they lived in Alaska. Crude mortality rates should not be used to draw conclusions about cause.

Prudence suggests that crude rates should be adjusted before comparisons are made. Regardless of which method of adjustment is used, it is important to remember that adjusted rates are *data transforms*, artificial rates that allow the epidemiologist to make comparisons between and among populations. Only populations adjusted to the same standard can be compared. Because of this limitation, it is important to read the footnotes to tables presenting adjusted rates. Some nations use their own populations as standards (e.g., Canada), whereas others use a regional standard such as the *Standard European Population,* or, for global comparisons, the *World Standard Population.* The WHO now recommends the *World Population Standard for 2000–2025* to reflect the average age structure of the global population for the millennial generation.[26]

Proportional Mortality Rates and Ratios

Proportional (proportionate) mortality is the proportion of deaths in a population ascribed to a particular cause compared to those overall. Although a fraction, proportional mortality may also be expressed as a percentage. Sometimes, proportional mortality is presented as a rate when a time interval is ascribed to the calculation:

$$Proportional\ Mortality\ Rate = \frac{Deaths\ from\ a\ given\ cause\ during\ a\ time\ interval}{Deaths\ from\ all\ causes\ during\ the\ same\ interval} \times 100$$

Consider two large cities of the same population size (1 million) in the same year with different crude death rates. The crude death rate for city A was 30 per 100,000 (300 total deaths) in that year and 10 per 100,000 for city B (100 total deaths). The risk of death from cardiovascular disease (the cause-specific rate) was the same for both cities at 5 per 100,000 (50 deaths), yet the proportion of deaths from cardiovascular disease in each city differed:

$$Proportional\ Mortality\ Rate_A = \frac{50}{300} \times 100 = 17\%$$

$$Proportional\ Mortality\ Rate_B = \frac{50}{100} \times 100 = 50\%$$

While residents in both cities were dying of cardiovascular diseases at the same rate, more were dying of other causes of death in city A compared to city B. Hence, the proportional mortality rate shows the epidemiologist the burden of a specific cause relative to the total mortality picture of a population or a specific stratum of that population. Examining age-, gender-, and race-specific proportional mortality rates can aid in identifying target populations and determining health planning priorities for population subgroups. However, they cannot substitute for comparable death rates.

The epidemiologist may use the *proportional (proportionate) mortality ratio* (PMR) when the information required for calculating proportional mortality rates is not available. Calculating a PMR is similar to computing an SMR that compares the observed proportion of deaths in a population or subgroup to the expected proportion based on a population standard. In the above example, the proportional mortality for cardiovascular disease in cities A and B were 17 percent and 50 percent, respectively. The proportion of deaths due to cardiovascular disease in the United States in 2000 was 29.6 percent.[28] The calculation of proportional mortality ratios for the two cities using the 2000 US standard would be as follows:

$$PMR = \frac{Observed\ proportionate\ mortality\ rate}{Expected\ proportionate\ mortality\ rate} \times 100$$

$$PMR_A = \frac{17.0\ per\ 1,000}{26.9\ per\ 1,000}\ 100 = 63\%$$

$$PMR_B = \frac{50.0\ per\ 1,000}{26.9\ per\ 1,000} \times 100 = 185.9\%$$

The results show that the proportion of deaths from cardiovascular disease was lower in city A than in the United States as a whole in the year 2000. In comparison, the proportion of deaths from cardiovascular disease in city B was almost double that for the United States as a whole in that same year. If the goal of the exercise was to suggest where to implement an intervention to reduce heart disease, absent other information, the epidemiologist would select city B rather than city A.

Years of Potential Life Lost

Average life expectancy is an estimate of the number of years a typical individual will live if the mortality experience of their birth cohort remains unchanged. Suppose, for example, that Mr. Smith develops a fatal condition and dies at age 40 years. If the average life expectancy for his birth cohort is 75 years, then Mr. Smith died 35 years before reaching that age. He sustained 35 *years of potential life lost* (YPLL), also known as *potential years of life lost* (PYLL). The epidemiologist calculates the YPLL for a population by subtracting the age of death of each individual from the average life expectancy and summing those lost years.

$$Years\ of\ Potential\ Life\ Lost = \sum \left(Average\ life\ expectancy - Age\ at\ death \right)$$

YPLL reflects the societal cost of premature mortality in a population. To compare the burden of early deaths for specific causes, however, the epidemiologist compares the proportion of years lost from each cause to the number of years lost for all causes. For instance, in 2010, the United States suffered a total of 11,043,870 YPLL to persons under age 65 years. When examined by cause, the major contributor to early death was unintentional injuries (2,083,297 YPLL at 18.9 percent).[29] Thus, unintentional injuries merit significant attention as a public health issue.

The epidemiologist can examine YPLLs by race, age, gender, or any other demographic characteristic by estimating the YPLL rate:

$$YPLL\ Rate = \frac{\substack{YPLL\ for\ a\ specific\ cause\ or\ subgroup \\ during\ a\ time\ interval}}{\substack{Number\ of\ individuals\ contributing\ to\ the \\ YPLL\ during\ the\ same\ interval}} \times 100,000$$

The CDC reports that the YPLL rate for unintentional injuries for whites in the United States in 2010 was 825.17 per 100,000 population; for blacks it was 629.21 per 100,000 population; for Asian/Pacific Islanders it was 238.92

per 100,000 population; and for American Indian/Alaskan Natives it was 1,074.14 per 100,000 population. The burden of early death from unintentional injuries in the United States clearly stands out for American Indian/Alaskan Natives. The epidemiologist may then advise those formulating public health injury prevention programs to target their efforts at American Indian/Alaskan Natives.

Natality

Natality statistics provide information about births and the period proximate to that event. These data are used by demographers to predict population growth or decline, but they are also used by epidemiologists to characterize both the women giving birth and the babies born to them, and to compare birth outcomes such as twinning, spontaneous abortion, and stillbirths among different populations and in different time periods. Are births to teenage mothers increasing or decreasing? Who is at elevated risk for having a low birth weight baby? How does the rate of birth defects differ from place to place? What is the risk to mothers of dying from childbirth? The epidemiologist seeks answers to such questions and, by using natality data, may identify health problems in the community. They may also generate hypotheses about the etiologic factors that are important for healthy mothers and babies.

Definitions

The terminology used to describe birth and its related phenomena differs widely among cultures and across time, and this occasionally makes it difficult to compare rates and trends for some natality measures. To address this issue, the WHO has standardized terminology within the ICD system. A *live birth* is defined as "the complete expulsion or extraction from its mother of a product of conception, irrespective of the duration of the pregnancy, which, after such separation, breathes or shows any other evidence of life, such as beating of the heart, pulsation of the umbilical cord, or definite movement of voluntary muscles, whether or not the umbilical cord has been cut or the placenta is attached."[30] This definition is conservative, designed to be as inclusive as possible. In contrast to a live birth is a *fetal death* (*stillbirth*), where the product of conception dies before being expelled or extracted from the mother. Nations vary in whether gestations (time since conception) of 20 or 28 weeks are required for registering fetal deaths.

The course of a pregnancy is divided into distinct time periods after conception. The developing fetus is said to have a *gestational age,* and the pregnancy is divided into *trimesters.* Human infants normally gestate between 37 to 42 weeks and end in a *term birth.* The newborn is called a *neonate* for the first 28 days, and then is considered an *infant* until reaching one year. A widely recognized predictor of infant survival is birth weight. Because of this, the WHO recommends that birth weights be entered into all vital statistics systems. In general, *low birth weight* is defined as less than 2500 grams, *very low birth weight* as less than 1500 grams, and *extremely low birth weight* as less than 1000 grams.[30] The epidemiologist uses these types of data and more to inform public health policies that may lead to improved birth outcomes.

Not all nations or regions have birth registration systems, and in such situations the United Nations may choose to create estimates of the number of births. The estimates are usually based on information gathered from household and various health surveys, which may or may not reflect a representative sample of the population. A second concern is that not all nations use the WHO definitions, making it difficult to compare measures related to birth among nations. For example, some reporting areas require a fetus to weigh at least 500 grams to be counted in their birth and infant mortality rates (Ireland, Poland). Others require the fetus to be at least 500 grams and 22 weeks gestation (Netherlands, France). At least one nation requires an additional measure to be considered—that the fetus be at least 500 grams, 22 weeks gestation, and survive at least 24 hours to be classified as a live birth (Czech Republic).[31] It is important when using natality data to understand these limitations.

Natality Measures

The *crude birth rate* is defined as the number of live births per 1,000 population, usually per year:

$$Crude\ birth\ rate = \frac{\begin{array}{c} Number\ of\ live\ births \\ during\ a\ time\ interval \end{array}}{\begin{array}{c} Total\ population \\ during\ the\ same\ interval \end{array}} \times 1,000$$

For populations where there might be disruption or uneven reporting due to social strife or natural disasters, the United Nations recommends calculating the average annual number of births over a five-year period for the numerator and the person-years lived by the population over the same time period in the denominator.[32]

The crude birth rate does not reflect the childbearing ability of a population, because it uses the total population as the denominator rather than the actual population at risk (the number of females of childbearing age). To account for this, the epidemiologist may use an alternative measure of natality focused on the population of women in their fertile years, the *general fertility rate* (GFR). The age range for the denominator in the GFR was originally 15 to 44 years, but as women (mostly in the developed world) are having babies later, the age range has increasingly been expanded to 15 to 49 years.

$$General\ Fertility\ Rate = \frac{Live\ births\ during\ a\ time\ interval}{\substack{Number\ of\ women\ ages\ 15-49\ years \\ during\ the\ same\ interval}} \times 1,000$$

The GFR is a crude measure of fertility, and a somewhat better understood fertility statistic is a standardized measure, the *total fertility rate* (TFR). The TFR is calculated by creating age-specific fertility rates for women aged 10 to 49 years and summing them up to approximate the number of children a typical woman in a population would bear over the course of her lifetime. Because it is standardized, the TFR is commonly used for making global fertility comparisons. Table 5.6 shows the natality measures for three nations in 2012. The United States is offered for comparative purposes. The TFR for Niger was the highest of any nation in 2012; Singapore's was the lowest.

TABLE 5.6 Natality Measures For the United States, Niger, and Singapore, 2012 (estimated)

NATALITY MEASURE	UNITED STATES	NIGER	SINGAPORE
Crude birth rate	13.7 live births/ 1,000 population	47.6 live births/ 1,000 population	7.72 live births/ 1,000 population
Total fertility rate	2.06 children/ woman	7.16 children/ woman	0.78 children/ woman
M/F ratio of live births	1.05/1	1.03/1	1.07/1
Gross reproduction rate	979 daughters/ 1,000 women	3,473 daughters/ 1,000 women	363 daughters/ 1,000 women

DATA SOURCE: CIA Factbook. https://www.cia.gov/library/publications/the-world-factbook/geos/us.html

Natality measures along with mortality measures are widely used to predict whether a population is likely to grow or contract. The epidemiologist may use that same information to determine whether public policies addressing contraception, assisted reproductive technologies, or cash supplements to families have yielded the desired effect. They may look for patterns in the number of infants born, whether those infants are born healthy, and whether women have healthy pregnancies and survive childbirth.

Mortality Related to Natality

Deaths occurring in the first year of life may reflect the overall health of a population. High infant mortality often indicates unmet public health needs for nutrition and prenatal care, as well as poor socioeconomic and environmental conditions. The *infant mortality rate* is easily calculated, but it must be remembered that the denominator will be influenced by the way in which live births are counted.

$$Infant\ mortality\ rate = \frac{\begin{array}{c} Number\ of\ deaths\ under\ one\ year \\ of\ age\ in\ a\ interval \end{array}}{\begin{array}{c} Number\ of\ live\ births \\ during\ the\ same\ interval \end{array}} \times 1,000$$

In the United States and many other countries, infant mortality records are linked to their matching birth records. This linkage allows the epidemiologist to examine the risk of infant death by both infant and maternal characteristics (i.e., age and pregnancy history).

Fetal deaths are a vital statistics measure that focuses on the period before birth (*prenatal period*). The number of deaths occurring early in pregnancy may not be reported because medical care for the loss was not sought. In addition, gestational age is often estimated—sometimes from the mother's report of her last menstrual period and in other instances by using fetal weight as a proxy. Areas with sparse populations may have small numbers of fetal deaths, with consequently unstable rates. It is important, therefore, for the epidemiologist to use information about fetal deaths with caution, as they are almost always underestimated.

Perinatal mortality is defined variously as beginning at 20 weeks (or 350 grams), 22 weeks (or 500 grams) or 28 weeks gestation, and ending either 7 days or 28 days (*neonatal period*) after birth. The epidemiologist must take care to assure that the same periods are used when comparing rates

from different populations. Both perinatal and neonatal mortality are public health indicators of adverse birth outcomes related to congenital anomalies, prematurity, and low birth weight.

The WHO defines the death of a woman who dies in pregnancy or within
42 days of the termination of a pregnancy as a *maternal death* or *death due
to puerperal causes*.[33] The *maternal mortality rate* uses all pregnancies in the
denominator (live births plus fetal deaths), and because fetal deaths are often
underreported, especially in places with limited vital registration systems,
this can be problematic. As an alternative, the epidemiologist may calculate
the *maternal mortality ratio* rather than the rate. The ratio uses as its denominator only live births. Maternal mortality ratios generally reflect the lack of
access to health care and poor socioeconomic circumstances and are widely
used for comparative purposes.

$$Maternal\ mortality\ ratio = \frac{Number\ of\ maternal\ deaths\ in\ a\ interval}{Number\ of\ live\ births\ in\ the\ same\ interval} \times 1,000\ live\ births$$

Estimating the Population at Risk

Most estimates of the population at risk come from population counts, or
census data. A census is typically conducted by a national government and
repeated on a regular basis. While it might seem logical that all individuals
should be counted, such has not always been the case. The first census of the
United States was done in 1790 for the purposes of allotting representation
in Congress. That census counted heads of households, not individuals, and
it is impossible to calculate rates from such information. It was not until
1850 that individual data replaced family data in the US census. When the
rules for enumeration change, calculating trends in health outcomes may
become challenging. For instance, changing from households to individuals,
changing categories of race/ethnicity, and shifting placements of geographic
boundaries will yield biased or at least different and noncomparable samples.

Population census data are gathered at varying times by various nations
and at varying scales (national, state/provincial, city/municipality, neighbor-
hood). For example, suppose the epidemiologist needs to calculate crude
death rates for two nations, one with a census from the prior year and the
other with a census from more than five years ago. They must rely on current
population estimates from those nations that may or may not be calculated

in the same way. It should be remembered that while census data enumerate the population at a given time, populations are dynamic. Thus, populations at risk are usually estimated from dated information, and all rates calculated using estimated data are estimated rates.

Summary

Vital statistics constitute a major source of information for epidemiologists. Birth and death statistics are most often expressed as rates, the number of events occurring in a given population over a specified period of time. Crude rates provide a metric that is inclusive of the total population and indicate the burden of an outcome on that population. When there is a variable of interest, such as a particular cause of death or birth weight category, the data set can be stratified and specific rates calculated (example, ASRs).

When whole populations are to be compared, differences in the distribution of potential confounders such as age, gender, or smoking status may skew results. To remove the problem of differences in distribution of the confounder, rates should be adjusted. Direct adjustment uses the stratum-specific rates from the study population and weights from a standard population to produce an adjusted rate (example, AARs). Indirect adjustment uses the numbers of persons in the study population at risk in each stratum of the confounder and a standard rate to calculate an expected number of outcomes. The number of observed outcomes is then compared to the number of expected outcomes and an SMR is calculated. The two methods differ in how they may be applied. Directly adjusted rates may be compared if they were calculated using the same population standard. Indirectly adjusted rates (SMRs) cannot be directly compared, but each SMR can be compared to the experience of the standard (100%).

Epidemiologists use ratios when it makes sense to exclude some subpopulations from the denominator (e.g., fetal death ratio and maternal mortality ratio). They use proportions to demonstrate the burden of one type of outcome relative to others (proportional mortality), and years of potential life lost to identify the burden of an outcome on society. While all of these calculations help set public health priorities, epidemiologists never lose sight of the potential problems posed in using vital statistics. Any observed trends may be due to changes in coding or reporting practices, the implementation of new diagnostic capabilities, or less than accurate estimates of the populations at risk.

References

1. Arthur Newsholme, *The Elements of Vital Statistics in Their Bearing on Social and Public Health Problems*. New York: D. Appleton and Company, 1924.
2. Alice M. Hetzel, *History and Organization of the Vital Statistics System*. Hyattsville, MD: National Center for Health Statistics, 1997. Available at http://www.cdc.gov/nchs/data/misc/usvss.pdf.
3. World Health Organization, *Improving the Quality and Use of Birth, Death and Cause-of-Death Information; Guidance for a Standards-Based Review of Country Practices*. Geneva, Switzerland: World Health Organization, 2010. Available at http://www.who.int/healthinfo/tool_cod_2010.pdf.
4. National Center for Health Statistics, Centers for Disease Control and Prevention, US Standard Death Certificate. Available at http://www.cdc.gov/nchs/data/dvs/DEATH11-03final-ACC.pdf.
5. Department of Health and Human Services: Centers for Disease Control and Prevention, CDC WONDER Online Databases, http://wonder.cdc.gov/.
6. Colin D. Mathers et al., "Counting the Dead and what They Died From: An Assessment of the Global Status of Cause of Death Data," *Bulletin of the World Health Organization* 83, no. 3 (2005): 171–177c.
7. George James, Robert E. Patton, and A. Sandra Heslen, "Accuracy of Cause-of-Death Statements on Death Certificates," *Public Health Reports* 70, no. 2 (1955): 39–51.
8. Iwao M. Moriyama, T. R. Dawber, and W. B. Kannel, "Evaluation of Diagnostic Information Supporting Medical Certification of Deaths from Cardiovascular Diseases," in *Epidemiological Approaches to the Study of Cancer and Other Chronic Diseases*, Ed. W. Haenszel, National Cancer Institute Monograph No. 19, 415–419. Washington, DC: US Government Printing Office, 1966.
9. Iwao M. Moriyama, William S. Baum, William M. Haenszel, and Berwyn F. Mattison, "Inquiry Into Diagnostic Evidence Supporting Medical Certification of Death," *American Journal of Public Health* 48, no. 10 (1958): 1376–1387.
10. Kurt Pohlen and Haven Emerson, "Errors in Clinical Statements of Causes of Death," *American Journal of Public Health* 32, no. 2 (1942): 251–260.
11. Kurt Pohlen, "Errors in Clinical Statements of Causes of Death: 2nd Report," *American Journal of Public Health* 33, no 5 (1943): 505–516.
12. Anne M. Hardy et al., "Review of Death Certificates to Assess Completeness of AIDS Case Reporting," *Public Health Reports* 102, no. 4 (1987): 386–391.
13. Leonard T. Kurland, Antonio Stazio, and Dwayne Reed, "An Appraisal of Population Studies of Multiple Sclerosis," *Annals of the New York Academy of Sciences* 122 (1965): 520–541.
14. Lee I. Corwin et al., "Accuracy of Death Certification of Stroke: The Framingham Study," *Stroke* 13, no. 6 (1982): 818–821.
15. F. G. Benavides, F. Bolumar, and R. Peris, "Quality of Death Certificates in Valencia, Spain," *American Journal of Public Health* 79, no. 10 (1989): 1352–1354.
16. Iwao M. Moriyama, "Problems and Measurement of Accuracy of Cause-of-Death Statistics," *American Journal of Public Health* 79, no. 10 (1989): 1349–1350.

17. Mohamed A. A. Moussa et al., "Reliability of Death Certificate Diagnoses," *Journal of Clinical Epidemiology* 43, no. 12 (1990): 1285–1295.

18. D. Mainland, "The Risk of Fallacious Conclusions from Autopsy Data on Incidence of Diseases with Applications to Heart Disease," *American Heart Journal* 45, no. 5 (1953): 644–651.

19. C. A. McMahan, "Age-Sex Distribution of Selected Groups of Human Autopsied Cases," *Archives of Pathology* 73 (January, 1962): 40–47.

20. S. O. Waife, P. F. Lucchesi, and Barbara Sigmund, "The Significance of Mortality Statistics and Medical Research: Analysis of 1000 Deaths at Philadelphia General Hospital," Annals of Internal Medicine 37, no. 2 (1952): 332–337.

21. Elizabeth C. Burton, "The Autopsy: A Professional Responsibility in Assuring Quality of Care," *American Journal of Medical Quality* 17, no. 2 (2002): 56–60.

22. Nadia Soleman, Daniel Chandramohan, and Kenji Shibuya, "Verbal Autopsy: Current Practices and Challenges," *Bulletin of the World Health Organization* 84, no. 3 (2006): 239–245.

23. World Health Organization, "Verbal Autopsy Standards: Ascertaining and Attributing Causes of Death. The 2012 WHO Verbal Autopsy Instrument." Available at http://www.who.int/healthinfo/statistics/verbalautopsystandards/en/.

24. Omar B. Ahmed et al., *Age Standardization of Rates: A New WHO Standard.* Geneva: World Health Organization, 2001 Available at http://www.who.int/healthinfo/paper31.pdf.

25. P. D. Sorlie et al., "Age-Adjusted Death Rates: Consequences of the Year 2000 Standard," *Annals of Epidemiology* 9, no. 2 (1999): 93–100.

26. R. N. Anderson, "Deaths: Leading Causes for 2000," *National Vital Statistics Reports.* 50, no. 16 (2002): 1–85.

27. National Center for Injury Prevention and Control. WISQARS™. *Years of Potential Life Lost (YPLL) Reports 1999–2013.* Atlanta, GA: Centers for Disease Control and Prevention. Available at http://webappa.cdc.gov/sasweb/ncipc/ypll10.html.

28. World Health Organization. *International Statistical Classification of Diseases and Related Health Problems, 10th Revision.* Geneva, Switzerland: World Health Organization, 2010. Available at http://apps.who.int/classifications/icd10/browse/2010/en.

29. K. S. Joseph et al., "Influence of Definition Based Versus Pragmatic Birth Registration on International Comparisons of Perinatal and Infant Mortality: Population Based Retrospective Study," *British Medical Journal* 344 (2012): e746, doi:10.1136/bmj.e746.

30. World Health Organization, *Improving the quality and use of birth, death and cause-of-death information: guidance for a standards-based review of country practices.* Geneva, Switzerland: World Health Organization Press, 2006. Available at http://www.who.int/healthinfo/tool_cod_2010.pdf.

31. Jiaquan Xu et al., *Deaths: Final Data for 2007.* Hyattsville, MD: National Center for Health Statistics, 2010. Available at http://www.cdc.gov/nchs/data/nvsr/nvsr58/nvsr58_19.pdf.

Problem Set: Chapter 5

1. The sovereign state of Academia's the newly installed Minister of Health, the Dean, is making a new budget for the Health Division. The governing political party promised during the last election to formulate health policy in as rational a way as possible. Naturally, the Dean thought of using mortality as guidance; whatever town had more deaths surely needed more funding to prevent future mortality. The ministry's chief vital statistician, the Department Chair, assembled all of Academia's vital records and health surveys for the past year and found that in one of the two major cities near Academia, All Knowing Senior, there were 20,400 deaths among 1.9 million people. In the other major city, Ignorant Freshman, there were 22,100 deaths among 2.17 million people.

    "Great," said the Dean, "I'll allocate more funding to programs in Ignorant Freshman."

    "Excuse me," protested the Department Chair, "but you need to look at death rates, not the number of deaths."

    "Do you have those rates?" asked the Dean.

    Help the Department Chair by calculating the crude death rates for these two major cities in the state of Academia. Which city has the higher burden of deaths?

2. Soon after the Department Chair left, the Dean realized that the overall crude death rates wouldn't provide all the information needed; only death rates by cause would provide the needed guidance. The Dean is most concerned about infectious disease and cancers, areas where the Academic Senate (consisting entirely of professors) has been critical of the Dean in the past. A quick email to the Department Chair got the Dean the following information:

    Help the Dean by creating a table with the cause-specific mortality rates for each of the causes for the two cities.

CAUSE	ALL KNOWING SENIOR		IGNORANT FRESHMAN	
	DEATHS	POPULATION	DEATHS	POPULATION
Infectious diseases	2,500	1,900,000	3,010	2,170,000
Cancers	2,700	1,900,000	2,900	2,170,000
All other	15,200	1,900,000	16,190	2,170,000
Totals	20,400	1,900,000	22,100	2,170,000

3. Later that night, the Dean was hosting a dinner at her home for a few members of the Department Chair's staff. She described how thankful she was for the Department Chair's efforts. One staff member, Underpaid Teaching Assistant, scowled at the Dean and asked, "Did you look at the age-specific rates? Even I know to look at those for each cause. We learned that our first year in my program."

The next day, the Dean asked the Department Chair about age-specific mortality rates for each town. The Dean was particularly interested in the rates for infectious diseases, as she wanted to impress Academia's President, whose mother lives in Ignorant Freshman and was recently hospitalized with pneumonia.

"I anticipated you might want that information, so I asked my assistant, Miss Taken, to assemble the data. She worked all night getting the ages of each case so you would have the data this morning."

Shortly afterward, a very tired Miss Taken walked into the Dean's office and said, "Here is the age information on each case that you asked for. I went to the census to look up the age structure of the populations in each town."

"But you didn't calculate the age-specific rates," said the Dean. "Oh," she said, "my error."

Help the tired Miss Taken by filling in the age-specific mortality rates for infectious diseases in the table below:

	CITY					
	ALL KNOWING SENIOR			IGNORANT FRESHMAN		
AGE (YEARS)			ANNUAL AGE-SPECIFIC MORTALITY RATE FOR INFECTIOUS DISEASES PER 100,000			ANNUAL AGE-SPECIFIC MORTALITY RATE FOR INFECTIOUS DISEASES PER 100,000
	DEATHS	POPULATION	PERSONS	DEATHS	POPULATION	PERSONS
<5	20	90,000		120	140,000	
5–24	180	300,000		910	650,000	
25–44	650	450,000		1,130	670,000	
45–64	950	650,000		650	520,000	
65+	700	410,000		200	190,000	
Totals	2,500	1,900,000		3,010	2,170,000	

4. Looking at the tabulations, the Dean could not find the age-adjusted rates.

"Where are the age-adjusted rates?" he asked, as Miss Taken was about to walk out of the room.

"Oh, yeah, right," she replied. "Here's a table so you can calculate them. I would have done it for you, but the Provost had an immediate need for some data about an outbreak of shingles at Old Fogies Village where the retired Professors live. You can use any standard population for the calculations, but I suggest you use one from a WHO population databook."

"Very well," said the Dean, and Miss Taken, wearily, left.

Help the Dean by completing in the empty cells and calculating the age-adjusted rates for infectious disease mortality for the two cities.

| | | CITY | | | |
| | | ALL KNOWING SENIOR | | IGNORANT FRESHMAN | |
AGE (YEARS)	STANDARD POPULATION (FROM A DATABOOK)	AGE-SPECIFIC MORTALITY RATES FOR INFECTIOUS DISEASES PER 100,000 PERSONS	EXPECTED DEATHS	AGE-SPECIFIC MORTALITY RATES FOR INFECTIOUS DISEASES PER 100,000 PERSONS	EXPECTED DEATHS
<5	3,000	22		86	
5–24	18,000	60		140	
25–44	40,000	144		169	
45–64	27,000	146		125	
65+	12,000	171		105	
Total	100,000				
Age-adjusted rate					

5. At Academia's Senate meeting that afternoon, the Dean presented the Ministry's budget (the "thesis" was the technical name for it) with more money for infectious disease control in Ignorant Freshman than in All Knowing Senior. The thesis defense was grueling, as the Senate president (the Provost) encouraged the back-bench professors to challenge the Dean about the findings.

"But Dean," one said, "what about survival? All that you've shown us are annual mortality rates. Once you're dead, you're dead."

The Provost smiled and added, "Professors, survival is measured by the case-fatality rate, and, given the differences in the age-specific mortality rates, there may well be differences in age-specific case-fatality. Can the Dean provide that information?"

The Professors quickly nodded their assent, hoping to see the Dean sweat, but she simply responded "We were fortunate that the Department Chair had the survey data needed to calculate the case fatality rates in both cities."

Unfortunately, Miss Taken hadn't had the time to fill in the needed data. Help the Dean defend her thesis on the spot by calculating the age-specific and total case-fatality rates for infectious diseases in both cities and entering them into the following table:

| AGE (YEARS) | ALL KNOWING SENIOR | | | IGNORANT FRESHMAN | | |
	DEATHS	NUMBER OF CASES OF INFECTIOUS DISEASE LAST YEAR	CASE FATALITY RATE PER 100 CASES OF INFECTIOUS DISEASE LAST YEAR	DEATHS	NUMBER OF CASES OF INFECTIOUS DISEASE LAST YEAR	CASE FATALITY RATE PER 100 CASES OF INFECTIOUS DISEASE LAST YEAR
<5	20	40		120	240	
5–24	180	400		910	2,275	
25–44	650	1,900		1,130	2,800	
45–64	950	3,600		650	1,625	
65+	700	4,000		200	2,000	
Total	2,500	9,940		3,010	8,940	

6. The Senate accepted the thesis and, as was traditional in Academia, all professors present at the thesis defense signed off on the budget. Walking with the Department Chair down Tenure Track Lane back to the Ministry of Health, the Dean said, "I'm glad we don't have to do that for another year. You and your colleagues are to be congratulated."

A few weeks later, however, the Department Chair and Miss Taken sheepishly went to the dean's office and said, "We have some bad news. We found a problem with those data you presented to the Senate. No one in the finance office can understand how you defended it as well you did."

"What's the problem?" the Dean snapped back angrily.

The Department Chair responded, "We found out that many of the death certificates in All Knowing Senior had incorrect ages on them. Because we can't rely on the age data, I suggest we use a different approach—the Standardized Mortality Ratio (SMR). To make things simple, we can use the mortality experience of Ignorant Freshman as the standard and apply it to All Knowing Senior's population."

Miss Taken presented a new chart to the Dean and said, "Here's a chart of what we found for infectious disease mortality. What we do know is that 2,500 people in All Knowing Senior died from infectious diseases last year."

Help Miss Taken complete the chart and calculate the SMR for infectious disease mortality for All Knowing Senior. What does the SMR indicate?

AGE (YEARS)	STANDARD RATE (INFECTIOUS DISEASE MORTALITY RATES PER 100,000 PERSONS IN IGNORANT FRESHMAN)	STUDY POPULATION (ALL KNOWING SENIOR)	EXPECTED NUMBER OF DEATHS IN THE STUDY POPULATION
<5	86	90,000	
5–24	140	300,000	
25–44	169	450,000	
45–64	125	650,000	
65+	105	410,000	
Total		1,900,000	

The Dean presented the revised findings to the Senate at noon. Though the back-bench professors were not pleased with the Dean's new thesis (some had already planned to move their infectious disease research agendas to Ignorant Freshman later in the year), they grudgingly assented to the new budget allotting equal funding to both cities.

7. Back-bench Professor B. A. Skeptic decided to move his infectious disease research to Ignorant Freshman because he was convinced the Dean's mortality study was flawed—he felt it focused on mortality outcomes rather than taking into account potential mortality risk. As the population of Ignorant Freshman was minimally vaccinated against infectious diseases, the risk of infectious disease mortality in that city was far higher than it was in All Knowing Senior.

"It's a time bomb waiting to happen," Professor Skeptic said to his staff.

The next year there was a measles epidemic in Ignorant Freshman and many young children who had not been vaccinated died of the disease or its complications. Eager to make his point about mortality risk, Professor Skeptic quickly put together the following table:

AGE (YEARS)	POPULATION	CASES OF MEASLES	ATTACK RATE (%)	DEATHS FROM MEASLES	CASE FATALITY RATE (%)
<1	29,184	1,291	4.4	94	7.3
2	28,472	1,497	5.3	75	5.0
3	29,050	1,682	5.8	67	4.0
4	28,793	1,786	6.2	69	3.9
5	24,501	10,013	40.9	201	2.0
Total	140,000	16,269	11.6	506	3.1

While each family grieved the loss of their own child, Professor Skeptic decided it was important to also speak to the community about the total loss suffered from this epidemic to show how important herd immunity is.

Help Professor Skeptic by calculating the rate of years of potential life lost to the population of Ignorant Freshman due to the measles outbreak. Assume the average life expectancy of Ignorant Freshman is 75 years.

6 | Using Vital Statistics

The tendencies of human beings to die are not constant;
diseases differ in their fatality; persons of different ages differ in
susceptibility to disease; sex, nationality, connubial condition are
likewise variable factors.[1]

George C. Whipple (1919)

V ITAL STATISTICS ALLOW THE EPIDEMIOLOGIST to examine patterns of
reproductive outcomes and causes of death, as they occur in *time*,
place, and among *persons*, from readily available data. This chapter
describes the ways in which the epidemiologist conducts and evaluates the
results of studies based on vital statistics. As with all other data sets, proper
consideration must be given to how those charged with collecting vital statistics gathered the information and whether there might be data artifacts
(biases) present that would influence any calculated rates.

Time

Trends over time are called *secular trends*. Figure 6.1 provides an example
of secular trends for mortality from cancer among US males, from 1930 to
2010. Note that lung cancer showed a marked increase from the beginning
of the period until it began to abate after 1990; stomach cancer showed a
continuous decline over the entire time period; as with lung cancer, the trend
for both prostate cancer and colorectal cancer also began to decline more
recently.

When a secular trend is observed, the epidemiologist must consider
whether it is real or artifactual. Table 6.1 lists several ways artifacts may

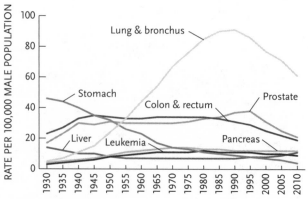

FIGURE 6.1 Age-adjusted (2000 US standard) cancer death rates per 100,000 US males by site, 1930–2010.

influence secular trends. Are the data gathered in the same way across time? Shifts in how data are gathered may cause discontinuities or changes in secular trends. For example, education and prenatal care data obtained from the 2003 revision of the US birth certificate are not comparable to the information drawn from earlier birth certificates. New medical imaging technologies may have improved diagnostic acumen over time, and improved access to medical care may impact mortality trends. As a result, more people may be correctly diagnosed, or even overdiagnosed with specific conditions, than in the past.

TABLE 6.1 Possible Explanations for Trends in Epidemiologic Rates

Trend may reflect data artifacts

Numerator

    Changes in the clinical recognition of outcomes

    Changes in the accuracy of reporting age

    Changes in the rules and procedures for reporting outcomes

    Changes in the coding system for classifying outcomes

Denominator

    Changes in enumeration of the population at risk

Trend may be real

Changes in the age distribution of the population

Changes in survivorship

Changes in the incidence of outcomes resulting from

    host factors

    environmental factors

An example of overdiagnosis was demonstrated by researchers examining the rise and then fall of prostate cancer mortality in the United States after the advent of the prostate-specific antigen (PSA) test for routine health screening in 1987. Feuer and colleagues split the prostate cancer mortality data into recently screened and other cases, and then compared the results for both groups.[2] They concluded that much of the increase in prostate cancer mortality could be explained by the presence of a data artifact—many recently screened patients were mislabeled as dying of prostate cancer when they actually died of other causes. The subsequent decline in prostate cancer mortality was explained as improved survival for screening-detected cases.

The International Classification of Diseases (ICD) system has been revised multiple times since its inception, with each revision expanding coding categories to improve diagnostic information that can be used by various standardized data collection systems, including vital statistics. The National Center for Health Statistics (NCHS) investigated the effect of ICD coding changes on the number of deaths coded to each cause from ICD-5 (1938 to 1948) through ICD-10 (1999 to 2015).[3] While each newer version allowed for better identification of specific conditions, the changes in the system also caused some confusion among coders and discontinuities in cause-of-death trends. The change from ICD-9 to ICD-10 may even have caused shifts in the rankings of the leading causes of death, particularly among the most common causes.

For example, Joyner-Grantham and colleagues examined mortality trends for heart disease, cardiovascular disease, and diabetes for 1994 to 1998 and from 1999 to 2005, the period before and after ICD-10 went into effect in 16 southeastern US states.[4] The researchers found that the change led to an underestimate of mortality from heart disease and cerebrovascular disease and an overestimate of mortality from diabetes. Cano-Serral and colleagues completed a comparative analysis of more than 88,000 death certificates in Spain, coding each death under both ICD-9 and ICD-10.[5] Under ICD-10, the same deaths were 3.6 percent higher for AIDS, 7.1 percent higher for arteriosclerosis, and 7.1 percent higher for drug overdose than under ICD-9. They were 3.2 percent lower for vascular disease and senile dementia. All other major causes of death were within 2 percent.

Each time the ICD system is updated, there will likely be discontinuities. For instance, ICD-11 includes title headings and disease classifications with structured definitions designed to improve coding and allow the information to be cross-mapped. The cross mapping uses *SNOMED CT*, a comprehensive and multilingual medical terminology system serving as the global standard for medical coding.[6] Under ICD-10, a death due to viral pneumonia

TABLE 6.2 Searchable Parameters under the ICD-11 Content Model

PARAMETER	DEFINITION
ICD entity title	Fully specified name
Classification properties	Disease, disorder, injury, etc.
Textual definitions	Short standard definition
Terms	Synonyms, other inclusions and exclusions
Body system/structure description	Anatomy and physiology
Temporal properties	Acute, chronic or other
Severity of subtypes properties	Mild, moderate, severe, or other scales
Manifestation properties	Signs, symptoms
Causal properties	Etiology: infectious, external causes, etc.
Functioning properties	Impact on daily life: activities and participation
Specific condition properties	Relates to pregnancy, etc.
Treatment properties	Specific treatment considerations: e.g., resistance
Diagnostic criteria	Operational definitions for assessment

SOURCE: World Health Organization. ICD Classifications: Content Model. See http://www.who.int/classifications/icd/revision/contentmodel/en/.

would fall within the category of respiratory disease and would be classified as viral pneumonia. Under ICD-11, that death would be classified similarly, but it would also be linked to a body part (lung) and a causative agent (virus). ICD-11 will have links to 13 parameters (Table 6.2) and more than 311,000 active concepts that can be organized into searchable hierarchies.

Changing the requirements or procedures for reporting or adding coding options has implications for coding accuracy. While coding may improve over the long term, the immediate effects may be problematic. Those responsible for reporting need to be trained or retrained on system changes and instructed on how to decide among codes when there are less than perfect coding options. For instance, a 2010 survey of 521 medical residents from 38 residency programs in New York City found that almost half admitted to knowingly reporting an inaccurate cause of death on a death certificate.[7] Cardiac disease was overreported, whereas septic shock and acute respiratory distress syndrome were underreported. The residents' purposeful miscoding was not because they did not know how to correctly complete a death certificate, but rather that they deemed the coding system inadequate for identifying the correct cause.

In places with established vital statistics systems, determining the age of a new mother or of the deceased is usually not difficult. There are, however, instances where vital records do not exist or ages are routinely under- or overestimated, especially among select groups. For example, young men may overestimate their age to meet the minimum age for employment or military service. Should they die on the job or in battle, their ages at death will be overestimated. Similarly, vital statistics systems often require that fetal deaths of 20 weeks gestation or more be reported. The results of pregnancies to women with lack of access to early prenatal care may not be captured by these statistics, and the result may be that adverse birth outcomes are underestimated.

Data artifacts may occur in the numerator or denominator of calculated rates, or both. For instance, many migration studies show a *healthy migrant effect* in which the mortality experience of migrants is lower than that of those in the host nation. Is this effect real or is it an artifact? In one study, the mortality rate for male migrants to Germany over the age of 65 years was underestimated by twofold, primarily due to *data censoring*, a situation where there is only partial information available on select individuals or groups in a population.[8] The denominator of the mortality rate for the migrants was overestimated because those who were less assimilated and less healthy tended to return to their countries of origin. While migrants registered with the German government upon entry, many did not de-register when leaving, thus inflating the population at risk. In addition, those who died after leaving the country were not counted in German mortality statistics. This created the illusion that many migrants were still alive and living in Germany.

Data censoring was first described as early as 1873 by William Farr, who explained that a data artifact exists when subjects are classified by their status at follow-up and analyzed as if they were in that category from the outset of the study.[9] An example of this is a published review of the lives of 86 noted jazz musicians. The investigator concluded that previous reports that jazz musicians usually died young, primarily from alcohol, drugs, and other lifestyle factors, were in error.[10] The conclusion was quickly challenged by epidemiologists who pointed out that comparing the longevity of jazz musicians with the average US citizen is inappropriate because the average citizen begins being counted at birth, whereas jazz musicians were unlikely to be recognized as prominent in their field before the age of 20.[11-12] In other words, the study was biased toward those jazz musicians that had survived youth, a status that could not be equally conferred upon the general population.

After data artifacts have been ruled out, the next step is to consider hypotheses for any observed trends. Has the population age distribution shifted? When populations live longer, their mortality patterns likely reflect increases from diseases of aging such as Alzheimer's disease or some cancers. Has survivorship changed? New treatments develop over time, and some, such as stem cell transplants and gene therapy, may offer increased survivorship and possibly even a cure. Has there been a change in health outcomes either because of changes in host factors or a change in the environment? Consider again the temporal trend in lung cancer mortality shown in Figure 6.1. The trend in lung cancer follows the rise in cigarette consumption, and thus is consistent with cigarette smoking being a major cause of lung cancer.

Place

Mortality and natality statistics are often used as indicators of the public health of nations or places within regions. In evaluating any differences observed, the epidemiologist follows the same sequence of reasoning used for examining secular trends. Are the differences the result of artifacts in the data? Are there differences among the places being compared, such as the availability of medical services, diagnostic and treatment practices of physicians, and classification procedures, that may introduce distortions? Some countries do not collect records of vital events or conduct a regular population census. For example, Lebanon has not had an official national census since 1932; the last population estimate was that three million people lived in Lebanon in 2001.[13] When places suffer from war and internal strife, how reliable is the estimate of their populations at risk or the coding of vital outcomes?

The degree of concern about artifacts in vital statistics data depends upon the outcomes being studied as well as the years and places compared. For instance, a US mortality study found that the proportion of coding disagreements about whether cancer was the underlying cause of death fell by 35 percent between ICD-8 and ICD-9, probably due to the new, more detailed rules for the coding of cancers. When the study was repeated using death certificates from seven countries, however, there were discrepancies in assigning cancer as the underlying cause of death in 54 percent of death certificates. The impact of coding differences was particularly acute when multiple cancer sites were mentioned in the medical record, when a decision had to be made as to whether heart disease or cancer was the underlying cause of death, or when there was difficulty interpreting the coding rules.[14]

Another study investigated large differences in diabetes mortality rates among European nations.[15] Approximately 220 randomly selected physicians in each of the participating countries (France, Germany, The Netherlands, Northern Ireland-UK, Republic of Ireland, Romania, Scotland-UK, and Switzerland) were asked to certify the causes of death for six case histories of patients dying with diabetes. Diabetes was under-coded as the underlying cause of death almost 40 percent of the time in Romania, 30 percent in Northern Ireland, and 25 percent in Switzerland. Over-coding of diabetes was 80 percent in The Netherlands and 60 percent in the Republic of Ireland. The study concluded that with such differences in coding practices, the published mortality rates for the disease were not directly comparable among European countries.

The epidemiologist must consider whether outcomes that differ among places are due to differences in environmental factors, the compositions of the populations, or both. For example, since the 1950s more than 200 studies linked multiple sclerosis with place of residence; populations residing farther from the equator have a higher incidence of the disease than those residing closer to it. Many studies investigated risk factors that might explain this geographic pattern, including prior exposure to Epstein-Barr virus, lack of vitamin D (from lesser sun exposures at higher latitudes), and genetic markers linked to the disease being more prevalent in populations residing at higher latitudes.[16] Disentangling the population versus environmental influences for multiple sclerosis has so far been difficult.

One way to separate population from environmental influences is through *migrant studies*. Such studies allow the mortality and natality experience of migrant groups in their current place of residence to be compared with those from their places of origin. Factors that influence migration include the pre-migration environment (severe poverty, endemic diseases, oppression, etc.), age at the time of migration (younger migrants or those who have a longer exposure to the new host country may have rates more similar to the host country), and selective factors (those who migrate may be healthier or more adaptable to new environments). One classic migrant study compared coronary heart disease (CHD) mortality among Japanese men 45 to 64 years of age in San Francisco, Honolulu, and Hiroshima/Nagasaki.[17] The researchers found that in all three places the age-specific CHD mortality rates were lower for Japanese subjects compared to whites. They also found the age-specific rates to be consistently lower in the group remaining in Japan compared to those relocating to Hawaii or San Francisco.

Whenever a mass migration takes place, there is the opportunity to examine the role of the original and new environments in the development of health-related outcomes. For instance, over the course of the twentieth century more than 6 million African Americans migrated from the southern region of the United States to other parts of the nation. One study examined patterns of mortality from diabetes among African Americans, finding that the southern-born migrants had significantly higher death rates from diabetes than their counterparts born elsewhere.[18] If the southern-born migrated to another US region, they retained the risk for diabetes mortality of their place of birth rather than taking on the risk of the region to which they migrated.

Migrant studies are also used to examine natality patterns. For example, a study of Caribbean migration after 1950 found that large-scale migrations, especially of young women, resulted in reduced birth and fertility rates in the sending countries and increased birth and fertility rates in the receiving countries. Even where migration remained within the Caribbean, immigrant women had significantly higher fertility rates compared with native women.[19] In contrast to the impact of female migration, a study of 314 municipalities in seven Mexican states found that where there was a large outmigration of men, fertility rates fell. As the investigators found no differences in fertility among married women across areas with different migration rates, they concluded that fewer men led to fewer marriages and thus lower fertility rates.[20]

Persons

In addition to time and place, person characteristics may influence the distribution of vital outcomes. The number of personal characteristics that can be analyzed is limited by the information available on vital registration certificates. These usually include age, gender, ethnicity, occupation, marital status, and birth cohort.

Age

Age is a major determinant of mortality. In general, there is high mortality in the first year of life, a decline in mortality at ages 1 through 5 years, the lowest mortality at ages 5 to 24 years, and then a steady upward increase with aging. Some health-related outcomes vary from the general pattern of increasing mortality with age. Maternal mortality, for instance, is age-limited, occurring in women of childbearing age but disappearing as women reach menopause. Mortality from homicide and suicide present age patterns as well; however, these may differ among various cultures. For instance, Figure 6.2 shows the age-specific homicide and suicide rates for the US population in 2009. Note that homicide peaked among young adults, whereas suicide peaked for those aged 45 to 55 years.

To demonstrate that age patterns may differ among populations, the age pattern for suicide among the Inuit residing in Greenland is shown in Figure 6.3. The figure shows that for the period 1990 to 1995, the highest

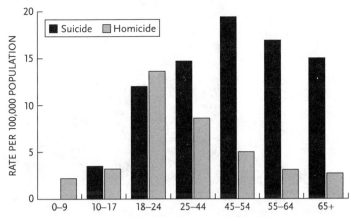

FIGURE 6.2 US suicide and homicide rates per 100,000, by age group, 2009.
SOURCE: MMWR 2012; 61(28):543.

suicide rate was among young men aged 15 to 24 years, with the rate declining with age.[21] This age pattern remained unchanged as of 2010, with Greenland maintaining the highest annual suicide rate of any country in the world at about 100 suicides per 100,000 population.[22] In contrast, the corresponding US rate was 12.4 per 100,000 population.[23]

Gender

Men generally have higher overall mortality than women at all ages and for many diseases. Even in the first year of life, male mortality is higher than female mortality, as first described by John Graunt in 1662 (Chapter 2). This

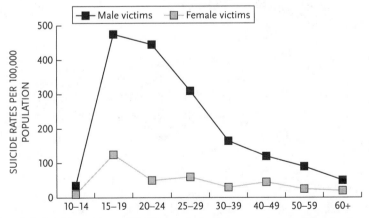

FIGURE 6.3 Suicide rates per 100.000 population by age and sex in Greenland, 1990–95, (N = 285).

SOURCE: Markus J. Leineweber, Doctoral Thesis, Katholieke Universiteit Nijmegen (2000).
http://mipi.nanoq.gl/~/media/2c79218a8db44635b61978c03685691c.ashx

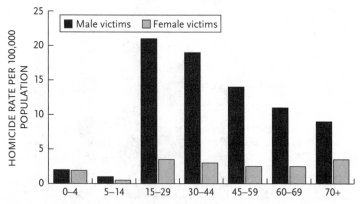

FIGURE 6.4 Global homicide rate by sex and age group, 2008.

DATA SOURCE: 2011 Global Study on Homicide. Copyright 2011 United Nations Office on Drugs and Crime. Reproduced with permission of the World Health Organization. See http://www.unodc.org/documents/data-and-analysis/statistics/Homicide/Globa_study_on_homicide_2011_web.pdf.

finding has been consistently confirmed historically, internationally, and across ethnic groups. The only exceptions are in places where selective abortion, infanticide, and gender-specific neglect are practiced.

Behavioral and occupational differences between the genders affect mortality trends. Mortality rates from accidents (motor vehicle and other), suicide, and homicide tend to be higher among men than among women. This may be partially explained by the tendency of males to participate in riskier behaviors (e.g., fail to use safety equipment, drive faster, use intoxicants), to hold jobs in hazardous occupations, and perhaps to be less socially engaged. Figure 6.4 demonstrates the gender disparity in global homicide rates.

Race and Ethnicity

In the United States, the race and ethnicity categories used to collect population data have changed over time. Consider the census, the usual resource for identifying populations at risk. Before 1960, US census takers determined the race and ethnicity of the individuals they counted. From 1960 forward, respondents to the census identified their own race and ethnicity but were restricted to only one selection for each variable. As of the 2000 census, individuals were allowed to identify themselves as multiracial and multiethnic by checking multiple boxes on the census form. These changes in the way people have been categorized require caution regarding populations at risk based on race and ethnicity categories in census data.

Historically in the United States, individual states created their own categories of race and ethnicity on their vital statistics forms, and these often did not match the census categories nor did they necessarily match the data gathered by the states. This situation changed in 1997, when the federal government required a minimum of two categories of ethnicity (Hispanic/Latino or not Hispanic/Latino) and five categories of race (white, black, Asian, American Indian/Alaskan Native, and Native Hawaiian/Pacific Islander).[24] Thus, the epidemiologist must carefully consider changes over time when using race and ethnicity variables contained in US vital statistics, as well as considering other potential data artifacts.

In nations other than the United States, ethnic and racial indicators such as national origin, tribe, clan, or religion might be recorded in vital records. These classifications are sometimes used as surrogate markers for genetic, cultural, or social class characteristics. For instance, blacks are the group most likely to die from sickle-cell anemia, Jews from Tay-Sachs disease. Under some conditions the surrogate markers may also be used to predict differences in diet, life style, education, occupations, and access to or use of health care.

With increasing migration, social mobility, intermarriage, and the reach of global media and marketing, questions arise about whether surrogate markers are becoming less useful. For instance, genetic makeup is highly correlated with ancestral geography but only modestly correlated with racial category. This is because the genetic variation within racial groups is so great that significant overlaps exist in the genetic makeup of those in different racial and ethnic categories.[25] With successful treatments for some diseases such as cancer now linked to genetic rather than racial or ethnic status, the importance of genetic markers for assessing risk will likely become greater than race and ethnicity.

Socioeconomic Status

Socioeconomic status (SES) or social class is an important variable when considering nonbiological factors that may contribute to health outcomes. Unfortunately, it is not recorded in US and many other nations' vital statistics and can only be inferred from other data sets. Occupation, education, and income are often used as indicators of social class, although these variables are often left blank on self-reported forms. An example of social class data is that gathered by Britain beginning in 1911. Its five social classes are categorized on the basis of occupation. These have changed every 10 years, so historical data may not be comparable, and time trends within a social class category may be the result of data artifacts. In 2001 the British began using the *National Statistics Socio-economic Classification* (NS-SEC) with 17 categories that can be collapsed into three.

Using SES to make international comparisons can be difficult, as nations use various measures and occupations may vary among national groups in their relative social standing, remuneration, and associated risks. An example is the physician who is well paid in the United States but poorly paid in Eastern European countries such as Hungary and the Czech Republic.

The distribution of advantages and disadvantages in life are often linked to SES, and these may in turn affect the distribution of health risks. The social epidemiologist, in particular, is concerned with the distribution of SES in order to predict where, when, and who is at greatest risk for various outcomes.[26] For example, Steenland and colleagues investigated SES and deaths due to injuries among employed persons aged 20 to 64 years.[27] They found that after adjusting for age, sex, year, and race, SES was strongly associated with mortality from injuries for men and, to a lesser extent, for women. The investigators estimated that 41 percent of deaths from injuries are attributable to having SES lower than the top 25 percent of a population.

Birth Cohorts

Analysis of data from a *cohort* (a designated population) can provide insight into the environmental influence of common exposures or experiences in time or place. In the mid-1800s, William Farr used the life table technique with successive birth cohorts (*longitudinal follow-up*) to examine the mortality experience of institutionalized mental patients. He found higher rates for those institutionalized for 0 to 1.5 years compared to 1.5 to 7.5 years. In the 1920s and 1930s, birth cohort analysis was used to examine the mortality experience from tuberculosis of successive generations and establish the importance of reactivated infections later in life.[28]

Epidemiologists may use data on birth outcomes (rates of low, normal, and high birth weight babies, as well as rate of stillbirths) for successive birth cohorts of mothers in order to monitor trends in public health. For instance, researchers examined the trend in stillbirths among successive cohorts of mothers in Italy from 1955 to 1979 (Figure 6.5).[29] They found the risk of stillbirth was consistently highest among mothers 45 to 49 years of age for the entire time period, and the risk of stillbirth trended steadily downward for mothers of all ages after 1920. The investigators anticipated that there might be a change in the downward trend of stillbirths among mothers born during

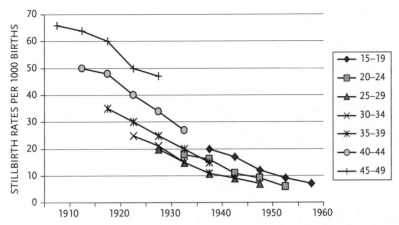

FIGURE 6.5 Trend in stillbirth rates in subsequent cohort of maternal birth, Italy, 1955–1979.

SOURCE: Parazzini et al. (1990).[29] Copyright 1990 by the BMJ Publishing Group. Reproduced with permission of BMJ Publishing Group, Ltd.

the economic depression of the early 1930s, but this was not the case. They suggested that this was perhaps because the economy of Italy was highly agricultural during that period, allowing many pregnant women to remain adequately nourished.

Birth and Infant Death Data

Some vital statistics systems have unique identifiers that allow birth and infant death certificates to be linked, thus providing a means of evaluating various risk factors and perinatal outcomes. Hermann and colleagues compared linked birth and infant death data sets from the United States (Georgia, Missouri, Utah, and Washington state), Israel, Norway, Scotland, and Western Australia.[30] While the methods for linking the data sets differed, and while the resultant data sets did not achieve a 100 percent match, the researchers concluded that the availability of these maternally linked data sets provides opportunities for expanded epidemiologic research. They point out the utility of these data sets for evaluating emerging and reoccurring risk factors that might lead to poor perinatal outcomes.

Identifying the risks for adverse perinatal outcomes, including infant mortality, is the first step toward lowering those rates. One of the newest risk factors for poor perinatal outcomes is the availability of *assisted reproductive technologies* (ART). ART has made pregnancy possible for large numbers of women who could not otherwise become pregnant for a variety of reasons or who choose to become pregnant by alternate means. ART pregnancies have now been shown to carry an increased risk of obstetrical complications, adverse perinatal outcomes, multiple gestations, structural congenital abnormalities, chromosomal abnormalities, genetic imprinting disorders, and childhood cancer.[31]

Multiple births, in particular, carry increased risks for prematurity, low birth weight, and perinatal mortality.[32] A study in Norway noted the triplet rate more than doubled during the past 40 years.[33] The investigators did not assign all of the increase in the Norwegian triplet rate to ART, but they did assign the risk of infant mortality for triplets as 10 times the risk for singletons. A global study in 2004 identified 2,184 clinics in 52 countries that reported initiating more than 950,000 cycles of ART that resulted in 237,809 babies born.[34] The average number of embryos implanted was 2.35, and the resultant deliveries were 25.1 percent twins and 1.8 percent triplets. The investigators noted that some countries have shifted to single embryo transfer, a practice that has and should improve perinatal outcomes.

Summary

Comparisons of mortality and natality by time, place, and persons have been useful in suggesting hypotheses about the causes of various health outcomes and in providing evidence to support or reject them. Population-based studies based on vital statistics often highlight directions for public health concerns. An increase in mortality from a disease may indicate the need for a change in health policy or research. Geographic comparisons of death rates and correlations with other factors that vary with geography, such as culture, diet, behavior, climate, or ethnicity, often suggest hypotheses for future research.

Death certificates contain general information about the person who died, including age at death, gender, ethnicity, occupation, marital status, and birth cohort. Comparisons by such characteristics provide much information about subgroups at risk for different causes of death and help target public health efforts. Birth certificates may provide information about prenatal care, maternal and paternal characteristics, birth weight, gender, and congenital anomalies. Following health outcomes of successive birth cohorts can yield information about trends in the overall public health of a population. In some instances, birth and death certificates can be linked in order to study risks for, and monitor trends related to, adverse perinatal outcomes. Linked data sets have been of particular use in identifying risk factors for infant mortality.

References

1. George Chandler Whipple, *Vital Statistics: An Introduction to the Science of Demography.* New York: John Wiley & Sons, 1919.
2. Eric J. Feuer, Ray M. Merrill, and Benjamin F. Hankey, "Cancer Surveillance Series: Interpreting Trends in Prostate Cancer—Part II: Cause of Death Misclassification and the Recent Rise and Fall in Prostate Cancer Mortality," *Journal of the National Cancer Institute* 91, no. 12 (1999): 1025–1032.
3. Robert N. Anderson et al., *Comparability of Cause of Death between ICD-9 and ICD-10: Preliminary Estimates,* National Vital Statistics Reports 49, no. 2. Hyattsville, MD: National Center for Vital Statistics, 2001. Available at http://www.cdc.gov/nchs/data/nvsr/nvsr49/nvsr49_02.pdf.
4. JaNae Joyner-Grantham et al., "The Impact of Changing ICD Code on Hypertension-Related Mortality in the Southeastern United States from 1994-2005," *Journal of Clinical Hypertension (Greenwich)* 12, no. 3 (2010): 213–222.
5. G. Cano-Serral, G. Perez, and C. Borrell, "Comparability between ICD-9 and ICD-10 for the Leading Causes of Death in Spain," *Revue d'Épidémiologie et de Santé Publique* 54, no. 4 (2006): 355–365.
6. Kathy Giannangelo and Jane Millar, "Mapping SNOMED CT to ICD-10," *Studies in Health Technology and Informatics* 180 (2012): 83–87.
7. Barbara A. Wexelman, Edward Eden, and Keith M. Rose, "Survey of New York City Resident Physicians on Cause-of-Death Reporting, 2010. Preventing Chronic Disease 10 (2014): E76, doi:10.5888/pcd10.120288.
8. Eva Kibele, Rembrandt Scholz, and Vladimir M. Shkolnikov, "Low Migrant Mortality in Germany for Men Aged 65 and Older: Fact or Artifact?" *European Journal of Epidemiology* 23, no. 6 (2008): 389–393.
9. William Farr, *A Memorial Volume of Selections from the Reports and Writings of William Farr.* Metuchen, NJ: Scarecrow Press, 1975.
10. Frederick J. Spencer, "Premature Death in Jazz Musicians: fact or fiction?" *American Journal of Public Health* 81, no. 6 (1991): 804–805.
11. John G. Haaga, "Jazz Musicians: 'Live Fast, Die Young' Stereotype Not Refuted," *American Journal of Public Health* 82, no. 5 (1992): 761.
12. Kenneth J. Rothman, "Longevity of Jazz Musicians: Flawed Analysis," *American Journal of Public Health* 82, no. 5 (1992): 761.
13. Lebanese Global Information Center, "General Information." Available at http://www.lgic.org/en/lebanon_info.php.
14. Constance Percy and Calum Muir, "The International Comparability of Cancer Mortality Data. Results of an International Death Certificate Study," *American Journal of Epidemiology* 129, no. 5 (1989): 934–946.
15. B. Balkau, E. Jougla, L. Papoz; EURODIAB Subarea C Study Group, "European Study of the Certification and Coding of causes of Death of Six Clinical Case Histories of Diabetic Patients," *International Journal of Epidemiology* 22, no. 1 (1993): 116–126.
16. Orhun Kantarci and Dean Wingerchuk, "Epidemiology and Natural History of Multiple Sclerosis: New Insights," *Current Opinion in Neurology* 19, no. 3 (2006): 248–254.

17. R. M. Worth et al. "Epidemiologic Studies of Coronary Heart Disease and Stroke in Japanese Men Living in Japan, Hawaii and California: Mortality," *American Journal of Epidemiology* 102, no. 6 (1975): 481–90.

18. Dona Schneider, Michael Greenberg, and Lisa (Li) Lu, "Early Life Experiences Linked to Diabetes Mellitus: A Study of African-American Migration," *Journal of the National Medical Association* 89, no. 1 (1997): 29–34.

19. Jerome McElroy and Klaus de Albuquerque, "Migration, Natality and Fertility: Some Caribbean Evidence," *International Migration Review* 24, no. 4 (1990): 783–801.

20. K. White and Joseph E. Potter, "The Impact of Outmigration of Men on Fertility and Marriage in the Migrant-Sending States of Mexico, 1995–2000," *Population Studies (Cambridge)* 67, no. 1 (2013): 83–95.

21. M. J. Leineweber, "Modernization and Mental Health: Suicide among the Inuit in Greenland," PhD dissertation, Katholieke Universiteit Nijmegen (Netherlands), 2000.

22. S. Soule, "An Evaluation of the Implementation of Greenland's National Strategy for Suicide Prevention with Recommendations for the Future," Greenland: PAARISA, Ministry of Health, Greenland Home Rule, 2007. Available at http://old.peqqik.gl/Sundhed/~/media/Paarisa/Evaluation_strategy_for_suicide_prevention_UK.ashx

23. Sherry L. Murphy, Jiaquan Xu, and Kenneth D. Kochanek, "Deaths: Final Data for 2010," *National Vital Statistics Reports* 61, no. 4 (2013): 1–117.

24. Office of Management and Budget, "Revisions to the Standards for the Classification of Federal Data on Race and Ethnicity," Washington, DC: Federal Register, 1997. Available at http://www.gpo.gov/fdsys/pkg/FR-1997-10-30/pdf/97-28653.pdf.

25. Mike Bamshad, "Genetic Influences on Health: Does Race Matter?" *Journal of the American Medical Association* 294, no. 8 (2005): 937–946.

26. Eric Jougla et al., "Death Certificate Coding Practices Related to Diabetes in European Countries—the 'EURODIAB Subarea C' Study," *International Journal of Epidemiology* 21, no. 2 (1992): 343–351.

27. Kyle Steenland et al., "Deaths Due to Injuries among Employed Adults: The Effects of Socioeconomic Class," *Epidemiology* 14, no. 1 (2003): 74–79.

28. M. Susser, "Commentary: The Longitudinal Perspective and Cohort Analysis," *International Journal of Epidemiology* 30, no. 4 (2001): 684–687.

29. Fabio Parazzini et al., "Maternal Cohort, Time of Stillbirth, and Maternal Age Effects in Italian Stillbirth Mortality," *Journal of Epidemiology and Community Health* 44, no. 2 (1990): 152–154.

30. Allen A. Herman et al., "Data Linkage Methods Used in Maternally-Linked Birth and Infant Death Surveillance Data Sets from the United States (Georgia, Missouri, Utah and Washington State), Israel, Norway, Scotland and Western Australia," *Paediatric and Perinatal Epidemiology* 11, Suppl. 1 (1997): 5–22.

31. V. M. Allen, R. D. Wilson, and A. Cheung, "Pregnancy Outcomes after Assisted Reproductive Technology," *Journal of Obstetrics & Gynaecology Canada* 28, no. 3 (2006): 220–250.

32. A. K., Henningsen et al., "The Prognosis for Children Born after Assisted Reproduction," *Ugeskrift for Laeger* 174, no. 41 (2012): 2462–2466.

33. Tandberg A, Bjorge T, Nygard O, et al. "Trends in Incidence and Mortality for Triplets in Norway 1967-2006: The Influence of Assisted Reproductive Technologies," *BJOG* 117, no. 6 (2010): 667–675.

34. E. A. Sullivan et al., "International Committee for Monitoring Assisted Reproductive Technologies (ICMART) World Report: Assisted Reproductive Technology 2004," *Human Reproduction* 28, no. 5 (2013): 1375–1390.

7 | Morbidity Statistics

> ... illness is a *datum* measurable in fairly exact terms of duration,
> degree of disability, symptoms, cause, and sequelae ... Statistics
> of illness can afford an indication of vitality ... more illuminating
> than mortality.[1]
>
> *Edgar Sydenstricker (1931)*

ORBIDITY STATISTICS ARE ESSENTIAL TO public health agencies attempting to control communicable diseases and eliminate health disparities. They also provide needed information for other entities. For example, nations monitor their citizens' health to estimate the potential for armed services conscription and to plan for and evaluate any tax-funded health and social services provided. Industry monitors the morbidity of its employees, particularly as it affects absenteeism and productivity. In recent years, increased reliance has been placed on a variety of morbidity statistics to maintain surveillance of the quality of medical care and to measure the utilization of health care facilities and services.

Sources of Morbidity Data

The epidemiologist must consider whether the definitions of illness used are consistent among data sets and which populations serve as the source of the information. Definitions of illness may be influenced by the nature of the program or activity for which the data were collected. For instance, statistics derived from disability programs will vary by agency or by a program's content and purpose. Some disability programs are concerned with specific forms of disability such as blindness, whereas others consider a person's physical or mental ability to support him/herself. Thus, disability may be

TABLE 7.1 Types and Sources of Morbidity Statistics

TYPE	SOURCE
Disease control	Communicable disease reporting systems
	Disease registries (birth defects, cancer, lead)
	Reportable injuries (domestic violence, child and elder abuse)
	Surveillance systems
Publicly financed	Aid to the blind or disabled
	Tax-funded medical care plans (Medicaid, Medicare)
	Workers' compensation programs
	Armed forces, including pre-induction records
	Department of Veterans Affairs
Employee and school	Pre-employment and periodic examinations
	Absentee records
Medical care	Group health and accident insurance
	Prepaid medical care and hospital insurance plans
	Life insurance companies
	Railroad retirement board
	Selective Service records
	Clinic and hospital records
Research programs	Clinical and other interventional trials
Morbidity surveys	Population samples for general health
	Population samples for specific diseases

defined differently and it may be scaled differently (temporary to permanent, or limited to total) in various data sets. Table 7.1 presents an overview of some sources of morbidity data.

Most sources of morbidity data only provide information on special population groups, such as those covered by a particular health insurance or retirement program. Some may pose significant problems with underreporting, especially for sexually transmitted[2-3] and other infectious diseases,[4] obstetrical conditions,[5] and birth defects.[6-7]

Screening Programs

Community-based or *case-finding* screening programs often use a single screening test (i.e., blood pressure or urinalysis) or survey (i.e., personal interview or self-reported questionnaire) to detect individuals with a high probability of having a specific disease. Unfortunately, response rates to questionnaires asking about chronic conditions are usually low.[8-9] Individuals who attend community-based screening programs or who respond to questionnaires may also differ in important ways from those who do not. As a result, epidemiologic measures derived from some screening results may result in biased estimates of disease frequency in the populations surveyed.[10]

It is important to remember that community screening and case-finding programs only provide information on individuals with a presumptive, not a definitive, diagnosis of illness. Diagnostic tests or other examinations are required to confirm whether an individual with a positive screening test actually has the condition. In contrast, morbidity data obtained from health care facilities usually provide a definitive diagnosis of illness. Health care data, however, may also be biased, as it may only include individuals who can afford treatment, have health insurance, or whose illness is so severe they must seek medical attention. Thus, the epidemiologist must consider the data source, the definitions of the illnesses used, and the methods of determining the presence or likely presence of illness before selecting a morbidity data set for epidemiologic studies.

Registries

Long-term population-based registration systems are extremely valuable for monitoring specific health conditions such as cancer or birth defects. A well-planned and well-operated registry not only furnishes information about the frequency of a disease, but it can also provide valuable data for epidemiologic evaluation. Registries attempt to collect as much information as is practical on all newly recognized cases of a condition in a population. To achieve the desired degree of completeness, information on some conditions may be collected from many sources including hospitals, pathology laboratories, practicing physicians, and official birth and death certificates.

Case-based registries, such as a hospital tumor registry, provide useful information about the characteristics of persons developing a given condition. They cannot be used to determine the frequency of that condition, however, because they lack reference to a population. For example, an individual may be visiting family in another state, become ill, and seek medical care in the host state rather than in their state of residence. If they are diagnosed with a disease that requires reporting to the host state's registry, their case would be assigned to the incorrect population-at-risk. Only a population-based registry or a population-based survey can provide appropriate reference population information. Examples of some population-based (total and regional) and hospital-based disease registries are shown in Table 7.2.

Some registries are legally mandated, requiring physicians, laboratories, and hospitals to report every diagnosed case to centralized public health

TABLE 7.2 Select Examples of Population-Based and Hospital-Based Disease Registries

DISEASE	POPULATION COVERAGE	LOCATION
Cancer	Total population	Australia, Canada, Cuba, Denmark, England and Wales, Finland, Iceland, Israel, New Zealand, Norway, Puerto Rico, Scotland, Sweden, and The Gambia
	Population-based registries that cover part of the total population	African Cancer Registry Network (19 nation members), Europe (EuroCan; 28 reporting members), India (NCRP), Italy, Japan Korea, Russia, Ukraine, and the United States (SEER)
	Hospital-based registries	Sudan, Thailand
Cardiovascular disease	Population-based registries that cover part of the total population	WHO Multinational Monitoring of Trends and Determinants in Cardiovascular Disease (MONICA; includes 21 countries)
	Hospital-based registries	United States (National Cardiovascular Disease Registry; 6 hospital-based registries and one outpatient registry)
Congenital anomalies	Total population	Canada, Costa Rica, Cuba, Czech Republic, Malta, United Arab Emirates
	Population-based registries that cover part of the total population	Chile; England and Wales (FASP); European Surveillance of Congenital Anomalies (EUROCAT), United States (select states)
	Hospital-based registries	China, Iran, Israel, Korea, Mexico, Palestine, South America Latin American Collaborative Study of Congenital Malformations (ECLAMC; 70 hospitals)
Stroke	Population-based registries that cover part of the total population	Australia, Canada, China, England and Wales, Germany, Japan, Korea, Paul Coverdell National Acute Stroke Registries (USA), Poland, Scotland, Sweden
	Hospital-based registries	Argentina, Brazil, Chile, Ecuador, Greece, Israel, Peru, Switzerland, Taiwan, Turkey

authorities. Despite legal mandates, some registries, especially if not automated for electronic reporting, suffer from underreporting. Other registries, such as the Nebraska Parkinson's Disease Registry, are voluntary. They depend upon the cooperation either of the patient to self-report, or of those diagnosing the case to report their findings. In a health care delivery system such as a health maintenance organization, diagnostic information may be administratively reported to a registry rather than individual health care providers being required to provide notification about a case. The ability for automated record linkage to a registry may improve the data quality of some voluntary registration systems.

Developing and maintaining a disease registry can be costly, whether the registry is population-based or case-based. It is, therefore, essential to compare the value of registry data for basic research, monitoring of clinical outcomes, or providing health and social services to patients. If the cost of a registry is too high, alternative measures for estimating the prevalence of select diseases may be preferable, such as surveillance systems, cross-sectional studies, and population-based morbidity surveys, especially for common health outcomes.

Surveillance

The concept of surveillance originated during the Napoleonic wars: to keep watch over a group of persons thought to be subversive.[11] The original goal of epidemiologic surveillance was to identify infected individuals, isolate them, and, in so doing, minimize disease transmission.[12-13] The focus of surveillance activities shifted during the latter half of the twentieth century when noninfectious diseases also began to be monitored through registries and population-based surveys. The information on chronic diseases was then disseminated for disease prevention and control efforts.[14] After September 11, 2001 and the anthrax terrorist episode that occurred in its immediate aftermath, the focus of surveillance again shifted, this time to address the hazards associated with bioterrorism. The goal became not only to find apparent cases but also to find suspected cases in order to minimize the potential of a catastrophic public health event[15-16] (see also Chapter 14).

A *surveillance system* includes the ongoing collection, analysis, and dissemination of data by a data center, with the goal of providing a public health response based on an identified need. Four types of surveillance systems are recognized: *active, passive, sentinel,* and *syndromic (clinical, enhanced).*[11,17]

Active surveillance depends on the periodic solicitation of case reports from health care providers or facilities. For example, members of the

Surveillance, Epidemiology and End Results (SEER) cancer registration system actively review hospital records for newly diagnosed (*incident*) cases of cancer and benign tumors; the same is true for many European cancer registries. The *Agency for Toxic Substances and Disease Registry* (ASDR) actively monitors chemical releases, evacuations, injuries, and other forms of victimization related to exposures to hazardous substances.[18] Active surveillance requires a significant effort by the data collection center and can be expensive to maintain, but it results in fairly complete and accurate data.

In contrast, passive surveillance relies upon the discretionary reporting of cases by health care professionals. While inexpensive to implement, it may suffer from underreporting. An example of passive surveillance is when physicians were asked to report cases of toxic shock syndrome in Wisconsin in the early 1980s.[19] Physicians and other community members (including patients) were asked to report cases to the state health department. One factor found to influence the level of reporting was media attention given to toxic shock syndrome.

In an evaluation of active and passive surveillance systems for notifiable diseases in two locations, Vermont[20] and Pierce County, Washington,[21] physicians in the active system reported far more cases compared to those in the passive-reporting locations. Similar results have been reported by other researchers in both the United States[22-23] and other countries.[24]

Sentinel surveillance relies on reports of cases of disease or other events whose occurrence suggests that prevention efforts or medical care needs to be improved. These cases, or *sentinel health events,* indicate that medical or public health professionals are seeing the earliest stages of a problem that requires intervention. Consider a sentinel health event—a case of measles in a public school. This single case indicates the need for attention to immunization in the community served by that school. Similarly, the first dead crow found in a community may serve as a warning that West Nile virus has arrived for the season. Appropriate responses may be to encourage the public to use insect repellent and wear protective clothing when outdoors. A spraying program to reduce the mosquito population may also be warranted.

Sentinel events may also be of concern for noninfectious diseases. For example, a rare outcome among a *healthy worker* cohort may indicate the need for changes to protect worker health and safety. Finding a case of mesothelioma among asbestos-exposed workers should signal the need for increased health and exposure monitoring in the workplace, including implementing workplace changes to improve occupational health and safety.

Active and sentinel surveillance systems gather information directly.[25] These forms of surveillance are limited, however, in that they rely on having a diagnosis or presumptive diagnosis of a known disease in order for a report to be generated. After September 11, 2001, it became apparent that existing reporting systems could not provide the information needed for rapid public health response in cases of a biological or chemical attack, or new diseases such as severe acute respiratory syndrome (SARS).[26] A system that could identify cases that suggested outbreaks before those cases had a definitive diagnosis, or which identified dangerous exposures before cases appeared, was needed. That information had to reach public health authorities quickly. The answer was *syndromic (enhanced) surveillance*.

Syndromic surveillance links and scans data systems for patterns. It does not require direct input from individuals, nor does it require that the data it scans include a diagnosis. For example, a slight increase in the number of patients presenting with respiratory distress in various emergency departments across a city could trigger a public health alert. The facilities simply need to be electronically linked to a centralized, real-time syndromic surveillance system. Despite the fact that the cases might present in different places, they could still be identified as a *cluster* in time.[27] Similarly, a spike in prescriptions for antibiotics or the purchase of over-the-counter medications at pharmacies linked to the system could trigger a public health alert. The real-time reporting advantage of syndromic surveillance allows preventive or response measures to be put into effect far more quickly than with other forms of surveillance. The system relies heavily, however, on coordinated efforts and computing systems that can handle inputs from multiple data sources.[16,28]

The advantages and disadvantages of the four types of surveillance are shown in Table 7.3. It is entirely possible that more forms of enhanced surveillance will emerge as technology and our ability to exploit it continues to improve. For example, the *CDC's Vision for Public Health Surveillance in the 21st Century* envisions infectious disease surveillance with global data available in real time.[29] *Electronic health records* (EHRs) and *health information exchanges* (HIEs) that are linked to centralized public health reporting while protecting individual's *protected health information* (PHI) and a knowledgeable, skilled, and effective public health workforce will be available to meet the needs of public health surveillance. This will be challenging but entirely achievable, as the epidemiologist learns to better use informal reporting systems such *HealthMap* or *ProMed* on the Internet, scan text data in systems such as *Google Flu Trends* (GFT),[30] and use mobile phones with *geographic positioning systems* (GPS) to report cases of malaria so that public health officials can target parasite reservoirs in an effort to control outbreaks.[31]

TABLE 7.3 Advantages and Disadvantages of Surveillance Systems

TYPE	CHARACTERISTIC	ADVANTAGES	DISADVANTAGES
Active	Regular periodic collection of case reports from health care providers or facilities	Provides the most accurate data of all types of surveillance	Expensive
Passive	Case reports given by health care professionals at their discretion	Inexpensive	Data are likely to underestimate the number of cases in the population
Sentinel	Case reports indicates a failure of the health care system or indicates that a special problem is emerging	Very inexpensive	Applicable only for a select group of diseases
Syndromic	Reports of potential cases based on signs and symptoms rather than diagnoses	Provides real-time reporting and the advantage for identifying potential health-related problems	Moderate cost; data may overestimate risk

Morbidity or Health Surveys

Morbidity (health) surveys elicit information from individuals or households about health outcomes in the population. They may also elicit data on risk and preventive behaviors, and exposure to potential etiologic agents. Some, such as the Demographic and Health Survey (DHS) Program from the United States Agency for International Development (USAID), provide global data for these purposes. A *cross-sectional (prevalence) study* utilizes morbidity survey data from a random sample of a population of interest at one point in time (a cross-section). The epidemiologist can use this information to estimate the frequency of various outcomes in the population as a whole and look for relationships between the outcomes and potential risk factors. When morbidity surveys are repeated periodically or continually using the same population, a *panel study* is established. Panel studies allow the epidemiologist to follow trends in population health, including the increase or decrease in select risk factors linked to various outcomes.

The US Public Health Service conducted the first US morbidity surveys in Hagerstown, Maryland between 1921 and 1924.[32] Surveillance of various health outcomes for the entire United States began in 1956 when the

National Center for Health Statistics (NCHS) implemented the *National Health Survey*. The survey remains active and contains three parts:

- National Health Interview Survey (NHIS)
- National Health and Nutrition Examination Survey (NHANES)
- National Health Care Surveys

The NHIS is based on a sample of the non-institutionalized population of the United States. Interviews of sample households are conducted each week and include questions on doctor visits and hospital stays, acute and chronic conditions, health status indicators, and limitations of activities. A supplemental set of questions is asked periodically on issues such as knowledge and attitudes about AIDS, health promotion practices, and smoking habits. The NHIS sampling framework has changed over time, allowing for the oversampling of select groups. In 2011, the NHIS included interviews of 35,000 households containing 87,500 persons, with an oversampling of Asians, blacks, and Hispanics.[33]

The NHANES consists of both interviews (including demographic, socio-economic, dietary, and health-related questions) and examinations (including physical, dental, and laboratory tests for specific conditions). Originally organized in the 1960s as the National Health Examination Survey, nutritional aspects were added to the program in 1970, and monitoring of the population became continuous in 1999. The program surveys a randomly selected group of 5,000 individuals from counties across the United States each year. Fifteen of those counties are the same each year, to provide for continuity of the findings. The NHANES provides the data for developing national standards against which measurements for height, weight, and blood pressure can be compared. Its utility for monitoring the public's health and informing public health policy is invaluable.[34]

The National Health Care Surveys sample various institutions or facilities that provide health or medical care services, including separate surveys for physicians' offices, hospital emergency and outpatient departments, inpatient hospital care, ambulatory surgical facilities, and long-term care settings. Surveys of home, hospice, and long-term care providers are also conducted. The surveys include questions about patient safety, disparities in health care provision, surgical procedures, the use of staffing and other resources, and the diffusion of technologies such as electronic medical records.[35]

Responders to morbidity surveys are usually anonymous, and information from such surveys is most often reported in the aggregate. Many nations (e.g., the United Kingdom, through the Office of Population Census and

Surveys; Canada, Health Canada; Japan, Health Statistics Office; the EU, Eurostat; and Australia, Australian Bureau of Statistics, among others) now have long-standing national health morbidity surveys, and some make these data available for epidemiological research. The World Health Organization reports that 80 percent of countries had national health survey systems (for both mortality and morbidity) in 2010, but only 21 percent of those countries has population-based morbidity data.[36]

Limitations of Morbidity Data

Data from various sources may under- or overestimate the prevalence of select diseases, conditions or disabilities, or exposure to risk factors. Screening data may overestimate disease prevalence because the data are based on presumptive rather than diagnosed disease status. They may also be biased if persons participating in the screening program are healthier or sicker than those not participating. Data obtained from registries or surveillance systems may underestimate the number of cases of disease in a population because there is no mechanism to enforce complete reporting. The epidemiologist must therefore consider the *validity* (*accuracy*) and *reliability* (*variability, reproducibility, or precision*) of the information obtained on morbidity before using it for epidemiologic studies.

Validity

Data from cross-sectional studies and morbidity surveys have some limitations. For example, multiple studies show some conditions as more or less likely to be documented in medical records, whereas others are more or less likely to be self-reported on questionnaires or in interviews. A study from the Netherlands, for example, showed that older male patients over-reported strokes and underreported both malignancies and arthritis. Older females over-reported malignancies and arthritis.[37] In Italy, investigators using data from the Italian Longitudinal Study of Aging (ILSA) documented significant under- and over-reporting issues, depending upon the condition. They concluded that the use of self-reported data could lead to inaccurate estimates of the prevalence of specific diseases in the population.[38]

Using self-reported data to assess the severity of a diagnosed disease or the extent of disability may also be problematic. A New Zealand study, for instance, showed that asthmatics who underused their inhalers over-reported use, whereas those who overused their inhalers tended to underreport such use.[39] Multiple studies from countries around the world show that individuals consistently underreport alcohol, tobacco, and other drug use/abuse. Many individuals deny the warning signs and symptoms of diseases such as hypertension or diabetes until the condition is severe enough to require medical intervention. If surveyed during the denial phase, these conditions will be underreported.

The epidemiologist must consider the potential for errors in self-reported data because the search for etiological factors requires information on both current and past exposures. If self-reported information is not accurate, the epidemiologic evaluation will be flawed. Thus, self-reported information on both disease and exposure status should be validated with medical or other records whenever possible.

Examination data (physical examination, laboratory tests, or other markers of disease) provide objective measures of morbidity, but these data sources must be assessed for both *validity* (measures what it purports to measure) and *reliability* (may be replicated). Three indices are used to evaluate the validity of both screening and diagnostic examination data—*sensitivity, specificity,* and *accuracy*. These three indices are characteristics of the test or observation and should not change when performed on various populations under standardized conditions.

To determine sensitivity and specificity, the examination is administered to a group of persons with and without the disease. Those results are then arranged in a 2 × 2 table (Table 7.4).

Individuals with known disease and who test positive are classified as *true positives* (a). Those without the disease and who test negative are *true negatives* (d). Only individuals in groups a and d had accurate test results. Individuals with the disease but who were classified as disease-free (*false negatives, c*) and

TABLE 7.4 Classifying the Results of Examination Data for Validity

TEST RESULT	DISEASE STATUS		TOTALS
	POSITIVE	NEGATIVE	
POSITIVE	A True positive	B False positive	A + B All those with positive tests
NEGATIVE	C False negative	D True negative	C + D All those with negative tests
TOTALS	A + C All those with disease	B + D All those without disease	A + B + C + D All those tested

those without disease who were classified as having the condition (*false positives, b*) had incorrect results.

Sensitivity measures the ability of the test to correctly identify those with disease (the proportion of those with disease that are correctly identified). Specificity measures the ability of the test to correctly identify those who are disease-free (the proportion of those without disease that are correctly identified). The accuracy (validity) of the test is simply the proportion of the population evaluated that had correct results.

$$Sensitivity = \frac{a}{a+c}$$

$$Specificity = \frac{b}{b+d}$$

$$Accuracy = \frac{a+d}{a+b+c+d}$$

Some tests are measured on a continuous spectrum (e.g., blood pressure or serum lipoprotein levels), and the distribution of their values for individuals with and without disease may overlap. Figure 7.1 shows two hypothetical distributions of blood glucose levels for normal and diabetic populations. Where there is no overlap, the results of a blood glucose test for diagnosing diabetes would be clear. The individual being tested would either be diabetic or not. Where there is an overlap in the distributions, however, the test results might not be definitive.

Figure 7.2 demonstrates how changing the cutoff value for a test measured on a continuous spectrum can influence test results. If the cutoff value is set low (Figure 7.2A), the blood glucose level becomes a very sensitive test for identifying all those who might have the disease. While every case will be identified (true positives), many normal subjects will be mistakenly thought to have the condition (false positives). If the cutoff limit is set high (Figure 7.2C), then the test becomes highly specific. This means that all those persons without diabetes will be correctly classified (true negatives), but many diabetics will have their diagnosis missed (false negatives). The minimum error of the test, the point where there are the fewest number of false positives and negatives, would be at the cutoff shown in Figure 7.2B.

Sensitivity and specificity measure the validity or accuracy of a test, but not the probability that test results will correctly identify an individual's disease status. Two additional indices are particularly helpful in this regard—*positive predictive value* and *negative predictive value*. Positive predictive value (sometimes called *yield*) is the probability that someone with a positive test actually

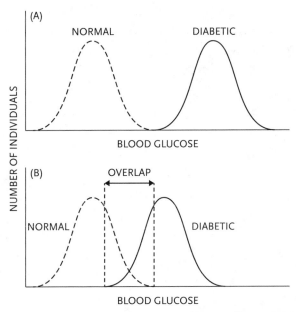

FIGURE 7.1 Hypothetical distributions of separate and overlapping blood glucose values in normal and diabetic individuals.

has the disease or condition. Negative predictive value is the probability that a negative test correctly identifies an individual's disease-free status.

$$Positive\,Predictive\,Value = \frac{a}{a+b}$$

$$Negative\,Predictive\,Value = \frac{d}{c+d}$$

Positive and negative predictive values may be as important as sensitivity and specificity when setting a cutoff point for a test. Incorrect test results have ramifications, including the psychological and economic costs borne by people who receive false positive tests and are burdened by unnecessary stress and follow-up examinations and procedures. Incorrect test results may also have ramifications for disease progression or transmission when persons are erroneously told they are disease-free. While sensitivity and specificity are characteristics of the test and do not change, positive and negative predictive values do vary with the prevalence of disease in the population being evaluated. As the prevalence of the disease in the population increases, the positive predictive value of the test will increase and the negative predictive value will decrease. In population-based screening programs where the prevalence of disease may be low, the positive predictive value will be low and the negative

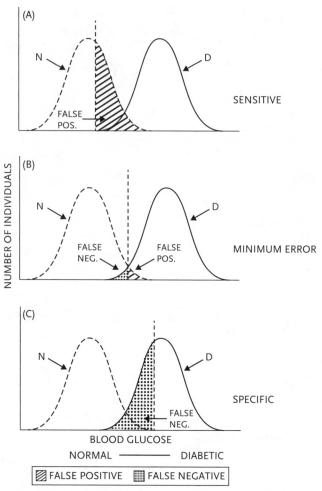

FIGURE 7.2 Effect of changing blood glucose cutoff levels on a hypothetical screening test for diabetes: (A) A low cutoff increases test sensitivity but also increases the number of false positives. (B) The point of minimal error. (C) A high cutoff increases test specificity but also increases the number of false negatives.

predictive value will be high. It is important for the epidemiologist to understand this relationship because it has implications for the allocation of public health dollars. It also assists clinicians when they counsel patients who are trying to make informed decisions about health care (see Chapter 13).

Reliability

Reliability is the ability of a test to provide the same results when repeated under the same conditions. In the case of self-reported data, it may be possible to have a subject complete more than one survey or to be interviewed by different observers to see if the results obtained are the same. For instance, investigators asked children referred to a urology clinic and their parents to complete three different survey instruments designed to elicit the severity of the child's lower urinary tract symptoms. The attending physician (a single observer) examined the patient and talked to the parents, but was masked as to the survey results. The physician's impression about the severity of the child's symptoms was then correlated with the surveys using a nonparametric statistical method (Kendall's tau-b), because the data did not fit a normal distribution. All of the survey instruments were reliably correlated with the physician's impression, so that no single survey was recommended as a "gold standard" for eliciting the severity of lower urinary tract symptoms in children.[40]

When surveys or interviews cannot be repeated, the investigator may use several questions in a single survey that are designed to elicit the same information, but that are posed in different ways. Consistency among the answers to questions posed on a *Likert-type scale* (e.g., 1 to 5, where 1 is strongly disagree, 3 is no opinion, and 5 is strongly agree) may be evaluated using a statistical technique called *Cronbach's α* (alpha), a measure of scale reliability.

Reliability may be challenged if there is variation among observers or if the instrumentation required for the test is unstable. The first report of problems with variation among observers dates to 1949, when Yerushalmy reported that individuals interpreting chest X-ray films for the diagnosis of tuberculosis differed in two distinct ways:[41]

1. *Inter-observer* variability was demonstrated by inconsistent interpretation among different readers of the films.
2. *Intra-observer* variability was demonstrated by the failure of a reader to be consistent with his/her own independent interpretation of the same set of films.

A study evaluating the cytological diagnosis of human papillomavirus (HPV) infection demonstrated both types of observer variability.[42] Between 1973 and 1981, two expert pathologists at a private cytological laboratory examined 87 cervicovaginal smears for the presence or absence of HPV infection. They then independently reexamined a sample of 24 of the specimens. The results of their evaluations were then compared using a statistic called *kappa* (κ). Kappa measures the degree of nonrandom agreement among observers where κ = 1 is perfect agreement, κ = 0 is what would happen by chance, and κ = −1 is perfect disagreement. The pathologists agreed with each other on a diagnosis 74 percent of the time ($\kappa = 0.38$), more than would be found by chance alone. Pathologist A agreed with his own diagnosis 96 percent of the time ($\kappa = .89$) and pathologist B agreed with himself 70 percent of the time ($\kappa = 0.40$). Similar results were found for other diagnostic tests.

Data Classification Schemes

There are several types of systems for classifying morbidity data. The first is a set of reference *nosologies* established by the World Health Organization as the WHO *Family of International Classifications* (WHO-FIC). The Family includes the *International Classification of Diseases* (ICD; see Chapter 5), the *International Classification of Functioning, Disability and Health* (ICF; endorsed by member states in 2001), and the *International Classification of Health Interventions* (ICHI; in adaptation).

The ICD system is widely used for many types of epidemiologic studies, but it was found insufficient in certain circumstances and additional classifications were developed to fill the gap. For example, to handle oncology-specific classifications that could identify characteristics and locations of specific tumors, the ICD-O (oncology) was developed. The ICF measures functional status and a specialized coding scheme—the ICF-CY now measures functional status among children and youth. The ICHI is currently under development to standardize the classification of preventive and curative interventions including those that are medical, surgical, and related to mental health. Other data classification schemes include the *Medical Dictionary for Regulatory Affairs* (MedDRA), used by pharmacoepidemiologists, and other specialized coding schemes not linked to the WHO-FIC.

Epidemiologists using data sets based on any particular nosology should familiarize themselves with the technical aspects of that coding scheme. In some instances, *personal identifiers* will allow the epidemiologist to link information from different data sets even if they use different coding systems (*record linkage*). Linked data produce a single comprehensive record for each case and are useful for epidemiologic investigations. For example, a disease registry that gathers personal identifiers can search medical insurance records, retirement records, and death certificates to provide a more complete history of a patient. A linked record can also benefit patients by providing their health care providers with a thorough compilation, in one place, of all the patient's examinations, laboratory findings, and therapeutics prescribed.

Protected (*Personal*) Health Information

Many local and national legislatures rely on information provided and recommended by the epidemiologic community. Societal concerns weigh on this relationship, however, especially those concerning individual privacy. In the United States, the Privacy Act of 1974 and, subsequently, the Health Insurance Portability and Accountability Act of 1996 (HIPAA) reflect these sensitivities. HIPAA recognizes that while select data elements must be gathered for legitimate purposes, failure to protect this information poses a threat to individual privacy. To address this threat, data sets containing personal identifiers are held by an *honest broker* (such as a disease registry). The honest broker then allows others access to the data for legitimate purposes (approved research protocols, billing of services, etc.). They may *de-identify* (recode) the information so that data records cannot be traced back to individuals. Alternatively, they may strip all identifying variables from the data set, thus creating an *anonymous* data set for general use.

In Sweden, concerns about unauthorized access to some elements of medical records, such as the dispensing of pharmaceuticals, resulted in the destruction of those records as soon as the prescriptions were filled. This prevented pharmacoepidemiologists from identifying new adverse events associated with use of prescribed medications. In Japan, too, privacy regulations have restricted access to medical data for legitimate research and quality assurance purposes. While regulations protecting personal information are clearly justified, society is perhaps better served if the regulations are balanced (allowing access for approved purposes) rather than totally prohibitive.

Morbidity Measures

Morbidity is characterized by the frequency with which a disease, injury, or required medical intervention occurs, or by the burden it places on a population. Incidence and prevalence are presented first, as these measures are the ones most frequently used by epidemiologists.

Incidence

Incidence is the number of outcomes of interest in a population that occur during a given time interval. Incidence can be presented as a simple count of occurrences, as a proportion (probability of risk), or as a rate, depending upon the target audience for the information.

For example, 1,296,070 babies were born by Cesarean section (the number of occurrences) in the United States (the population) in 2012 (the time period).[43] While the above sentence describing incidence as a count is informative, the information might be even more useful if presented in a different way. Suppose a hospital administrator is interested in knowing whether the proportion of births delivered by Cesarean section in his or her institution is the same as the national average. How would this information be determined? The answer lies in the calculation of the *incidence proportion*, sometimes called *cumulative incidence*, of an event.

$$Incidence\ proportion\ (cumulative\ incidence) = \frac{Number\ of\ new\ occurrences\ in\ a\ time\ period}{Total\ population\ at\ risk\ in\ that\ time\ period}$$

The National Vital Statistics System (NVSS) reports that there were 3,952,841 live births in the United States in 2012.[44] The proportion of babies born by Cesarean section was 1,296,070/3,952,841 = 0.328, or 32.8 percent of live births in that year. Proportions are equated with probability, the likelihood or *risk* that an event will occur. Probability is limited by having a range of values between 0 and 1, reflecting the risk of an outcome from no chance (0 percent) to certainty (100 percent). In the above example, the administrator might note that the *risk* of Cesarean section at their hospital was greater or less than the 32.8 percent for all US live births in 2012.

In contrast to incidence proportion, *incidence rates* are not bound by probability limits. To address the needs of multiple audiences, the NVSS reports both the incidence proportion (32.8 percent in 2012) and the incidence rate (327.9 per 1,000 US live births in 2012) of Cesarean sections annually. It is not uncommon for reporting agencies to provide both calculations, as risk can be equated with rate when the time period of observation is relatively short (as per year) and everyone in the population is considered equally exposed (as in a live birth).

Populations, however, are not always static. Sometime the epidemiologist has to take into account that there is population change from the beginning of an interval to its end. Consider a population that has experienced in- or outmigration over the period of a year. This is a common problem in public health, so the midpoint or average population at risk becomes the denominator in the incidence calculation.

$$\text{Incidence rate} = \frac{\begin{array}{c}\text{Number of new occurrences}\\\text{in a time period}\end{array}}{\begin{array}{c}\text{Average population at risk}\\\text{in that time period}\end{array}} \times 10^n$$

Another concern that the epidemiologist must take into account is that individuals making up the population at risk may not be exposed to the risk or observed for the outcome for equal amounts of time. Consider the risk of traumatic brain injury for football players. Not all players play for the same number of years, nor do they necessarily play every game of every season nor have the same amount of field time when they do play. Another example is that of the relationship of smoking to cardiopulmonary disease. Not every-one who smokes does so in the same intensity or for the same amount of time. To address the problem of different amounts of exposure or different times of observation for the individuals in the study population, the epide-miologist may choose to use an *incidence density* (*interval incidence density, person-time incidence rate, hazard rate,* or *force of morbidity*) calculation.

$$\text{Incidence density} = \frac{\begin{array}{c}\text{Number of new occurrences}\\\text{in a time period}\end{array}}{\begin{array}{c}\text{Total person - time units observed}\\\text{in the same time period}\end{array}}$$

As an example, the Occupational Safety and Health Administration (OSHA) weights the numerator in the incidence density calculation by 200,000 to produce an *incident rate* (200,000 hours being the number of hours worked by 100 employees who each work 40 hours a week for 50 weeks a year—taking a two-week vacation).[45] Assume that a construction company has 12 full-time employees who work a 40-hour week and four part-time employees who each work 20 hours per week. All employees are given a two-week vacation. In the last year, three employees suffered back injuries that prevented them from returning to work in construction. What was the incident rate (incidence density) of back injuries at the construction com-pany for the past year?

$$\text{Incident rate} = \frac{3 \times 200,000}{\left(12 \times 40 \times 50\right) + \left(4 \times 20 \times 50\right)} = \frac{600,000}{13,600} = 44.12 \text{ per 100 employees}$$

Weighting the rate allows OSHA to compare standardized incident rates among companies with the same types of workers, as well as among workers from different types of industries.

Prevalence

In contrast to incidence, *prevalence* measures the amount of disease in a population, that is, how many cases of the disease are present at or during a specified time period. It provides a measure of the burden of an outcome on a population (the proportion of existing disease) by taking into account not only new cases but also existing ones.

$$\text{Prevalence} = \frac{\textit{Total cases at or in a time period}}{\textit{Population at risk at or in that time period}}$$

Prevalence can be estimated as *point prevalence* (a cross-section at a single point in time) or *period prevalence*. Period prevalence is sometimes reported as *prevalent cases per unit time* or *lifetime prevalence,* situations where the calculated measure is sometimes reported in the literature as a *prevalence rate.* The *Dictionary of Epidemiology, 6th Edition* is clear, however, that prevalence is a proportion and not a rate.[46]

In a stable population, the relationship between incidence and prevalence is such that if either the incidence or duration of a disease changes, it will impact prevalence. This is often written as:

$$P \cong I \times D$$

Assume, for instance, that disease X is endemic in a stable population, occurring at the same rate each year. Persons with the disease suffer for several months, and then they all die. A new treatment for disease X is developed. If the treatment provides a cure, then the duration of disease will be cut short and the prevalence of disease in the population will decrease, though the incidence rate will be unchanged. If the treatment does not provide a cure but prolongs life, the duration of the disease will be longer and the prevalence of disease in the population will increase; again, the incidence rate would be unchanged. If the population is not stable, perhaps because of rapid in- or outmigration, this may not hold.

The *incidence proportion* (referred to as the *attack rate* in Chapter 1) estimates the probability of developing a disease. It is possible to calculate how transmissible a disease agent is by evaluating how fast it spreads among closed groups (families, friends, co-workers, or classmates) who have come into contact with a primary case of the disease. In some instances, the *secondary attack rate* is calculated to reflect the transmissibility of the infectious agent. It may indicate possible modes of transmission, and may even be used to evaluate the efficacy of preventive measures or treatments. For example, the risk for developing Kaposi's sarcoma among homosexual and bisexual men with AIDS was shown to be 10 times as great as among groups with other modes of HIV transmission.[47] Investigators also noted that British AIDS patients who had sexual partners from the United States or Africa (secondary attack rate) had a significantly higher risk for Kaposi's sarcoma than did those whose sexual partners came from Britain or other areas.[48] These findings led to the search for an infectious agent. Guided by this information, researchers identified herpes simplex virus type 6 (HSV-6) as the agent associated with Kaposi's sarcoma.

Incidence and prevalence measures have different uses. Assume a hospital is concerned about an infectious disease outbreak. The epidemiologist would want to know the incidence of the disease (how fast each case is occurring), because each new case will require a separate isolation room. Will there be enough rooms available? The epidemiologist also has to consider the prevalence of the disease, defined by how long the disease is infectious. How long will each case require an isolation room? Both measures are required for dealing with the outbreak. Now assume a health maintenance organization wants to know how many people need diabetic testing and treatment supplies so they can mail these items each month and minimize emergency room use due to uncontrolled diabetes. In this case, the epidemiologist needs to know how many people have the disease, not how fast the disease is increasing. The appropriate calculation in this instance is prevalence.

DALYS and QALYS

The burden a disease places on a population can be assessed by two related yet distinctly different measures: *disability-adjusted life years* (DALYs) and *quality-adjusted life years* (QALYs). The former measures health loss due to a specific disease or disability, whereas the latter measures functional gain from an intervention.

Disability-Adjusted Life Years

DALYs require the epidemiologist to calculate two measures: years of potential life lost (YPLL; see Chapter 5) and years of life with the disability (YLD) leading to premature death from particular health-related conditions. These two measures are then summed to yield DALYs.

$$DALY = YPLL + YLD$$

The epidemiologist calculates the YLD as the number of incident cases in the population (I) times the disability weight (DW ranging from 0.0 for perfect health to 1.0 for death) and the average number of years until remission or death (YR):

$$YLD = I \times DW \times YR$$

Disability weights are established by panels of experts and may differ depending on the specific circumstance. An example of calculating YLD is shown in Table 7.5. In this example, the World Health Organization developed the disability weights.[49]

Used by the WHO *Global Burden of Disease Project* (GBDP), DALYs allow the impact of diseases in different countries to be assessed and compared; public health resources can be allocated accordingly. The GBDP and its utility for targeting select populations or specific disease outcomes are discussed further in Chapter 8.

Quality-Adjusted Life Years

QALYs can be considered the mirror image of DALYs. Rather than measuring loss, QALYs assess the gains achieved by various therapeutic interventions and preventive efforts. For instance, the National Institute for Health and Clinical Excellence uses QALYs to determine whether they should recommend that the English National Health Service pay for specific services and treatments. To be recommended, a service or treatment must be balanced in terms of both expected benefits and costs.

QALYs differ from DALYs in that the weights used are reversed (1.0 for perfect health to 0.0 for death). Rather than the weights being developed by a panel of experts, they are derived from survey data comparing those with and without a specific condition or disease. A wide variety of survey instruments are available for measuring health-related quality of life, both for specific diseases and for general health status. An example of a disease-specific

TABLE 7.5 Example of Calculating Years of Life with Disability

CLASS	ACTIVITY	DISABILITY WEIGHT*	NUMBER OF CASES	AVERAGE DURATION (YEARS)	YLD [+]
1	Limited ability to perform at least one activity among recreation, education, procreation, or occupation.	0.096	100	20	192
2	Limited ability to perform most activities in any one of recreation, education, procreation, or occupation.	0.220	200	15	660
3	Limited ability to perform activities in two or more of recreation, education, procreation, or occupation.	0.400	400	5	800
4	Limited ability to perform most activities in recreation, education, procreation, and occupation.	0.600	300	3	540
5	Needs assistance with instrumental activities of daily living such as meal preparation, shopping, or housework.	0.810	400	2	648
6	Needs assistance with activities of daily living such as eating, personal hygiene, or toilet use.	0.920	20	.5	9.2
Total YLD					2,849.2

* DISABILITY WEIGHTS FROM C. J. Murray (1996).[49]
[+] YLD = (Disability Weight) × (Number of Cases) × (Average Duration in years).

instrument used to evaluate quality of life of individuals with breast cancer is the *Functional Assessment of Cancer Therapy, Breast* (FACT-B). Among the more widely used instruments used to measure quality of life are the *Short Form Health Survey* (SF-36) developed in the Medical Outcomes Study, and the EQ-5D developed by the EuroQoL Group. Once weights are generated from these survey data, the epidemiologist calculates QALYs similarly to the calculation for YLDs.

Although DALYs and QALYs are widely used in the formulation of health policy, these indices are not without their limitations.[50-51] DALYs rely on weights developed by experts without the input of the population impacted by the condition of interest. This means they may not accurately measure disability. The weights for calculating QALYs depend upon the choice of the survey instrument selected. This may affect the calculation of QALYs and limit their comparability, potentially a major deficiency.

Summary

The epidemiologist must consider the data source, the definitions of the illnesses used, and the methods of determining the presence or likely presence of illness before selecting a morbidity data set for epidemiologic studies. Data sets for epidemiologic studies of morbidity are available from a variety of sources, including registries and surveillance systems that allow for the routine collection, analysis, and dissemination of information on disease occurrence. Registries can be voluntary or mandatory. Voluntary registries are less expensive to maintain than mandatory registries, but they tend to underreport cases of disease. Surveillance systems can be active, passive, sentinel, or syndromic. Active surveillance is more expensive than passive surveillance, but it provides more complete data on cases of a specific disease. Sentinel surveillance relies on the occurrence of sentinel events to signify the potential of a public health problem. Syndromic (enhanced) surveillance can scan multiple electronic databases in real time and identify patterns that indicate potential health issues even before a diagnosis is obtained. Additional forms of surveillance are likely to emerge as technology improves.

Data on morbidity can also be obtained by cross-sectional studies and morbidity surveys. Whether these data are based on self-reports, interview data, or examinations (physical and laboratory examinations, and other measures of health and disease), they should be evaluated for validity (Did the surveys measure what they were intended to measure?) and reliability (Do questions designed to measure the same outcome give consistent results?). Measures of validity for examination data (including screening) include sensitivity and specificity. Sensitivity measures the proportion of diseased persons detected by a test; specificity measures the proportion of those the test correctly identifies as negative for the disease. These indices are characteristic of the test and do not change from population to population. Positive predictive value measures the probability that someone with a positive test result actually has the disease, and negative predictive value measures the probability that someone with a negative test result does not have the disease. These indices will vary according to the prevalence of disease in the populations being tested.

Whenever examinations require the judgment of observers, there is the potential for variability in the results. Inter-observer variability can be tested using kappa statistics to measure whether the levels of agreement rendered by the observers could be expected by chance alone.

Measures of morbidity include the risk of developing a disease over a given period of time (the incidence rate) and the proportion (prevalence) of a population having a disease at a particular point or period of time. There is a relationship between incidence and prevalence whereby the prevalence of disease in a population roughly equals the incidence rate for that disease multiplied by its average duration. A special type of incidence rate, the secondary attack rate, describes the transmissibility of a disease among a particular group (such as a family) that has been exposed to a primary (or index) case. Secondary attack rates can also be used to evaluate the efficacy of preventive treatments.

Measures of the burden of diseases on populations include DALYs and QALYs. DALYs measure health loss in a population due to a specific disease or disability. QALYs measure health improvement in a population due to a specific therapy or preventive actions.

References

1. Edgar Sydenstricker, "The Incidence of Influenza among Persons of Different Economic Status during the Epidemic of 1918," *Public Health Reports (1896–1970)* 46, no. 4 (1931): 154–170.
2. L. M. Calzavara et al., "Underreporting of AIDS Cases in Canada: A Record Linkage Study," *Canadian Medical Association Journal* 142, no. 1 (1990): 36–39.
3. M. Pacheco, T. Sentell, and A. R. Katz, "Under-Reporting Of Pelvic Inflammatory Disease in Hawaii: A Comparison of State Surveillance and Hospitalization Data," *Journal of Community Health* 39, no. 2 (2014): 336–338, doi:10.1007/s10900-013-9766-x.
4. J. D. Young, "Underreporting of Lyme Disease." *New England Journal of Medicine* 338, no. 22 (1998): 1629.
5. Abraham M. Lilienfeld et al., "Accuracy of Supplemental Medical Information on Birth Certificates," *Public Health Reports* 66, no. 7 (1951): 191–198.
6. S. J. Milham, "Underreporting of Incidence of Cleft Lip and Palate," *American Journal of Diseases of Children* 106 (1963): 185–188.
7. S. L. Boulet et al., "Sensitivity of Birth Certificate Reports of Birth Defects in Atlanta, 1995–2005: effects of maternal, infant, and hospital characteristics," *Public Health Reports* 126, no. 2 (2011): 186–194.
8. P. L. Colsher and R. B. Wallace, "Longitudinal Application of Cognitive Function Measures in a Defined Population of Community-Dwelling Elders," *Annals of Epidemiology* 1, no. 3 (1991): 215–230.

9. Lorene M. Nelson et al., "Proxy Respondents in Epidemiologic Research," *Epidemiologic Reviews* 12 (1990): 71–86.

10. Marian Knight, Sarah Stewart-Brown, and Lynn Fletcher, "Estimating Health Needs: The Impact of a Checklist of Conditions and Quality of Life Measurement on Health Information Derived from Community Surveys," *Journal of Public Health Medicine* 23, no. 3 (2001): 179–186.

11. W. J. Eylenbosch and N. D. Noah, *Surveillance in Health and Disease.* New York: Oxford University Press, 1988.

12. Alexander D. Langmuir, "The Surveillance of Communicable Diseases of National Importance," *New England Journal of Medicine* 268 (1963): 182–192.

13. Stephen B. Thacker and R. L. Berkelman, "Public Health Surveillance in the United States," *Epidemiologic Reviews* 10 (1988): 164–190.

14. William Halperin, Edward L. Baker, and Robert R. Monson, *Public Health Surveillance.* New York: Van Nostrand Reinhold, 1992.

15. "Syndromic Surveillance for Bioterrorism Following the Attacks on the World Trade Center—New York City, 2001," *Morbidity and Mortality Weekly Report* 51, Special Issue (2002): 13–15.

16. J. W. Buehler et al. "Framework for Evaluating Public Health Surveillance Systems for Early Detection of Outbreaks: Recommendations from the CDC Working Group," *MMWR – Recommendations and Reports* 5, no. 3 (2004): 1–11.

17. Peter Nsubuga et al., Public Health Surveillance: A Tool for Targeting and Monitoring Interventions, in *Disease Control in Developing Countries, 2nd edition,* eds. D. T. Jamison et al. Washington, DC: World Bank, 2006. Available at http://www.ncbi.nlm.nih.gov/books/NBK11770/.

18. H. I. Hall et al. "Surveillance of Hazardous Substance Releases and Related Health Effects," *Archives of Environmental Health* 49, no. 1 (1994): 45–48.

19. Jeffrey P. Davis and James M. Vergeront, "The Effect of Publicity on the Reporting of Toxic-Shock Syndrome in Wisconsin," *Journal of Infectious Diseases* 145, no. 4 (1982): 449–457.

20. Richard L. Vogt et al., "Comparison of an Active and Passive Surveillance System of Primary Care Providers for Hepatitis, Measles, Rubella, and Salmonellosis in Vermont," *American Journal of Public Health* 73, no. 7 (1983): 795–797.

21. Miriam J. Alter et al., "The Effect of Underreporting on the Apparent Incidence and Epidemiology of Acute Viral Hepatitis," *American Journal of Epidemiology* 125, no. 1 (1987): 133–139.

22. Robert Marier, "The Reporting of Communicable Diseases," *American Journal of Epidemiology* 105, no. 6 (1977): 587–590.

23. Stephen B. Thacker et al., "A Controlled Trial of Disease Surveillance Strategies," *American Journal of Preventive Medicine* 2, no. 6 (1986): 345–350.

24. Daniel Brachott and James W. Mosley, "Viral Hepatitis in Israel: The Effect of Canvassing Physicians on Notifications and the Apparent Epidemiological Pattern," *Bulletin of the World Health Organization* 46, no. 4 (1972): 457–464.

25. Denise Koo and Stephen B. Thacker, "In Snow's Footsteps: Commentary on Shoe-Leather and Applied Epidemiology," *American Journal of Epidemiology* 172, no. 6 (2010): 737–739.

26. Michael St. Louis, "Global Health Surveillance," *MMWR Surveillance Summaries* 61, Supplement (2012): 15–19.
27. Katherine M. Hiller et al., "Syndromic Surveillance for Influenza in the Emergency Department—A Systematic Review," *PLoS One* 8, no. 9 (2013): e73832. doi:10.1371/journal.pone.0073832.
28. H. S. Burkom et al., "Public Health Monitoring Tools for Multiple Data Streams," *Morbidity and Mortality Weekly Report* 54, Supplement (2005): 55–62.
29. Centers for Disease Control and Prevention, "CDC's Vision for Public Health Surveillance in the 21st Century," *Morbidity and Mortality Weekly Report* 61, Supplement (2012): 1–40.
30. Donald R. Olson et al., "Reassessing Google Flu Trends Data for Detection of Seasonal and Pandemic Influenza: A Comparative Epidemiological Study at Three Geographic Scales," *PLoS Computational Biology* 9 no. 10): (2013): e1003256, doi:0.1371/journal.pcbi.1003256.
31. Aniset Kamanga et al., "Rural Health Centres, Communities and Malaria Case Detection in Zambia Using Mobile Telephones: A Means to Detect Potential Reservoirs of Infection in Unstable Transmission Conditions," *Malaria Journal* 9, April (2010): 96, doi:10.1186/1475-2875-9-96.
32. *The Challenge of Facts: Selected Public Health Papers of Edgar Sydenstricker*, ed. Richard V. Kasius. New York: Taylor & Francis, 1974.
33. Centers for Disease Control and Prevention, National Center for Health Statistics, *National Health Interview Survey*. Available at http://www.cdc.gov/nchs/nhis.htm.
34. Centers for Disease Control and Prevention, National Center for Health Statistics, "National Health and Nutrition Examination Survey." Available at http://www.cdc.gov/nchs/nhanes.htm.
35. Centers for Disease Control and Prevention, National Center for Health Statistics, "National Health Care Surveys." Available at http://www.cdc.gov/nchs/dhcs.htm.
36. World Health Organization, Global Health Observatory, "Health system response and capacity to address and respond to NCDs." Available at http://www.who.int/gho/ncd/health_system_response/en/.
37. D. M. Kriegsman et al., "Self-Reports and General Practitioner Information on the Presence of Chronic Diseases in Community Dwelling Elderly. A Study on the Accuracy of Patients' Self-Reports and on Determinants of Inaccuracy," *Journal of Clinical Epidemiology* 49, no. 12 (1996): 1407–1417.
38. Italian Longitudinal Study on Aging Working Group, "Prevalence of Chronic Diseases in Older Italians: Comparing Self-Reported and Clinical Diagnoses," *International Journal of Epidemiology* 26, no. 5 (1997): 995–1002.
39. Mitesh Patel et al., "Accuracy of Patient Self-Report as a Measure of Inhaled Asthma Medication Use," *Respirology* 18, no. 3 (2013): 546–552.
40. Dona Schneider, Akira Yamamoto, and Joseph G. Barone, "Evaluation of Consistency between Physician Clinical Impression and 3 Validated Survey Instruments for Measuring Lower Urinary Tract Symptoms in Children," *Journal of Urology* 186, no. 1 (2011): 261–265.
41. J. Yerushalmy, "Problems in Radiological Interpretation," *California Medicine* 70, no. 1 (1949): 26–30.

42. P. L. Horn et al., "Reproducibility of the Cytologic Diagnosis of Human Papillomavirus Infection. *Acta Cytologica* 29, no. 5 (1985): 692–694.

43. J. A. Martin et al., "Births: Final Data for 2012," *National Vital Statistics Report* 62, no. 9 (2013): 1–87.

44. J. A. Martin et al., "Births, Final Data for 2012," *National Vital Statistics Report* 62, no. 9 (2013): 1–87.

45. Occupational Safety and Health Administration, "Calculating Injury and Illness Incidence Rates," in *OSHA Forms for Recording Work-Related Injuries and Illnesses* (online booklet). Available at http://www.osha.gov/recordkeeping/new-osha300form1-1-04.pdf.

46. Miquel Porta, ed., *A Dictionary of Epidemiology, 6th Edition.* New York: Oxford University Press, 2014.

47. Valerie Beral et al., "Kaposi's Sarcoma among Persons with AIDS: A Sexually Transmitted Infection?" *Lancet* 335, no. 8682 (1990): 123–128.

48. Valerie Beral et al., "Is Risk of Kaposi's Sarcoma in AIDS Patients in Britain Increased if Sexual Partners Came from United States or Africa?" *British Medical Journal* 302, no. 6777 (1991): 624–625.

49. C. J. Murray, "Quantifying the Burden of Disease: The Technical Basis for Disability-Adjusted Life Years," *Bulletin of the World Health Organization* 72, no. 3 (1994): 429–445.

50. Marthe R. Gold, David Stevenson, and Dennis G. Fryback, "HALYS and QALYS and DALYS, Oh My: Similarities and Differences in Summary Measures of Population Health," *Annual Review of Public Health* 23 (2002): 115–134.

51. Franco Sassi, "Calculating QALYs, Comparing QALY and DALY Calculations," *Health Policy and Planning* 21, no. 5 (2006): 402–408.

Problem Set: Chapter 7

1. The local veterinarian of Heifer Place, Dr. Salmon Run, noticed that during the past four months, eight young dogs presented at his clinic with hypothyroidism. Two of the dogs died soon after the disease had been diagnosed. Dr. Run reviewed the clinic's records and found only three similar occurrences over the previous 15 years. Thinking this situation odd, Dr. Run decided to consult the closest veterinary school in Farmerville, some 100 kilometers downstream from his clinic. The head of the veterinary school's endocrinology department, Dr. Ox R. Bull, suggested that Dr. Run contact each of the veterinary practices in the county in which his clinic was located and ask how many cases of hypothyroidism had come to their attention during the past 15 or so years, when the cases were diagnosed, as well as other helpful information such as breed and age. With those data, they could estimate the incidence of the condition and assess whether it was increasing in occurrence. Dr. Bull also stated that for the past two decades, the school had conducted a countywide census of standard poodles. As five of the eight cases Dr. Run had seen were standard poodles, Dr. Bull suggested the canvas be limited to cases of hypothyroidism diagnosed in that breed. The results of Dr. Run's data collection effort appear in the following table:

YEARS	2000–2004		2005–2009		2010–2014	
AGE (MONTHS)	NEW DIAGNOSES	NUMBER OF STANDARD POODLES	NEW DIAGNOSES	NUMBER OF STANDARD POODLES	NEW DIAGNOSES	NUMBER OF STANDARD POODLES
<2	10	230	8	180	11	250
2–11	18	1,000	14	750	13	700
12–23	17	1,520	22	2,000	28	1,400
24 +	45	3,450	9	1,200	42	1,600

Create a new table showing the *average annual* age-specific incidence rates per 1,000 standard poodles in each of the three time periods. What trends might be observed in these data?

2. Dr. Run presented these data at a seminar at the veterinary school, at which Professor Red Herring, the school's epidemiologist-in-chief, objected. Specifically, Professor Herring said, "I remember that half of the dogs who are at least two years old recently spent only half a year in the county; the other half of the year they lived on the Mediterranean coast basking in the sunshine. You need to use the incidence density, not the incidence rate *per se*, to account for that difference."

   Dr. Bull agreed with Professor Herring, but Dr. Run was puzzled. "How much difference could that possibly make?"

   Professor Herring responded, "Potentially, quite a lot."

   Help Dr. Run understand the significance of Professor Herring's observation by calculating the incidence density for the oldest dogs for the years 2010–2014.

3. With the knowledge about the incidence of hypothyroidism in standard poodles, Dr. Bull thought it a good time to consider the prevalence of the condition. This would help the veterinary school estimate how many veterinarians should be trained to care for these additional cases. The average duration of untreated hypothyroidism among dogs two years (24 months) of age and older was known to be about 1.5 years (18 months). Dr. Bull suggested taking a sample of dogs with the disease and calling their owners to find out what had happened to them. The veterinary students made multiple calls and determined that the average duration of untreated hypothyroidism in the most recent time period for dogs less than 2 years of age was 2.5 years. What is the prevalence of untreated hypothyroidism among standard poodles in this county for the time period 2010–2014? Given the county is fairly isolated, assume the population of standard poodles is stable.

4. During a presentation of these incidence and prevalence data at the veterinary school, Dr. Ima Boar, a visiting faculty member on sabbatical, objected to the

way terms such as "incidence" and "prevalence" were bandied about. Dr. Bull responded by projecting the following Figure 7.3 in his slide presentation:

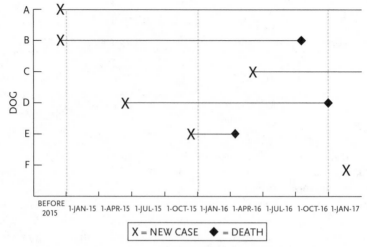

FIGURE 7.3 Dates of diagnosis and death from hypothyroidism for six standard poodles from Heifer Run

After explaining that each of the six dogs is shown in terms of having been diagnosed with hypothyroidism (shown with "X") or death ("◆"), Dr. Bull asked:

a. Which dogs would be included in the numerator for period prevalence during 2015? 2016?

b. Which dogs would be included in the numerator for period prevalence during the first six months of 2015? The last six months of 2016?

c. Which dogs would be included in the numerator for point prevalence on 1 January 2015? 1 January 2016? 1 January 2017?

5. Dr. Bull closed the presentation with an announcement: "One of our school's benefactors, the renowned banker Fat Cat, gave our school a grant to survey all of the standard poodles in the county for hypothyroidism. We quickly realized that we would not be able to have veterinarians conducting the survey, so we trained a number of veterinary assistants to quickly examine all standard poodles during a door-to-door campaign. Any dog with symptoms suggestive of hypothyroidism would be brought to their local vet for further work-up. We think this will work because we tried it in a pilot of 300 dogs, and the results were good. Arranging for examinations of the 300 dogs by a veterinarian provided useful information about what I call the 'Standardized Surveyor Assessment Exam.' Take a look."

Dr. Bull presented this table:

	VETERINARY DIAGNOSIS		TOTAL
SURVEY ASSESSMENT	HYPOTHYROIDISM	NO HYPOTHYROIDISM	
Hypothyroidism	36	9	45
No Hypothyroidism	4	251	255
Total	40	260	300

a. What is the sensitivity and specificity of the standardized surveyor assessment?

b. What are the positive and the negative predictive values?

c. What is the accuracy of the exam?

6. Dr. Bull knows the average life expectancy of a standard poodle is 12 years, but those with untreated hypothyroidism have many medical problems and tend to die early. He also knows that treatment can extend the lives of many of these dogs, but it does carry the burden of veterinary and medication costs. To get a better idea of how to counsel the owners of standard poodles with hypothyroidism, Dr. Bull challenged the veterinary students to use the data from Dr. Run's county for the most recent time period to help him put together information for the owners of dogs diagnosed with hypothyroidism, so he can encourage them to put their dogs into treatment.

The veterinary students decide to calculate the years of lost companionship (YPLL) suffered by the owners of the standard poodles with untreated hypothyroidism. Help the students by completing the following table (the mean age of cases over two years of age was 72 months):

AGE GROUP OF CASES (MONTHS)	NUMBER OF CASES	MEAN AGE OF CASES (MONTHS)	MEAN SURVIVAL TIME IF UNTREATED (MONTHS)	EXPECTED AGE AT DEATH IF UNTREATED (MONTHS)	YEARS OF COMPANION— SHIP LOST (YPLL)
<2	11		6		
2–11.9	13		6		
12–23.9	28		6		
24+	42	72	18		
Total	94				

The students proudly bring Dr. Bull their years of companionship lost calculation but he is not fully satisfied. "You're only halfway there," he snarled. "I want to make a case for the burden this disease has on the dog's and family's quality of life. These dogs sometimes get seizures and are prone to infections. They gain weight, have a slowed heart rate, and they are very intolerant to cold. Imagine your dog not being able to play with your children or frolic in the snow!"

The students slipped away and met later that evening to discuss what to do next. They decided to pursue a DALY calculation, and after much discussion they determined that not being able to play with children and frolic in the snow equated to a disability weight of 0.6. Help the students calculate the DALY for standard poodles with untreated hypothyroidism in Dr. Run's county.

8 | Using Morbidity Statistics

> The epidemiologist must study in the field the way in which disease
> is caused. He must use the statistical method, and the application
> of statistical methods to epidemiology is more difficult and less
> attractive than laboratory experiment.[1]
>
> *Charles V. Chapin (1910)*

S WITH MORTALITY, EPIDEMIOLOGISTS ARE interested in the occurrence of morbidity by *time, place, and persons.* The reasoning processes used in interpreting the results of morbidity studies are similar to those applied when evaluating studies on mortality. The similarity stops there. Mortality studies are limited by the information available on death certificates, and mortality data sets are free and readily available. Morbidity studies can ask a far greater range of questions, but building a morbidity data set requires significant planning and resources (time and costs). One way to gather information on persons and their exposures is to collect the information directly from individuals, from entire communities, or from population samples using *cross-sectional surveys*. The additional information on exposures may be particularly relevant to finding the underlying causes (*etiologies*) of the specific health outcomes under consideration.

Time

Chapter 3 presented one aspect of time that pertains to morbidity, that of *incubation periods* or the time distribution of the onset of disease after exposure to an etiological agent. Another aspect of time, *mortality trends,* or how patterns of mortality change over time, was introduced in Chapter 6. This

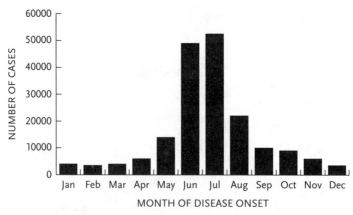

FIGURE 8.1 Confirmed Lyme disease cases by month of disease onset—United States, 2001–2010.

SOURCE: Centers for Disease Control and Prevention, National Center for Emerging and Zoonotic Infectious Diseases, Division of Vector-Born Diseases; see http://www.cdc.gov/lyme/stats/chartstables/casesbymonth.html.

same characteristic applies to *morbidity trends*, specifically how the occurrence of health outcomes varies over time.

An aspect of time not discussed previously is the seasonal distribution of disease. Many diseases, particularly infectious ones, occur more frequently during particular times of the year (i.e., in the warm months, during the rainy season, when clearing fields, etc.). An example of this seasonal pattern of disease is Lyme disease. Figure 8.1 shows that there is an *endemic level* of Lyme disease year-round; however, disease onset peaks during the summer months (when the agent and host are more likely to come into contact).

Place

The time distribution of disease is often influenced by place, and it may be appropriate to consider both variables contemporaneously. For instance, Gessner examined the occurrence of influenza in sub-Saharan Africa and noted that the time distribution of new infections varied by country.[2] Figure 8-2 shows the activity level (*frequency*) of influenza cases by week for three countries: Madagascar, Senegal, and South Africa. The first two countries have tropical climates, and the frequency of cases varied little over the course of the year. The pattern differed for South Africa, a country with more seasonality. During the winter (weeks 14 to 27), the frequency of influenza cases increased and then began to decline, returning to essentially no

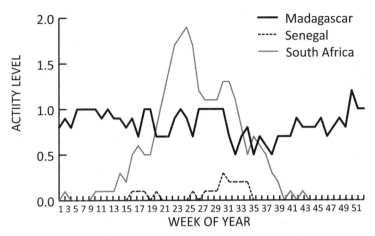

FIGURE 8.2 Average weekly activity levels of influenza virus cases in three sub-Saharan African countries that reported to the WHO FluNet between 2000 and 2009.

SOURCE: Gessner and Shindo (2011).[2] Copyright 2011, Lancet Publishing Group. Reproduced with permission of Elsevier Health Science Journals, Ltd.

cases by summer (weeks 39 to 52). This pattern makes sense, as during the colder weeks people tend to spend more time indoors where they are in close proximity to others and are more likely to transmit the virus from person to person.

A classic example of the use of place in deriving etiological inferences about a disease is Maxcy's 1926 study of Brill's disease (*endemic* typhus) in the Southeastern United States.[3] At the time of the study, Old World typhus (the *epidemic* form) was understood as being transmitted from person to person by lice. As the clinical, serological, and experimental evidence all showed the endemic and epidemic forms of typhus to be similar, many investigators inferred that both forms of the disease were transmitted by lice. Maxcy noted that the incidence of cases in Romania (Rumania, Roumania) and the southeastern United States (Figure 8.3) differed in their time distributions, suggesting that the diseases were not the same. He then went about analyzing the cases by place.

Maxcy plotted each endemic typhus case on a map of Montgomery, Alabama (a *spot map*) by place of residence and found no distinct localization of cases. He then examined the same cases by place of employment and found a focus of the disease in the heart of the business district. A more detailed analysis indicated a high attack rate among those working at food depots, groceries, feed stores, and restaurants. This suggested a rodent *reservoir* for the disease, with transmission of the agent by fleas, mites, or lice. He

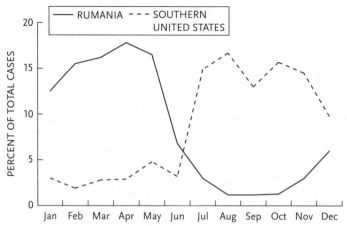

FIGURE 8.3 Seasonal distribution of endemic typhus (Brill's disease) based on 197 cases in Alabama and Savannah, Georgia, 1922–1925 compared with typhus in Rumania, 1922–1924.

SOURCE: Maxcy (1926).[3]

also noted the lack of evidence of communicability from person to person. Maxcy's inferences about the etiology of endemic typhus were subsequently shown to be correct. The rat is the *reservoir* of the disease, and the rat flea is the *vector* that transmits the etiological agent, *Rickettsia mooseri (R. typhi),* to humans via an insect bite.[4]

Another example of the use of place in epidemiologic investigations is Gordis's classic study of rheumatic fever in Baltimore, Maryland. In the period 1960 to 1964, the incidence rate of rheumatic fever in that city was much greater for black children than for white children. By 1968 to 1970, the incidence rate of rheumatic fever among black children was much closer to that for white children (declining by 35 percent), while for white children it remained essentially unchanged. Could the decline in the incidence of the disease among the black children be explained by the availability and effectiveness of comprehensive health care programs? To examine this possibility, Gordis compared the incidence of rheumatic fever among black children in Baltimore who resided both in and outside census tracts with comprehensive health care programs. Those residing in the census tracts with comprehensive care experienced a 60 percent decline in rheumatic fever between the two time periods, while those residing in the census tracts without the programs experienced a 2 percent increase. The findings suggested that the comprehensive health care programs were effective in promptly diagnosing and treating streptococcal infections, the precursor of rheumatic fever. Their early intervention halted the natural progression of the disease.[5] The study was important in documenting a relatively rare public health success in eliminating a health disparity.

Time and Space Clusters

The term used to describe the increase in the number of cases of a disease in time, place, or both is *cluster*. A clustering of cases in time might indicate that certain etiological factors were introduced into the environment at a particular time, such as an infectious agent, drug, or environmental pollutant. An example is the food-poisoning outbreak discussed in Chapter 1, a clustering of cases of gastroenteritis due to exposure to contaminated food. The clustering of cases in Maxcy's spot maps showed the focal distribution of endemic typhus by place (of employment), thus providing the evidence that incriminated an animal reservoir and the mode of infection for that disease.

The investigation of time-space clusters has proven to be an invaluable epidemiologic tool for unraveling the etiology of infectious diseases. It is not surprising, then, that interest developed in studying clusters of noninfectious diseases, especially those with unknown etiologies. For example, a veterinary practitioner noted a time-space cluster of lymphoma among cats during the early 1960s. That observation was followed by laboratory experiments that led to the identification of the feline leukaemia virus (FeLV) and launched the field of feline retrovirology.[6] Could viruses be the trigger for some human cancers, as well?

During the early 1980s, a cluster of childhood leukemia and lymphoma cases appeared near a nuclear reprocessing plant in Sellafield, England. Studies of environmental contamination did not support the notion that discharges from the plant could be the cause. Kinlen noted that the clusters appeared in Dounreay and Sellafield, isolated places where *herd immunity* to viral infections might be lower than average. If leukemia was a rare response to one or more viral infections, then large influxes of people to work in the plants might have triggered viral epidemics in the susceptible population. To test the hypothesis, he examined a rural area of Scotland that received a large population influx at the same time as the area around Sellafield. Results showed a significant increase in leukemia among persons under age 25 years, with a greater increase among those under age five, the age groups presumed most susceptible to novel viral infections.[7]

Gardner and colleagues also examined the Sellafield cluster and noted that the childhood cancer cases were more likely than control subjects to have fathers who had been exposed to ionizing radiation before their conception.[8]

These findings were challenged, however, as they conflicted with the results from the studies of the progeny of the survivors from Hiroshima and Nagasaki.[9] Over the next two decades, multiple studies examined the incidence of childhood cancers near nuclear facilities throughout Europe. Although the numbers of cases were small, many of the studies documented elevated but not statistically significant rates. Baker and Hoel evaluated the results of these studies using *meta-analysis* techniques (see Chapter 15 for more discussion of meta-analysis) and found an increase in childhood leukemia near nuclear facilities. The investigators did not find a dose-response for living near the plant, nor could they offer a hypothesis to explain the excess of the disease.[10]

A major problem for many time-space cluster studies is that they deal only with a small number of cases and generally do not take into consideration the population densities of the communities where the cases appear. The cases are variously aggregated in time-space to look for a cluster effect, and the resultant clusters may be artifactual in nature. Schneider and colleagues demonstrated this problem in their study of patterns of childhood cancer in New Jersey.[11] Using the SEER cancer registry for the years 1979 through 1985, the investigators manipulated geographic scale to look for clusters. They found no clusters at the county scale or at the urban/rural/ most rural scales, but they did find clusters at the minor civil division (local) scale. Their study demonstrated the importance of using multiple geographic scales and considering population densities when investigating clusters.

Cluster detection methods have also been evaluated for their sensitivity and specificity (see Chapter 7), and they are recognized for having low statistical power for detecting small numbers of cases.[12] When a true cluster is identified, it is important to determine whether the cases have been exposed to a potential etiologic agent. Epidemiologic studies may be instituted that examine the homes, neighborhoods, schools, and workplaces where the cases may have been exposed. For instance, Kurtze and colleagues investigated a cluster of cases of multiple sclerosis (MS) in the Faroe Islands that appeared between 1943 and 1960. These investigators suggested that the disease might be infectious in origin, based on the fact that the cases resided primarily in locales where British troops were stationed during World War II.[13] After multiple follow-up studies, the investigators concluded that MS is the result of a systemic infectious disease acquired by susceptible persons between the ages of 11 and 45 years, that transmission of the agent ends by age 27 years or younger, and that clinical disease affects only a small portion of those infected.[14]

Frequently, the epidemiologist does not have access to information about the exposures of interest among the cases in a cluster. That information might be estimated, however, by comparing survey responses about exposures obtained from individuals living within and outside the cluster zone. Pugliatti and others used this technique to examine the rising incidence and prevalence of MS in Sardinia, an island off the coast of Italy. The Sassari province of Sardinia has among the highest rates of MS in the world. Because the population is genetically stable, the authors concluded that the sudden increase in MS among this population was likely due to environmental rather than genetic factors.[15] After looking at the time-space clustering of the cases, they found patterns in the seasonality of births among the cases, along with temporal trends linked to childhood that supported the role of viruses as potential etiological factors for the disease.[16]

When diseases seem to run in families, it is important to disentangle the roles of genetics and environment. One of the ways to do this is through the use of twin studies. For instance in Finland, Kuusisto and colleagues examined the role of genetics in MS by examining the concordance of MS in twins.[17] They found that over the course of two decades the rate of MS among monozygotic twins had not changed, while the rate for dizygotic twins increased. As the genetic variance of the twins was low but their environmental variance was high, the researchers attributed the rise in MS among the dizygotic pairs to unique environmental factors.

Persons

Epidemiologists are interested in variables that may influence morbidity such as age, gender, ethnicity, occupation, personal behaviors (such as travel, smoking habits, or sexual activities), and social status. Sometimes the epidemiologist is interested in the distribution of these variables in the community as a whole. This is particularly true when risk factors for specific health outcomes have already been identified and data about them can be obtained from population-based surveys. For example, smoking is an established risk factor for lung cancer. Smoking habits are captured in various population-based surveys such as the Australian Health Survey, the Canada Health Survey, the Health Survey for England, and the Behavioral Risk Factor Surveillance Survey (BRFSS) in the United States. The information on smoking gathered by these population-based surveys can be used to estimate the prevalence of smoking for the nation and to identify subpopulations at highest risk for lung cancer. It can also aid health care systems in estimating the economic burden on their budgets that lung cancer will pose if smoking habits do not change.

Age

Many infectious diseases such as measles and chickenpox are considered childhood diseases; that is, their frequency of occurrence is highest among those in the youngest age groups. Before the widespread use of measles vaccination in the United States, the incidence rate of measles increased sharply from about one to four years of age. This pattern probably results from low *herd immunity* among the very young, along with increasing levels of socialization that result in elevated risk of exposure to the measles virus. After age four, the incidence rate for measles gradually decreased until it neared zero at 12 to 15 years of age. Since an attack of measles conferred lifelong immunity, the increasing incidence rate up to age four resulted in a high proportion of immune individuals in the age group from four to about 13 years, with few persons at older ages remaining susceptible to the infection.

Older ages may serve as a proxy for increased or decreased risk, depending upon the outcome of interest. For example, the 2003–2007 unadjusted incidence rate for uterine cancer in Germany was about 80 per 100,000 women. When the researchers accounted for the one-third of older German women who had undergone a hysterectomy and were not therefore susceptible to developing uterine cancer, the corrected rate became 133 per 100,000 women, an increase of 67 percent.[18] In this instance, increasing age removed many women from the pool of susceptibles for uterine cancer. A similar phenomenon has been reported in other countries, including the United Kingdom and the United States.

Age-related factors also influence morbid outcomes related to natality. Perhaps the most consistently observed relationship is the marked ascendance in the incidence of Trisomy 21 (Down's Syndrome) with increasing maternal age. This relationship has been shown across cultures as diverse as Sweden, New York, and West Jerusalem,[19,20] leading some researchers to suggest a biological rather than environmental cause for the observation.

Gender

Biological and behavioral factors related to gender contribute to differences in the prevalence or incidence rates of a variety of conditions, including heart disease, accident-related disabilities, and autoimmune diseases. The initial observation that Kaposi's sarcoma and pneumocystis pneumonia occurred only among gay men provided one of the clues to determining the means of disease transmission for acquired immune deficiency syndrome (AIDS), even before the disease agent (human immunodeficienty virus or HIV) was identified.[21] Men continue to demonstrate a higher prevalence of HIV infection except in sub-Saharan Africa where the incidence is more prevalent among women. Factors to explain the gender disparity in HIV infection in different regions are complex, involving the nature of disease transmission (including the presence of co-infections) as well as behavioral and cultural practices, such as varying rates of circumcision and the sexual preference of older men for young girls.[22]

Kuru is a degenerative neurologic disorder found to be endemic in the New Guinea highlands during the 1970s. Gajdusek noted that women and children were at much greater risk of developing the disease than were men.[23] Subsequent investigations revealed the cause to be an infectious protein (*prion*) transmitted during a cannibalistic funeral ritual. The women of the tribe prepared the body for burial and may have become infected through open cuts or sores on their hands while completing the task. During the ritual, the men consumed the preferred muscle cuts whereas the women and children consumed the brains, the organ where the infectious prions were concentrated. This epidemiologic characterization of kuru provided important prevention information for the tribes, as well as insights for researchers investigating the prion etiology of Creutzfeldt-Jakob disease (CJD, or human spongiform encephalopathy) and Mad Cow disease (BSE, or bovine spongiform encephalopathy).

Race and Ethnicity

Factors such as race and ethnicity (clan, tribe) may be associated with some genetic traits such as sickle-cell anemia, glucose-6-phosphate dehydrogenase (G6PD) deficiency, or Tay-Sachs disease. They can also be associated with a wide range of lifestyle characteristics (smoking, alcohol consumption, and childbearing patterns) and educational, environmental, or occupational exposures, all of which can be related to health outcomes.

An example of the significance of race and ethnicity in formulating etiological hypotheses and identifying high-risk populations is a survey done in Copiah County, Mississippi. Mortality data from the 1970s suggested that blacks were at lower risk of death from dementia than were whites. Could this difference be the result of variation in exposures to etiological agents? Could it be from incomplete diagnosis of dementia cases among blacks, in part because of reduced access to health care? Schoenberg and colleagues sought to answer these questions by assessing whether the prevalence and clinical features of dementia were the same for blacks and whites living in the same Southern county.[24] Specially trained surveyors went door-to-door, collecting information about whether persons with dementia lived in that home (including their own assessment about the presence of the condition). The investigators found that the prevalence of the condition was the same in blacks and whites. Subsequent studies confirmed the finding, suggesting that the risk factors for dementia are distributed approximately equally in both racial populations.

The racial and ethnic minority status of pregnant women in the United States has been linked to low birth weight in repeated studies. During the earlier part of the twentieth century this outcome was assumed to be the result of young maternal age, poor education, poverty, and lack of prenatal care. By the end of the century, however, the complexities of the relationship had become apparent.[25] Of particular interest were studies on *weathering*, the hypothesized impact of holding minority status and accumulating the slights of racism and the stresses of assimilation over time.[26] One study showed that African-American women who were older, had high educational achievement and family incomes, and who had good access to medical care (including prenatal care) carried a higher risk for a low birth weight (LBW) baby than younger and less affluent minority women.[27] This presented a paradox, as rates for LBW among white women generally decline as maternal age increases. The weathering hypothesis was supported by an additional study that LBW rates for African-American women increase as maternal age increases.[28] In addition, Vang and Eo found that LBW rates for recent African and Latina immigrants to the United States had a lower risk of an LBW baby than those who had come earlier and supposedly assimilated.[29] The researchers suggested that while time may allow for better assimilation, it also allows for more weathering to exact its toll on the mother.

While the weathering hypothesis holds promise for explaining the patterns of some health outcomes, the use of race and ethnicity for epidemiologic research must be treated with care. The definitions accorded to each may vary from country to country and may shift to accommodate sociological or political trends. Hispanic ethnicity, for example, is less useful for predicting health risks than whether a person is from Spain, where the gene pool has a large European influence, Puerto Rico, where the gene pool has a large African influence, or Mexico, where there is a large Native American influence. Sehgal reported that some treatments, such as the use of β-blockers and ACE inhibitors for the treatment of hypertension, work better in European Americans than African Americans.[30] On the other hand, the treatments do work well for many African Americans and poorly for some European Americans. In other words, diversity of response to drug treatment exists within racial categories, and race is a poor predictor of a response to treatment. Bamshad used Sehgal's work as an example of how socially constructed racial and ethnic categories include a wide distribution of genetic factors. Specifically, a person's genetic ancestry (linked to their geographic ancestry) better predicts their risk for developing a disease or their response to a particular treatment than does their racial or ethnic category.[31] Unfortunately, the epidemiologist often does not have ancestral data available unless these data were specifically gathered in a purposeful survey.

Religion

Though religion may serve as a proxy for genetic disease etiologies (for instance, a variety of diseases among the Old Order Amish), it most frequently serves as a proxy for cultural factors associated with increased or decreased exposure to etiological agents. For example, Jews historically demonstrated a low prevalence of cervical cancer.[32] One hypothesis to explain this outcome was that male circumcision reduces the risk of viral transmission, a potential etiological agent for cervical cancer.[33] The hunt to identify the virus took several decades until the human papilloma virus (HPV) was identified during the 1980s. This allowed for the subsequent development of a vaccine and a population-based prevention program against HPV infection.[34]

Another example was a small epidemic of tapeworm infestation due to *D. latum* among Jewish housewives in the 1940s. Knowing the ethnic group and its eating habits, the investigators were able to trace the epidemic to contaminated fish. Housewives became infected by sampling uncooked gefilte fish as they tasted its seasoning during preparation.[35]

Epidemiologic studies have used religion as a variable to identify risk and protective factors that might explain patterns of health outcomes. Examples of some of these patterns are the lower risk of suicide among Catholics,[36] the lower risks of cancers and cardiovascular diseases among Seventh Day Adventists,[37] and the lower incidence of cancers among Mormons.[38] The former may perhaps be explained by religious training, and the latter two by dietary restrictions and the prohibition of alcohol and tobacco use.

Personal Behaviors

Personal behaviors may affect the manner by which an individual interacts with an etiological agent. Changes in personal behaviors at the population level may provide the epidemiologist with insights into why patterns of disease vary. For instance, the pattern of drug abuse was shown to be different among the urban and rural populations in Kentucky. Urban subjects were more likely to abuse crack, whereas rural subjects were more likely to begin abusing drugs at an earlier age and had higher odds of nonmedical opiod abuse.[39]

Sexual behaviors and mores change over time, and these may also have public health consequences. When the rates of sexually transmitted infections (STIs) began to rise and HIV became of epidemic concern, public health officials issued recommendations that condoms be used for sexual activity, although it was not explicitly specific for which types of sexual activity. For instance, a study of STI clinics in Spain compared gonorrheal infections among men who have sex with men (MSM), men who have sex with women (MSW), and women. They found that women with gonorrhea were generally younger than the men, mostly foreigners (51 percent), and often in the sex trade (41 percent). Thirty percent were infected via the pharynx.[40] A study of STI clinics in California showed the incidence of gonorrhea to be highest among those 15 to 24 years of age. The researchers suggested that this is due to the high prevalence of oral sex among this population, the low prevalence of condom use for oral sex, and the difficulty eradicating pharyngeal gonorrhea with the current available treatments and increasingly resistant forms of the disease.[41]

Disability

Chapter 7 described how DALYs assess the burden of diseases whereas QALYs provides a means of valuing an intervention. An example of the use of DALYs comes from the Global Burden of Disease (GBD) Study. Begun in the 1990s, this massive effort determined that the global burden of disease shifted over the course of two decades, from being defined by premature mortality to being defined by increasing disability. In the 1990s the largest burdens of disease were communicable, perinatal, and nutritional disorders that primarily affected children. The top three risk factors for disease were childhood underweight, tobacco smoke, and household air pollution from solid fuels.[42] By 2010, the largest burdens were from noncommunicable diseases, primarily due to the aging of the global population, decreased mortality among children under five years of age, and changes in exposures to potential etiological factors. The top three risk factors became high blood pressure, tobacco smoking, and alcohol consumption.[43] Researchers also documented significant increases in mental health issues and substance abuse, especially for those 10 to 29 years of age.[44]

QALYs assist health policy makers with decisions about which interventions can best improve the quality of life for a population. The measure takes into account reductions in pain as well as improvements in mobility and general mood. For instance, suppose there are two treatments for a given disease. The first treatment costs more than the second, but it is also more effective in prolonging life. Which treatment should health insurers agree to cover? The UK's National Institute for Clinical Excellence (NICE) uses QALYs for valuing and comparing treatments. If the cost per QALY is too high, NICE will not recommend that the National Health Service cover the treatment. Such recommendations are not without controversy, as where to set the cost threshold for refusal to cover a treatment is widely debated. What is an incremental increase in quality of life worth? The answer might be different for the individuals in need of treatment, their health insurers, and governments.

Summary

As with mortality, demographic studies of morbidity are concerned with the characteristics of time, place, and persons. *Time* may be viewed from the perspective of temporal trends in disease, but it can also be viewed in terms of seasonality. Some diseases occur more often in the fall or winter; others in the spring or summer.

Both *time* and *place* variables have the potential to convey information about the etiology and natural history of a disease. The epidemiologist may create a spot map of variables related to place (e.g., residence and place of employment) and use the results to formulate hypotheses about disease etiology and modes of transmission. Time and space clusters of disease may reflect a common exposure to the etiologic agent, but they may also occur by chance alone. Epidemiological efforts to evaluate clusters should be undertaken with care, as the methods to detect small numbers of cases have low statistical power.

The characteristics of *persons* with a particular disease (in comparison with those who have not developed it) provide further information about the epidemiologic profile or pattern of the disease. Variation in the risk of disease with age may suggest endogenous and exogenous influences on the development of the condition. Gender, ethnicity, religion, and other personal characteristics may help identify those at high risk for a disease, leading to etiologic hypotheses and screening programs.

Other measures of disease burden in the population include DALYs and QALYs. Public health planners and health policy makers/analysts use DALYs as a basis for allocating resources to achieve the maximal health status possible for all populations. QALYs provide a means for comparing the effectiveness of different therapeutic and preventive activities relative to cost.

References

1. Charles V. Chapin, *Sources and Modes of Infection*. New York: John Wiley and Sons, Inc., 1910.
2. B. D. Gessner, N. Shindo, and S. Briand, "Seasonal Influenza Epidemiology in Sub-Saharan Africa: A Systematic Review," *Lancet Infectious Diseases* 11, no. 3 (2011): 223–235.
3. Kenneth F. Maxcy, "An Epidemiological Study of Endemic Typhus (Brill's disease) in the Southeastern United States: With Special Reference to Its Mode of Transmission," *Public Health Reports (1896-1970)* 41, no. 52 (1926): 2967–2995.
4. T. E. Woodward, "Typhus Verdict in American History," *Transactions of the American Clinical and Climatological Association* 82 (1971): 1–8.
5. Leon Gordis, "The Virtual Disappearance of Rheumatic Fever in the United States: Lessons in the Rise and Fall of Disease; T. Duckett Jones Memorial Lecture," *Circulation* 72, no. 6 (1985): 1155–1162.
6. B. J. Willett and M. J. Hosie, "Feline Leukaemia Virus: Half a Century Since Its Discovery," *Veterinary Journal* 195, no. 1 (2013): 16–23.
7. Leo Kinlen, "Evidence for an Infective Cause of Childhood Leukaemia: Comparison of a Scottish New Town with Nuclear Reprocessing Sites in Britain," *Lancet* 2, no. 8624 (1988): 1323–1327.
8. M. J. Gardner et al., "Results of Case-Control Study of Leukaemia and Lymphoma among Young People Near Sellafield Nuclear Plant in West Cumbria," *British Medical Journal* 300, no. 6722 (1990): 423–429.
9. G. M. Watson, "Leukaemia and Paternal Radiation Exposure," *Medical Journal of Australia* 154, no. 7 (1991): 483–487.
10. P. J. Baker and D. G. Hoel, "Meta-Analysis of Standardized Incidence and Mortality Rates of Childhood Leukaemia in Proximity to Nuclear Facilities," *European Journal of Cancer Care* 16, no. 4 (2007): 355–363.
11. Dona Schneider et al., "Cancer Clusters: The Importance of Monitoring Multiple Geographic Scales. *Social Science & Medicine* 37, no. 6 (1993): 753–759.
12. Daniel Wartenberg and Michael Greenberg, "Detecting Disease Clusters: The Importance of Statistical Power," *American Journal of Epidemiology* 132, no. 1, Supplement (1990): S156–S166.
13. John F. Kurtzke and Kay Hyllested, "Multiple Sclerosis in the Faroe Islands: I. Clinical and Epidemiological Features. *Annals of Neurology* 5, no. 1 (1979): 6–21.

14. John F. Kurtzke and Kay Hyllested, "Multiple Sclerosis in the Faroe Islands: III. An Alternative Assessment of the Three Epidemics," *Acta Neurologica Scandinavica* 76, no. 5 (1987): 317–339.

15. Maura Pugliatti et al., "Increasing Incidence of Multiple Sclerosis in the Province of Sassari, Northern Sardinia," *Neuroepidemiology* 25, no. 3 (2005): 129–134.

16. Maura Pugliatti et al., "Environmental Risk Factors in Multiple Sclerosis," *Acta Neurologica Scandinavica* 188, Supplement (2008): 34–40.

17. H. Kuusisto et al., "Concordance and Heritability of Multiple Sclerosis in Finland: Study on a Nationwide Series of Twins," *European Journal of Neurology* 15, no. 10 (2008): 1106–1110.

18. Andreas Stang, "Impact of Hysterectomy on the Age-Specific Incidence of Cervical and Uterine Cancer in Germany and Other Countries," *European Journal of Public Health* 23, no. 5 (2013): 879–883.

19. Susan Harlap, "A Time-Series Analysis of the Incidence of Down's Syndrome in West Jerusalem," *American Journal of Epidemiology* 99, no. 3 (1974): 210–217.

20. Ernest B. Hook and Agneta Lindsjo, "Down Syndrome in Live Births by Single Year Maternal Age Interval in a Swedish Study: Comparison With Results From a New York State Study," *American Journal of Human Genetics* 30, no. 1 (1978): 19–27.

21. "Kaposi's Sarcoma and Pneumocystis Pneumonia among Homosexual Men—New York City and California," *Morbidity and Mortality Weekly Reports* 30, no. 25 (1981): 305–308.

22. World Health Organization, *Gender, Women and Health: Gender Inequalities and HIV*. Available at http://www.who.int/gender/hiv_aids/en/.

23. D. Carlton Gajdusek, "Urgent Opportunistic Observations: The Study of Changing, Transient, and Disappearing Phenomena of Medical Interest in Disrupted Primitive Human Communities," *Ciba Foundation Symposium* 49 (1977): 69–94.

24. Bruce S. Schoenberg, Dallas W. Anderson, and Armin F. Haerer, "Severe Dementia: Prevalence and Clinical Features in a Biracial US Population," *Archives of Neurology* 42, no. 8 (1985): 740–743.

25. Michal D. Kogan, "Social Causes of Low Birth Weight," *Journal of the Royal Society of Medicine* 88, no. 11 (1995): 611–615.

26. Arline T. Geronimus, "Black/White Differences in the Relationship of Maternal Age to Birthweight: A Population-Based Test of the Weathering Hypothesis," *Social Science & Medicine* 42, no. 4 (1996): 589–597.

27. Paul A. Buescher and Manjoo Mittal, "Racial Disparities in Birth Outcomes Increase With Maternal Age: Recent Data from North Carolina," *North Carolina Medical Journal* 67, no. 1 (2006): 16–20.

28. Catherine Love et al., "Exploring Weathering: Effects of Lifelong Economic Environment and Maternal Age on Low Birth Weight, Small for Gestational Age, and Preterm Birth in African-American and White Women," *American Journal of Epidemiology* 172, no. 2 (2010): 127–134.

29. Z. M. Vang and I. T. Elo, "Exploring the Health Consequences of Majority–Minority Neighborhoods: Minority Diversity and Birthweight Among Native-Born and Foreign-Born Blacks," *Social Science & Medicine* 97 (2013): 56–65.

30. A. R. Sehgal, "Overlap Between Whites and Blacks in Response to Antihypertensive Drugs," *Hypertension* 43, no. 3 (2004): 566–572.
31. Mike Bamshad, "Genetic Influences on Health: Does Race Matter?" *Journal of the American Medical Association* 294, no. 8 (2005): 937–946.
32. Barbara S. Hulka, "Risk Factors for Cervical Cancer. *Journal of Chronic Diseases* 35, no. 1 (1982): 3–11.
33. Brian J. Morris, "Why Circumcision is a Biomedical Imperative for the 21st Century," *Bioessays* 29, no. 11 (2007): 1147–1158.
34. M. Adams, B. Jasani, and A. Fiander, "Human Papilloma Virus (HPV) Prophylactic Vaccination: Challenges for Public Health and Implications for Screening," *Vaccine* 25, no. 16 (2007): 3007–3013.
35. Robert S. Desowitz. *New Guinea Tapeworms and Jewish Grandmothers: Tales of Parasites and People.* New York: W. W. Norton & Company, 1987.
36. M. J. Kelleher et al., "Religious Sanctions and Rates of Suicide Worldwide," *Crisis* 19, no. 2 (1998): 78–86.
37. W. L. Beeson et al., "Chronic Disease Among Seventh-Day Adventists, a Low-Risk Group. Rationale, Methodology, and Description of the Population," *Cancer* 64, no. 3 (1989): 570–581.
38. Ray M. Merrill and Joseph L. Lyon, "Cancer Incidence in Mormons and Non-Mormons in Utah (United States) 1995-1999," *Preventive Medicine* 40, no. 5 (2006): 535–541.
39. A. M. Young, J. R. Havens, and C. G. Leukefeld, "A Comparison of Rural and Urban Nonmedical Prescription Opioid Users' Lifetime and Recent Drug Use," *American Journal of Drug and Alcohol Abuse* 38, no. 3 (2012): 220–227.
40. Asuncion Diaz et al., "Gonorrhoea Diagnoses in a Network of STI Clinics in Spain During the Period 2006-2010: Differences By Sex and Transmission Route," *BMC Public Health* 23, Nov. 25 (2013), 13, 1093. doi:10.1186/1471-2458-13-1093.
41. M. Javanbakht et al., "Prevalence and Correlates of Rectal Chlamydia and Gonorrhea among Female Clients at Sexually Transmitted Disease Clinics," *Sexually Transmitted Diseases* 39, no. 12 (2012): 917–922.
42. C. J. Murray and A. D. Lopez, "Global Mortality, Disability, and the Contribution of Risk Factors: Global Burden of Disease Study," *Lancet* 349, no. 9063 (1997): 1436–1442.
43. S. S. Lim et al., "A Comparative Risk Assessment of Burden of Disease and Injury Attributable to 67 Risk Factors and Risk Factor Clusters in 21 Regions, 1990-2010: A Systematic Analysis for the Global Burden of Disease Study 2010," *Lancet* 380, no. 9859 (2012): 2224–2260.
44. H. A. Whiteford, et al., "Global Burden of Disease Attributable to Mental and Substance Use Disorders: Findings from the Global Burden of Disease Study 2010," *Lancet* 382, no. 9904 (2013): 1575–1586.

III | Analytic Studies

Epidemiology is in large part a collection of methods for finding
things out on the basis of scant evidence, and this by its nature is
difficult.[1]

Alex Broadbent (2011)

PART I (LAYING THE FOUNDATIONS) described how epidemiologic
study designs that use aggregate (group) data to determine statistical associations may be subject to *ecological fallacy*. Epidemiologic
studies that use individual observations may suggest an association between a risk factor and a health outcome, but they fail to
fulfill the criteria for showing cause. Part II explained how the
epidemiologist uses descriptive studies based on vital and morbidity statistics to uncover trends in health outcomes and generate hypotheses about their potential etiologies. Part III moves one
step further, presenting the *analytic study designs* the epidemiologist uses to confirm statistical associations and test etiological
hypotheses.

Analytic study designs are based on the scientific method in
that they compare groups of similar individuals for either their
outcomes or past exposures. Such studies may be either *observational* or *experimental* by design. In an observational study design,
the epidemiologist can only observe, but not control, the exposure. There are two observational study designs: *cohort studies*
(Chapter 9) and *case-control studies* (Chapter 10). These differ in
the variable known at the time the study commences. Specifically,
subjects in a cohort study are grouped by their observed exposure
status and followed forward from time of exposure to determine
the incidence of one or more outcomes. In a case-control study,

subjects are grouped by their observed outcome status, and their prior exposures are then reconstructed to determine the statistical association between exposure and outcome.

In contrast to observational designs, the epidemiologist controls the exposure in experimental designs. This is done by assigning subjects to either a treatment or comparison group, often through a process of random allocation (*randomized controlled trial*) (Chapter 11). When whole communities are assigned to a treatment or control group, the experimental study design is known as a *community trial* (Chapter 12). As with a cohort study, individuals are then followed forward in time to determine their incidence of the outcomes of interest.

The experimental study design is recognized as the *gold standard* in epidemiology, the design most supportive of a causal relationship. Experimental designs, however, are not always feasible. In these instances, observational study designs provide the best available information on associations between exposure and outcome. Because the epidemiologist has no control over exposure assignment in an observational study, its results are open to challenge. A common alternative explanation for the findings of observational studies is *confounding*, a concept introduced in Chapter 4. Methods of controlling confounding are described throughout Part III, as this is a major activity of the epidemiologist.

Reference

1. Alex Broadbent, University of Johannesburg philosopher commenting on epidemiology in *The Epi Monitor*, 2011.

9 | Observational Studies

COHORT STUDIES

How else but by observation upon man himself can one hope to
find clues to the etiology of his diseases?[1]

Harold F. Dorn (1959)

C OHORT STUDIES (VARIOUSLY CALLED *INCIDENCE studies, follow-up studies, forward-looking studies, longitudinal studies, panel studies,* or *prospective studies*) are both observational and prospective in design. They are observational because the epidemiologist does not control subjects' exposures. Rather, the epidemiologist observes health outcomes based on each subject's exposure status. Cohort studies are prospective in design because exposure is always assessed before health outcomes are observed.

A cohort study begins when the epidemiologist identifies a population to study (the *cohort*), verifying that each subject is at risk of developing one or more outcomes of interest. At the time of enrollment, information is collected about each subject's exposure status and potential confounding variables. The subjects are then followed forward from the time of exposure to observe whether the exposed and unexposed groups demonstrate differences in the relative frequency of the outcome(s) of interest. While the design is simple, the terminology used to describe cohort studies may be confusing. Figure 9.1 demonstrates how the terminology often appears in the epidemiologic literature.

At the top of the figure is the *retrospective (nonconcurrent, historical)* design which allows the epidemiologist to identify subjects' exposures at a time in the past and observe health outcomes at one or more time periods after exposure. For example, investigators studied the carcinogenic effects of in-utero

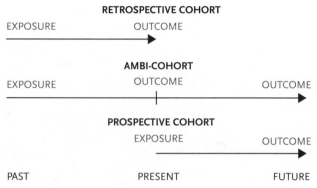

FIGURE 9.1 Three types of cohort study designs.

exposure to short-lived radioactive fallout from the Chernobyl nuclear power plant accident in 1986. Between February 1998 and December 2000, children at all schools within 150 km of the plant were screened for thyroid abnormalities. The children were separated into three groups: those born before the incident and who were exposed to the fallout (n = 9,720), those with at least some in-utero exposure to the fallout (n = 2,409), and those born after the incident without exposure to the fallout (n = 9,472). The first group exhibited 31 cases of thyroid cancer, the second group had one case, and the third group had none. After adjusting for age and sex, the investigators found a statistically significant ($p = 0.006$) difference between groups. They concluded that the increased risk of thyroid cancer detected in these children could be attributed to exposure to the short-lived radioactive fallout from the Chernobyl accident.[2]

At the bottom of Figure 9.1 is the *prospective* (*concurrent*) cohort design that identifies exposure status in the present and follows the subjects into the future to determine their health outcomes. An example of the prospective cohort design is the Birth to 20 Study (also known as the "Mandela's Children Study," given its temporal proximity to the release of Nelson Mandela from prison), perhaps the largest pediatric cohort study in Africa. The study focuses on environmental influences and nutrition (among many other factors) in the growth and development of 3,273 urban children during the first two decades of their life. Recruitment of began in 1989 with the identification of all singleton children born to women resident in Soweto-Johannesburg during a 7-week enrollment period. These children were then followed using a variety of techniques. As of 16 years later, more than 70 percent of the cohort was still active in the study, and for much of the cohort, data collection has continued through the participants' 23rd birthday.

Finally, the *ambi-cohort* design shown in the middle of Figure 9.1 allows the investigator to identify a cohort with an exposure in the past, determine outcomes of interest in the present, and follow subjects into the future to monitor additional outcomes. The Pediatric Anesthesia NeuroDevelopment Assessment (PANDA) project provides an example of this design. The study enrolled 28 sibling pairs, ages 6 to 11 years, in which one child had a single episode of anesthesia before 36 months of age (the exposed) and the other did not (the unexposed). Neurodevelopmental testing was conducted when the subjects enrolled in the study. The children will be followed into adulthood to look for differences in neurological development possibly related to early-life anesthesia exposure.[3]

Regardless of when a cohort study begins, exposure status is always determined before information about outcomes is obtained. This makes the design flexible, as multiple exposures can be assessed at the time of enrollment and multiple outcomes can be observed prospectively, as in the *Framingham Heart Study*. Beginning in 1948, the Framingham Heart Study enrolled 5,209 men and women between the ages of 30 and 62 years. Epidemiologists collected information on multiple exposures for each subject including smoking and obesity status, blood pressure, physical activity, serum cholesterol levels, and prevalence of diabetes.[4] To date, the data gathered on outcomes following these various exposures has proven valuable not only for the study of cardiovascular diseases but also the study of many other outcomes such as arthritis, dementia, diabetes, hearing disorders, lung diseases, nutritional outcomes, osteoporosis, and genetic patterns of common diseases.[5] Examples of other well-known cohort studies are listed in Table 9.1.

Measuring Association in Cohort Studies

The epidemiologist calculates the incidence of the health outcome(s) of interest for the exposed and unexposed groups and compares them. If the incidence rates differ, a statistical association exists between the exposure and the outcome, although that statistical association in and of itself does not prove cause (see Chapter 4).

Data on the exposure status and outcome for each subject in a cohort study are commonly aggregated into a 2 × 2 table (Table 9.2). The total number of subjects in the exposed group (top row) is a + b; that for the non-exposed group (bottom row) is c + d. The columns correspond with the outcomes. The total number of subjects with positive outcomes (left column) are represented by a + c and those without the outcome (right column) b + d. Hence,

TABLE 9.1 Examples of Well-Known Cohort Studies

TYPE OF COHORT STUDY	DESCRIPTION
Prospective	
British Birth Cohort Studies National Survey of Health and Development National Child Development Study 1970 British Cohort Study Millennium Cohort Study	Birth cohorts were enrolled from 1946 to 2000 to explore relationships between social class, education, and various exposures on child development, health, and other outcomes.
British Doctors' Cohort Study	Beginning in 1951, 34,439 male doctors were recruited to examine the relationship between smoking habits and lung cancer.
Framingham Heart Study	Beginning in 1948, 5,209 subjects were recruited to examine the relationship between various risk factors and cardiovascular disease.
Whitehall Study I and II	Beginning in 1967, Whitehall I enrolled 18,000 male civil servants to examine the role of social determinants in health. Whitehall II began in 1985 and enrolled 10,308 male and female civil servants, again for the role of social determinants of disease and mortality.
Bogalusa Heart Study	Beginning in 1972, 3,524 black and white children were enrolled to investigate the natural history of coronary artery disease and essential hypertension.
Study of Men in Taiwan	Beginning in the late 1970s, 22,707 Chinese male civil servants were enrolled to examine the relationship between hepatitis B and liver cancer.
Nurses' Health Study	Beginning in 1976, 122,000 nurses were recruited to examine the long-term effects of oral contraceptives (and later lifestyle, fertility/pregnancy, environment, and nursing exposures) on health outcomes.

Birth to 20	Beginning in 1989, 3,273 newborns were enrolled in a birth cohort study of child and adolescent health and development in South Africa.
European Prospective Investigation into Cancer and Nutrition (EPIC Study)	Beginning in 1992, 521,457 adults were recruited in multiple European countries to examine the relationship between diet and cancer.
Millenium Cohort Study	Beginning in 2001, more than 150,000 military personnel were recruited to evaluate the long-term health effects of US military service, including deployments.
Retrospective	
Dutch Famine Birth Cohort Studies	Dutch citizens born during the "Hunger Winter" of 1944-45 were enrolled to examine how experiencing famine *in utero* affected their subsequent life course.
Atomic Bomb Casualty Commission (ABCC) Studies	Survivors of the 1945 atomic bomb blasts in Hiroshima and Nagasaki were enrolled to examine the relationship of exposure to varying levels of radiation on their subsequent health.
Air Force (Ranch Hand) Health Study	Vietnam veterans were enrolled to examine the relationship of exposure to herbicides (Agent Orange) on their subsequent health.
Seveso Women's Health Study	Women exposed to dioxin from a 1976 chemical explosion in Sevaso, Italy were enrolled to examine the relationship of dioxin exposure on their reproductive health and cancer risk.

TABLE 9.2 Setting Up a 2 × 2 Table

GROUP	OUTCOME OF INTEREST		TOTAL
	YES	NO	
EXPOSED	a	b	a + b
UNEXPOSED	c	d	c + d
Total	a + b	c + d	a + b + c + d

the incidence rate for the outcome in the exposed group (I_e) is calculated as $\dfrac{a}{a+b}$; the incidence rate for the non-exposed group (I_n) is $\dfrac{c}{c+d}$.

Relative Risk

Relative risk (*risk ratio, rate ratio*) is used to measure the strength of association in a cohort study. It is estimated by dividing the incidence rate in the exposed group by the incidence rate in the non-exposed group.

$$RR = \frac{I_e}{I_n}$$

If the incidence rate for the exposed group is higher than that for the non-exposed group, the relative risk will be greater than 1.0. The epidemiologist must then consider whether the exposure may be a *risk factor* for that outcome. Conversely, if the incidence is lower among the exposed than the non-exposed, the relative risk will be less than 1; therefore, the exposure might be a *protective factor* for the outcome.

The magnitude of the relative risk reflects the strength of the association between the exposure and the outcome of interest (Table 9.3). Epidemiologists generally consider an increased risk of less than 50% (RR = 1.0 to 1.5) or a risk reduction of less than 30 percent (RR = 0.9 to 0.7) to be a weak association.[6]

An example of a strong positive association is the relative risk between cigarette smoking and lung cancer. That risk has been demonstrated in multiple studies, even after adjusting for potential confounders.[7] Conversely, the strong protective effect of an exposure has been demonstrated in some vaccine trials. For instance, a vaccine campaign against meningococcal meningitis was instituted in Mali after an outbreak of the disease.[8] The incidence of meningococcal meningitis over the 5-week period following the vaccine campaign differed significantly among those vaccinated and those who were

TABLE 9.3 Strength of Association Based on Relative Risk

RELATIVE RISK	DEFINED AS	STRENGTH OF ASSOCIATION
>1.5	Risk increased more than 50%	Moderate to strong
1.2–1.5	Risk increased 20% to 50%	Weak
0.9–1.2	Risk increased up to 20% **or** Risk decreased up to 10%	None
0.7–0.9	Risk decreased 10% to 30%	Weak
<0.7	Risk decreased more than 30%	Moderate to strong

SOURCE: Adapted from Monson (1990).[6]

not (0.7 vs 4.7 per 10,000 persons, respectively; RR = 0.15). The 0.15 relative risk indicates that the exposed (those vaccinated) had only 15 percent of the risk of developing the outcome (meningococcal meningitis) compared to the non-exposed (those not vaccinated), suggesting a strong protective effect of the vaccine. Otherwise stated, those vaccinated reduced their risk of developing meningitis by 85 percent compared to those not vaccinated.

The epidemiologist can assess the statistical significance of relative risks in different ways. One way is to test whether a relative risk is statistically significantly different from 1.0 (i.e., no difference) by calculating a p-value.[9] Reporting relative risks with p-values has been criticized, however, as it restricts the interpretation of findings to the dichotomous decision made in hypothesis testing based on a single level of statistical significance.[10] Accordingly, many peer-reviewed journals require investigators to report relative risks with confidence intervals to enhance understanding of the data.

It is a simple task for the epidemiologist to interpret relative risks and confidence intervals. In hypothesis testing, the null value indicates no difference between groups. If the confidence interval for a relative risk overlaps the null value (RR = 1.0), then the rates of outcomes for the exposed and unexposed groups are not statistically significantly different from each other. If the confidence interval does not overlap the null value, however, the rates are significantly different (the null hypothesis is rejected).

An example of interpreting relative risks and confidence intervals comes from the Oxford Family Planning Association (Oxford-FPA) contraceptive study. Between 1968 and 1973, researchers enrolled 25- to 39-year-old white married women from family planning clinics in England and Scotland. Of the 17,032 women enrolled, 6,838 had given birth to at least one child and used oral contraceptives (OCs; the exposed group); 3,154 had given birth to at least one child and used an intrauterine device (IUD; the non-exposed group). All of the women were followed for 20 years, and their causes of death were recorded. After 20 years of observation, 238 of the women in the cohort had died and their mortality data were reviewed. Results indicated that the risk for death from ovarian cancer for OC users was reduced by 60 percent compared to IUD users (RR = 0.4). The relative risk suggested that OC use provides a strong protective effect against mortality from ovarian cancer; however, the 95% confidence interval clarified this interpretation (95% CI = 0.1, 1.2). Because the confidence interval overlapped 1.0, the researchers reported that the association was too small to suggest a protective effect for OCs at that time.[11]

In 2010, the investigators repeated their evaluation of outcomes from the Oxford-FPA cohort study, this time based on 1,715 deaths rather than the original 238. The relative risk for all-cause mortality comparing OC users to never users was 0.9 (95% CI = 0.79, 0.96) and for ovarian cancer, 0.4 (95% CI = 0.3, 0.6). The investigators concluded that OC use reduces all-cause mortality (a weak association) and strongly protects against death from ovarian cancer.[12]

Person-Time

Subjects in cohort studies may be observed for varying lengths of time as a result of loss to follow-up, withdrawal from the study, or other reasons. When this happens, each subject does not contribute equally to the risk associated with developing the outcome of interest, and the epidemiologist will calculate *incidence density* rates using *person-time* (*person-years* or *person-months*) units (see Chapter 7 for use of ID in morbidity studies). The sum of the units of observation for all subjects is used as the denominator of the incidence density calculation.

$$ID = \frac{Total\ new\ outcomes\ in\ a\ time\ period}{Sum\ of\ person\text{-}time\ units\ in\ the\ cohort}$$

An example of the use of incidence density comes from a study of the lifetime risk of stroke for Americans.[13] At the time the study was undertaken, 4,897 subjects from a large cohort study in Framingham, Massachusetts had not yet suffered a stroke. These individuals were followed prospectively for the development of stroke, but each subject was observed for a different amount of time (some were lost to follow-up, others died, etc.). To accurately measure the risk of stroke for this cohort, the researchers tallied 115,146 person-years of follow up for the 4,897 subjects and calculated the incidence density. The result reported was the lifetime risk of stroke as 1 in 6 for Americans over age 55.

The epidemiologist using person-years makes two assumptions: (1) the risk of the outcome is constant per unit time of observation, and (2) the risk of the outcome is the same for similar persons in the cohort.[14-15] If either of these two assumptions does not hold (if risk increases with age or with higher levels of exposure, for example), then the incidence density strategy is not appropriate for cohort analysis. The epidemiologist may then move to a different analytical technique, such as *life tables (actuarial tables, mortality tables)*.[15-17] Life tables provide direct estimates of the probability of developing an outcome in a given time period, and relative risks can be computed as the ratio of these probabilities. The methods are beyond the scope of this introductory text.

Dose-Response

Inferences about the statistical association between an exposure and a disease are strengthened if the epidemiologist observes a dose-response relationship (Chapter 4). The dose-response relationship can be explored by setting up a series of 2 × 2 tables for varying levels of exposure and calculating a relative risk for each level. An excellent example comes from the final report of the Oxford-FPA contraceptive study discussed above.[18] Because subjects in the study were followed for different amounts of time for various reasons (loss to follow-up, becoming ineligible for some outcomes because of hysterectomy, oophorectomy, etc.), incidence density was calculated using women-years of follow-up. After adjusting for confounders, the results showed that OC use was not associated with the incidence of breast cancer (RR = 1.0; 95% CI = 0.9, 1.1). OC use was, however, associated with an increased incidence of cervical cancer (RR = 3.4; 95% CI = 1.6, 8.9) and demonstrated a protective effect against the incidence of both uterine body (RR = 0.5; 95% CI = 0.3, 0.7) and ovarian cancers (RR = 0.5; 95% CI = 0.4, 0.7). Dose-response effects (defined as total duration of OC use in months) were then explored and the ovarian cancer mortality rates by levels of exposure appear in Table 9.4.

The ovarian cancer mortality rate for those who had not used OCs was 9.2 per 100,000 women-years (the referent group). Those using OCs for less than four years had a 32 percent higher risk of ovarian cancer (RR = 1.32) compared to those with no OC use, yet among those using OCs for a longer period, the mortality rates from the disease dropped precipitously. Note the 80 percent lower mortality rate from ovarian cancer for women using OCs for at least four years (RR = 0.20), and the 84% lower mortality rate among those using OCs for eight years or more (RR = 0.16). The results suggested that OC use of four years of more might be protective against ovarian cancer mortality.

TABLE 9.4 Mortality Rates and Relative Risks of Ovarian Cancer by Duration of Oral Contraceptive Use

TOTAL DURATION OF USE	OVARIAN CANCER MORTALITY RATE PER 100,000 WOMEN-YEARS	RELATIVE RISK
None	9.2 ($n = 10$)	1.00
<47 months	12.1 ($n = 5$)	1.32
48–95 months	1.8 ($n = 1$)	0.20
>95 months	1.5 ($n = 1$)	0.16

SOURCE: Data from Vessey et al. (1989).[11]

Attributable Risk

Sometimes the epidemiologist wants to know more about the relationship between an exposure and an outcome than simply the magnitude of the relative risk. The *attributable risk* (*excess risk, causal risk difference*) is an absolute measure obtained by subtracting the risk of the outcome among those not exposed from that among persons exposed. As risk is defined as the probability of an occurrence, a risk difference of zero indicates that the exposure imparts no additional risk. As attributable risk increases, the likelihood that an exposed individual will have the outcome increases.

$$AR = I_e - I_n$$

The epidemiologist may find it preferable to calculate the *attributable rate* (*causal rate difference*) rather than the attributable risk, because rates can be adjusted whereas probabilities cannot. An example comes from the British Doctors Study conducted by Doll, Hill and Peto.[19] After 20 years of observation, the age-adjusted death rates for lung cancer were 140 deaths per 100,000 physicians for the smokers in the study and 10 deaths per 100,000 physicians for the nonsmoking subjects (RR = 14.0). The lung cancer mortality attributable to smoking was 130 deaths per 100,000 physicians (AR = 140 deaths per 100,000 physicians – 10 deaths per 100,000 physicians). Otherwise stated, 130 deaths from lung cancer among every 100,000 physicians in the study would not have occured had the physicians not smoked.

The British Doctors Study ended in 2001. Findings from the 50 years of observation confirmed the strong association between smoking and a variety of vascular, neoplastic, and respiratory diseases.[20] For members of the cohort born between 1900 and 1909, the probabilities of dying in middle age (35–69 years) were 42 percent for smokers and 24 percent for nonsmokers (a twofold mortality rate ratio and an 18 percent excess risk of dying young from smoking). For those born in the 1920s, the probabilities of dying were 43 percent for smokers and 15 for nonsmokers (a threefold mortality rate ratio and a 28 percent excess risk if dying young from smoking). The researchers concluded that the risks from smoking cigarettes were underestimated in the previous reports. Almost half of all persistent cigarette smokers in the cohort died from smoking-related diseases; about one-quarter of the smokers died by the time they reached middle age. Nonsmoking members of the cohort lived, on average, 10 years longer than their smoking counterparts. Those who ceased smoking at age 60, 50, 40, or 30 years gained additional life expectancies of 3, 6, 9, or 10 years, respectively.

Attributable Fraction

It is sometimes important to know the *proportion* of an outcome that can be attributed to an exposure. The *attributable fraction* (*etiologic fraction, attributable proportion, attributable risk percent*) for the exposed group, and the *population attributable fraction* (*population attributable risk percent*) for the population as a whole are measures calculated by the epidemiologist to address the probability that an exposure is a likely cause of an outcome. If an exposure serves as a preventive agent (such as a vaccine), the term used is *preventive fraction*.

The epidemiologist may be called upon by the courts to use the attributable fraction as a means of assessing whether a given outcome was "more likely than not" the result of an exposure (see Chapter 4). If the attributable fraction is more than 50 percent, the epidemiologist would report the exposure as the likely cause of that individual outcome, assuming the criteria for causality has been met.

Consider again the British Doctors Study, with lung cancer mortality rates of 140 deaths per 100,000 physicians for smokers and 10 deaths per 100,000 physicians for nonsmokers.[19] These rates yield a relative risk of 14.0 and an attributable risk of 130 deaths per 100,000 physicians. The attributable fraction can be calculated from this information in two algebraically equivalent ways:

$$AF = \frac{I_e - I_n}{I_e} = \frac{AR}{I_e} = \frac{130\,deaths\,per\,100,000\,physicians}{140\,deaths\,per\,100,000\,physicians} \times 100 = 92\%$$

or

$$AF = \frac{RR-1}{RR} = \frac{14-1}{14} \times 100 = 92\%$$

For the epidemiologist, this means that up to 92 percent of the lung cancer deaths observed in the British Doctors Study could have been prevented if the smokers in the study (the exposed group) did not smoke. As the 92 percent exceeds the 50 percent threshold, the epidemiologist could conclude that smoking was "more likely than not" the cause of lung cancer mortality among the exposed group.

Attributable fractions are helpful in developing strategies for both epidemiologic research and health policy development. In general, if a very high proportion of a disease is attributable to only one factor, the search for additional etiological factors may not be worthy of additional research efforts. On the other hand, when diseases are multifactorial, identifying the etiologic factors associated with the highest attributable fractions may serve to focus clinicians' efforts in counseling their patients about risk reduction. This information may similarly assist public health professionals in developing multipronged strategies for improving public health and communicating the importance of those strategies to the general public.

Policymakers and those planning public health interventions are often guided by both the attributable fraction and the *population attributable fraction,* measures that estimate the burden of disease that is directly related to a causal exposure.[21] Assume cancer registry data show the incidence of lung cancer in the total population as 120 cases per 100,000 population. When stratified by smoking status, the rates are 330 cases per 100,000 population for smokers and 30 cases per 100,000 population for nonsmokers (RR = 11.0). While the relative risk shows the epidemiologist that smoking is a strong risk factor for developing lung cancer, policymakers might need to know what proportion of lung cancer cases would be prevented if they were to fund programs or pass laws designed to reduce or eliminate smoking. To answer this question, the epidemiologist must know the prevalence of smoking in the total population. Assume that the epidemiologist finds prevalence data from a national survey showing that 30 percent of the overall population smokes. Two mathematically equivalent formulas for calculating the population attributable risk are shown below (P representing the prevalence of smoking and I_p representing the lung cancer incidence rate for the total population):

$$PAF = \frac{P(I_e - I_n)}{I_p} = \frac{P(AR)}{I_p}$$

$$= \frac{0.3\ (300\ cases\ per\ 100,000\ population)}{120\ cases\ per\ 100,000\ population} \times 100$$

$$= 75\%$$

or

$$PAF = \frac{P(RR-1)}{P(RR-1)+1} \times 100 = \frac{0.3(11.0-1)}{0.3(11.0-1)+1} \times 100 = 75\%$$

The results indicate that up to 75 percent of all new lung cancer cases could be prevented if smoking in the overall population was reduced or eliminated. Such findings provide a strong case for policymakers to support smoking prevention and cessation programs. Standard error and confidence limits for the attributable fraction[22-23] and methods for stratifying attributable fractions by varying levels of exposure are also available.[24]

Designing a Cohort Study

Select Subjects

If the outcome(s) of interest has a high prevalence in the general population, and if there are resources available to follow a sufficient number of subjects until they manifest the outcome(s) of interest, a prospective cohort design may be feasible. Consider the Framingham Heart Study. The town of Framingham, Massachusetts was chosen for its population stability, cooperation with previous community studies, presence of a local community hospital, and proximity to a large medical center. The initial cohort included approximately 5,000 persons aged 30 to 62 years who, followed over a period of 20 years, would experience enough new cases or deaths from cardiovascular disease (estimated at approximately 2,150) to ensure statistically reliable findings.[4]

Using the general population for prospective cohort studies can prove challenging for the long-term follow-up of subjects. In such instances it might be preferable to select a special population that would be easier to follow, especially those that can be identified from an occupational or administrative data set. For instance, the British Doctors' Cohort Study[25] and the Nurses' Health Study[26] were strengthened by the fact that the subjects were medical personnel who could be tracked through medical licensure and their professional associations. Despite the fact that these cohorts differ from the general population in various ways, they were considered likely to experience a high prevalence of the outcomes of interest.

Other special populations providing the opportunity for long-term follow-up are civil servants, college alumni, union members, and veterans. An example of the use of a special population is the Study of Men in Taiwan. That study recruited a cohort of more than 21,000 male Taiwanese civil servants identified through a government health clinic. The men were tracked through their job placements and, after retirement, through their benefits. Each subject was tested for the presence hepatitis B surface antigen upon enrollment and classified as exposed if he tested positive. Both groups (with and without hepatitis B surface antigen) were followed, and their incidence and mortality rates for hepatocellular carcinoma compared. The results indicated a particularly strong association (RR = 223) between the exposure to hepatitis B and the subsequent development of the carcinoma.[27]

Civil servants also served as subjects for the Whitehall prospective cohort studies. Whitehall I began in 1967, enrolling 17,530 male British civil servants and classifying them by employment grade (I—IV). Grade I was the highest, representing administrators. Grade IV was the lowest, representing job titles such as messenger. Incidence and mortality from coronary heart disease and other causes were observed over a 10-year period. Subjects employed in Grade IV had rates three times higher than those in Grade I, even after adjusting for confounders such as smoking. The steep inverse relationship suggested that psychosocial stressors related to social class might contribute to the increased health risks.[28] Whitehall II began in 1985, enrolling 10,308 subjects, this time both male and female. Longitudinal findings from Whitehall II confirmed the social gradient of risk for a variety of physical illnesses and mental health conditions.[29] These studies have influenced the clinical approach to heart disease and spurred research into the underlying biological mechanisms associated with psychosocial stressors.

Using special populations for a cohort study may facilitate tracking subjects, but it can challenge the study's *external validity*; that is, the results may not be generalizable to the population as a whole. For instance, special populations may include only one gender. Cohorts based on professional licensure or alumni status may have socioeconomic (SES) or social class status that differs from the general population. On the other hand, special populations that have experienced a rare exposure are well suited to the cohort design. For instance, the Life Span Study in Japan was a prospective cohort study of atomic bomb survivors from Hiroshima and Nagasaki that continued for more than 50 years.[30] A second example is another investigation associated with the Chernobyl nuclear accident, the Estonian Study of Chernobyl Cleanup Workers. The cohort consisted of almost 4,900 men aged 20–39 years who were sent to assist in cleanup activities after the nuclear reactor accident. Each worker spent more than three months in the Chernobyl area and experienced various levels of exposure to ionizing radiation. Study results yielded new information about cancer risks from protracted radiation exposure. The subjects will continue to be followed in order to evaluate future health outcomes.[31]

The retrospective cohort study design is rarely conducted with samples of the general population; however, it is well suited for studies where records are available for special populations, such as the Medicare database. For occupational cohorts, past exposures may be estimated from employment or medical records, or from environmental or personal monitoring devices. An example is an occupational study examining the relationship between exposure to benzene and leukemia mortality.[32] The cohort included 1,165 white male employees who worked in the rubber hydrochloride department in one of three Ohio manufacturing plants for at least one day between January 1, 1940 and December 31, 1965. These workers were presumed to have been exposed to benzene. An industrial hygienist, unaware of each subject's vital status (that is, whether the subject was alive or dead), estimated the cumulative occupational exposures to benzene for each subject by using company work records. Vital status through the end of 1981 was determined for each subject using data from the Social Security Administration, the Ohio Bureau of Motor Vehicles, and a commercial tracing service. Death certificates were obtained for all deceased members of the cohort. As the entire cohort was exposed, the group's leukemia mortality experience was compared with that of the US population for the same time period (generally assumed to be unexposed to benzene). The results demonstrated a strong association between cumulative occupational exposure to benzene and leukemia mortality.

While using an occupational cohort allows select exposures to be evaluated efficiently, such studies may be biased by the *healthy worker effect*. The healthy worker effect recognizes that cohorts of employed individuals often exhibit lower overall death rates than the general population because severely ill or chronically disabled persons are likely excluded from employment. The healthy worker effect has also been recognized in many cohorts such as military personnel, migrants, and other select groups.[33]

Determine Exposure

Exposure status can be determined directly by clinical testing, interviews, questionnaires, personal monitoring, or physical examinations of subjects.

For example, direct mail questionnaires were used to ascertain each subject's smoking status in the British Doctors Study. In the Nurses' Health Study, direct mail questionnaires were used to ascertain each subject's medical conditions and lifestyle practices. Indirect methods of determining exposure may also be used. These include interviews or questionnaires of subjects' family members, friends, or work supervisors; reviews of medical records or administrative data sets; job or travel histories; or other means. Sometimes multiple means of determining exposure are implemented. For instance, the Framingham Heart Study used clinical testing to determine cholesterol levels, physical examinations to determine blood pressure levels, and questionnaires to determine physical activity and smoking status.

When a cohort study is designed to evaluate a *dose-response* effect, accurately measuring the amount of the exposure is critical. The epidemiologist must first determine whether the *reference population* (*control group*, the comparator) had no exposure (zero dose) or a background level (baseline or low dose) of exposure to the potential etiologic agent. Various levels of exposure will then be examined to determine whether there is a *threshold exposure* above which an effect might be observed. Consider that most everyone is exposed to some level of particulate matter (PM_{10}) in ambient air. Most healthy adults show little to no effect from these low levels of exposure, but as PM_{10} increases, a threshold may be crossed whereby sensitive individuals such as children and asthmatics are likely to manifest respiratory symptoms. The field of *exposure assessment* deals with how individuals come into contact with environmental contaminants, as well as how to quantify the dose received. Good study design practice requires that the epidemiologist specify the methods of quantifying exposure before the study begins.

Study Procedures

Bias is a systematic error that can creep into a study design and lead the epidemiologist to inaccurate findings. It is best dealt with preventively, by carefully designing study procedures that can minimize its effects. Two types of bias are recognized as problematic for cohort studies: *selection bias* and *information bias*.

Selection Bias

Selection bias may happen if persons who agree to be in an epidemiologic study (volunteers) differ significantly from those who decline to participate. Indeed, participants in an epidemiologic study may differ from nonparticipants in their personal characteristics, exposure status, or their willingness to complete the study. Selection bias may also happen due to *loss to follow-up* of subjects. If the proportion of subjects lost to follow-up is high and if information on their outcomes is not available, the analysis may yield incorrect conclusions.

Efforts to minimize loss to follow-up must be part of the study protocol. Methods for keeping in contact with each subject and determining his/her health outcome(s) may include periodic physical exams or clinical tests, home visits, telephone calls, mailed questionnaires, a review of administrative or insurance databases, and more. One technique to minimize loss to follow-up in a prospective cohort study is to obtain the names and addresses of several friends and relatives at the beginning of a study, so that they may be contacted if the subject moves out of the community. Additional personnel may be needed who can track the subjects by phone or social media, and a budget may be required that includes incentives to encourage subjects to continue to participate.

Selection bias in a cohort study can be evaluated by comparing information gathered on all subjects at the beginning of the study to determine if those lost to follow-up differ in some way from the ones who completed the study. If the groups do not differ with respect to individual characteristics, exposure status, or outcomes (if known), then the study results are less likely to be biased.

Information Bias

All subjects in a cohort study should be followed in the same manner, for the same outcomes, and at the same time intervals. If not, two types of information bias, *observer bias* and *surveillance bias*, may occur. Observer bias occurs if those responsible for gathering outcomes information approach subjects who are exposed and unexposed differently. This problem can be minimized if the study design includes strict protocols for data collection. The protocols may be as simple as listing the elements required for a clinical evaluation, setting monitoring guidelines for equipment accuracy, or having the subjects take their shoes off when measuring height and weight. Sometimes, though, a more complicated method needs to be used, such as requiring two or more physicians to evaluate the same radiographic studies or specifying that clinical specimens be evaluated in duplicate or at independent laboratories. If information on outcomes is obtained through interview, the use of a script may be necessary. When multiple observers are used, a training period should be instituted so that all observers are equally able to evaluate exposures and outcomes.

Surveillance bias can happen if the exposed group is followed more closely than the unexposed group. Outcomes may then be identified more quickly in the more closely watched group so they become apparent at an earlier time in the study. This means that an interim analysis of the data would provide a biased view of the relationship between the exposure and the outcomes of interest. Again, a good study design that includes monitoring protocols can minimize surveillance bias by assuring that the subjects are evaluated in similar time frames regardless of exposure status.

Ascertain Outcomes

The outcomes of the study need to be carefully specified before the study begins. For example, if the outcome of interest is diabetes, does the specification include insulin-dependent diabetes, non-insulin-dependent diabetes, or both conditions? How will the diagnosis be verified (from laboratory test results, from physician records, or from diagnostic coding on an insurance form)? These decisions need to be carefully considered to assure they do not introduce information bias. Suppose the epidemiologist is interested in the relationship between serum cholesterol level and the risk of stroke. Some 1,000 subjects are enrolled in a study, and each subject's exposure is defined as their serum cholesterol level upon enrollment. How will the epidemiologist ascertain whether any of the subjects suffered a stroke? Should each subject be sent an annual survey and ask whether they have experienced a stroke? Should the epidemiologist monitor each subject's health insurance claims for hospital admissions due to stroke? How long should this study continue? Must the epidemiologist wait until all the subjects have died, and then check their death certificates for cause?

The length of a cohort study is dependent upon the *latency period* for subjects to develop the outcome(s) of interest. If the exposure is defined demographically, such as becoming a widow or widower, and if the outcome of interest is early mortality, then perhaps the cohort could be followed for as short a time as one year. In contrast, the atomic bombs dropped on Japan in 1945 instantly killed about 200,000 persons and left many survivors exposed to radiation. In one of the largest cohort investigations ever undertaken, the Life Span Study was launched in 1950 to evaluate the late mortality effects of radiation on the survivors. The cohort of about 110,000 persons are grouped as exposed to radiation close to ground zero, exposed at sufficient distance that radiation exposure was reduced, and controls who were not exposed.[31] The study required lifetime follow-up, as the latency of some outcomes could not be known at the time the study commenced. While some of the associations with specific diseases were expected (such as cancers), others (such as heart disease) were not.

Analyze Results

The epidemiologist approaches the analysis of cohort data similarly to that of any other data set (Chapter 3). The first task is to consider the role of data artifacts. Was there bias in the study design (the way subjects were enrolled, the way exposure and outcomes were determined, or the way data were gathered and entered into the study)? If the answers to these questions are "no," then the next step is to evaluate the role of potential confounders. This can be done through the construction of a series of 2 × 2 tables, one for each strata of the potential confounder. For example, suppose the epidemiologist is interested in a study of suicidal behavior and anticipates that gender might be a confounder in this study. Separate 2 × 2 tables would be assembled for males and females and their relative risks compared. If the results for the two groups differ, then gender may be a confounder. If the results are similar, however, gender did not confound the results and the epidemiologist can calculate one relative risk for the entire cohort.

When there are many groups to compare, as 10-year age groups (0 to 100+ years) for large populations, the interpretation of the overall study results may be difficult. Chapter 5 described the process of adjusting rates. Similarly, it is possible to adjust risks. An overall (*adjusted*) risk can be calculated from the strata by using a statistical technique that takes into account all of the relative risks.[34] Adjusted relative risks may be reported in the literature as *Mantel-Haenszel relative risks* (RR_{MH}), *adjusted relative risks* (RR_{adj}), or *adjusted risk ratios*.

Sometimes the epidemiologist wishes to model the risk of developing outcomes based on varying levels of exposure. Advanced statistical techniques beyond the scope of this text, such as *logistic, log-linear,* and *proportional hazards* models can be used in these instances. An example of the use of the proportional hazards model comes from the Diet, Cancer and Health cohort study in Denmark. That study enrolled 57,053 Danes aged 50 to 64 years between December 1993 and May 1997. Each subject's home address was mapped, and the geologic data for radon at that location was identified. Their lifetime levels of exposure to radon (the sum of the exposures based on the proportion of time spent in residence at each location) were compared to their risk for developing a primary brain tumor.[35] Statistical modeling allowed the investigators to adjust the relative risks for age, sex, consumption of fruits and vegetables, employment in the chemical industry, and levels of the air pollutant nitrous oxide at the various residential addresses. The study results showed a dose-response relationship, and the researchers reported a significant association between long-term residential radon exposure and the risk of primary brain tumor.

Summary

Cohort studies are both observational and prospective in design. They are observational because investigators do not allocate the exposure; rather, subjects are recruited based on their exposure status. Cohort studies are prospective in that all subjects are followed after time of exposure to determine the study outcomes. This establishes the single required criterion for causation—temporality.

The primary measure of association between exposure and outcome in a cohort study is the relative risk, calculated from incidence rates for outcomes experienced by the groups being compared. The larger the relative risk, the greater the strength of the association—a second criterion for building a case for a causal relationship (Chapter 4). The epidemiologist approaches data analysis for a cohort study similarly to that for other study designs, examining the data first for bias and then for any confounding effects. Confounding variables may be related to the exposure, to the disease, or both, and may influence the magnitude of the relative risk. To test for effects of confounding, the epidemiologist may calculate stratum-specific relative risks or construct a statistical model of the data. Adjusted risk calculations may be appropriate to estimate, depending upon the circumstances. The attributable risk and the attributable risk fraction are additional outcome measures that may be calculated from the data in cohort studies. The larger the attributable risk fraction for a given factor, the more difficult it becomes to study other possible etiologies for the outcome.

Most challenges to launching a cohort study can be handled with careful planning and execution. Clearly defining exposures and anticipated outcomes begins the process. Ensuring sufficient resources to follow up all subjects (exposed and unexposed) equally, for the relevant amount of time to cover the latency period, is critical. This is because inadequate follow-up may cause biased data and can lead to spurious associations or missed relationships. Monitoring and documenting changes in exposure status and diagnostic criteria over time are important, so that person-years of exposure can be calculated and the data stratified according to dose. When these challenges are addressed, the well-designed cohort study can provide invaluable information on the associations between exposures and outcomes.

References

1. Harold F. Dorn, "Some Problems Arising in Prospective and Retrospective Studies of the Etiology of Disease," *New England Journal of Medicine* 261 (1959): 571–579.
2. Yoshisada Shibata et al., 15 Years after Chernobyl: New Evidence of Thyroid Cancer. *Lancet* 358, no. 9297 (2001): 1965–1966.
3. L. S. Sun et al., "Feasibility and Pilot Study of the Pediatric Anesthesia NeuroDevelopment Assessment (PANDA) Project," *Journal of Neurosurgical Anesthesiology* 24 no. 4 (2012): 382–388.
4. Thomas R. Dawber, Gilcin F. Meadors, and Felix E. Moore, Jr., "Epidemiological Approaches to Heart Disease: The Framingham Study," *American Journal of Public Health and the Nation's Health* 41, no. 3 (1951): 279–286.
5. Framingham Heart Study, 2014. Available at http://www.framinghamheartstudy.org/.
6. Robert Monson, *Occupational Epidemiology.* Boca Raton, FL: CDC Press, 1990.
7. US Surgeon General, *The Health Consequences of Smoking. Cancer.* Washington, DC: US Government Printing Office, 1982.
8. Nancy Binkin and Jeffrey Band, "Epidemic of Meningococcal Meningitis in Bamako, Mali: Epidemiological Features and Analysis of Vaccine Efficacy," *Lancet* 2, no. 8293 (1982): 315–318.
9. W. G. Cochran, "Some Methods of Strengthening the Common $\chi 2$ Tests," *Biometrics* 10 (1954): 417–451.
10. M. J. Gardner and D. G. Altman, "Confidence Intervals Rather Than *P* Values: Estimation Rather Than Hypothesis Testing," *British Medical Journal (Clinical Research Edition)* 292, no. 6522 (1986): 746–750.
11. M. P. Vessey et al., "Mortality among Oral Contraceptive Users: 20 Year Follow Up of Women in a Cohort Study," *British Medical Journal* 299, no. 6714 (1989): 1487–1491.
12. M. Vessey, D. Yeates, and S. Flynn, "Factors Affecting Mortality in a Large Cohort Study with Special Reference to Oral Contraceptive Use," *Contraception* 82, no. 3 (2010): 221–229.
13. Sudha Seshadri and Philip A. Wolf, "Lifetime Risk of Stroke and Dementia: Current Concepts, and Estimates from the Framingham Study," *Lancet Neurology* 6, no. 12 (2007): 1106–1114.
14. Mindel C. Sheps, "On the Person Years Concept in Epidemiology and Demography," *Milbank Memorial Fund Quarterly* 44, no. 1 (1966): 69–91.
15. N. E. Breslow and N. E. Day, *The Design and Analysis of Cohort Studies.* Lyon: International Agency for Research on Cancer, 1987.
16. Chin Long Chiang, "A Stochastic Study of the Life Table and Its Applications. III. The Follow-Up Study with the Consideration of Competing Risks," *Biometrics* 17 (1961): 57–78.

17. Harold A. Kahn and Christopher T. Sempos, *Statistical Methods in Epidemiology*. New York: Oxford University Press, 1989.

18. M. Vessey and D. Yeates, "Oral Contraceptive Use and Cancer: Final Report from the Oxford-Family Planning Association Contraceptive Study," *Contraception* 88, no. 6 (2013): 678–683.

19. Richard Doll and Richard Peto, "Mortality In Relation To Smoking: 20 Years' Observations on Male British Doctors," *British Medical Journal* 2, no. 6051 (1976): 1525–1536.

20. Richard Doll, Richard Peto, et al., "Mortality In Relation To Smoking: 50 Years' Observations on Male British Doctors," *British Medical Journal* 328, no. 7455 (2004): 1519.

21. M. E. Northridge, "Public Health Methods—Attributable Risk as a Link between Causality and Public Health Action," *American Journal of Public Health* 85, no. 9 (1995): 1202–1204.

22. S. D. Walter, "The Distribution of Levin's Measure of Attributable Risk," *Biometrika* 62 (1975): 371–374.

23. S. D. Walter, "The Estimation and Interpretation of Attributable Risk in Health Research," *Biometrics* 32, no. 4 (1976): 829–849.

24. D. G. Kleinbaum, L. L. Kupper, and Hal Morgenstern, *Epidemiologic Research: Principles and Quantitative Methods (Industrial Health & Safety)*. Wiley, 1982.

25. Richard Doll and Austin Bradford Hill, "Mortality in Relation to Smoking: Ten Years' Observations of British Doctors," *British Medical Journal* 1, no. 5395 (1964): 1399–1410.

26. C. H. Hennekens, et al., "Use of Permanent Hair Dyes and Cancer among Registered Nurses," *Lancet* 1, no. 8131 (1979): 1390–1393.

27. R. P. Beasley et al., "Hepatocellular Carcinoma and Hepatitis B Virus. A Prospective Study of 22,707 Men in Taiwan, *Lancet* 2, no. 8256 (1981): 1129–1133.

28. M. G. Marmot, M. J. Shipley, and Geoffrey Rose, "Inequalities in Death—Specific Explanations of a General Pattern?" *Lancet* 1, no. 8384 (1984): 1003–1006.

29. M. G. Marmot, "Understanding Social Inequalities in Health," *Perspectives in Biology and Medicine* 46, no. 3 Supplement (2003): S9–23.

30. Yukiko Shimizu et al., "Radiation Exposure and Circulatory Disease Risk: Hiroshima and Nagasaki Atomic Bomb Survivor Data, 1950-2003," *British Medical Journal*. 340 (2010): b5349.

31. Mare Tekkel et al., "The Estonian Study of Chernobyl Cleanup Workers: I. Design and Questionnaire Data," *Radiation Research* 147, no. 5 (1997): 641–652.

32. Robert A. Rinsky et al., "Benzene and Leukemia. An Epidemiologic Risk Assessment," *New England Journal of Medicine* 316, no. 17 (1987): 1044–1050.

33. Miquel Porta, Ed., *A Dictionary of Epidemiology, 6th Edition*. New York: Oxford University Press, 2014.

34. Nathan Mantel and William Haenszel, "Statistical Aspects of the Analysis of Data from Retrospective Studies of Disease," *Journal of the National Cancer Institute* 22, no. 4 (1959): 719–748.

35. E. V. Brauner et al., "Residential Radon and Brain Tumour Incidence in a Danish Cohort," *PLoS One* 8, no. 9 (2013): e74435.

Problem Set: Chapter 9

1. In the East Eagle's Neck School District, the superintendent of public education, O. B. Kwiet, was concerned with a series of suicides among students starting in 7th grade and continuing through high school. During the past decade, at least 10 students had committed suicide during the school year. The superintendent called the commissioner of the local health department, Dr. Wright Now, for help. When the two met, it became clear to Dr. Now that the district needed to conduct an observational study to determine what factors were involved in these students deciding to commit suicide. Since psychological profiles would be a key element in the study, and since such information would be impossible to obtain from the deceased, the district would need to conduct a cohort study—the only means of providing the information needed to address this outbreak of suicides. Thus, The East Eagle's Neck Health Evaluation and Learning Project (TEEN HELP) was conceived.

   Twice during each school year, each student in grades 4 and above would complete a series of assessments regarding stress levels, social involvement and relationships, affect, and so on. Health department epidemiologists would analyze the data to discern risk factors that could assist the district in combating this outbreak.

   By the end of the third year, six assessments had been completed and 11 students were either confirmed or suspected of committing suicide. Dr. Now contended that parental pressure placed on children to excel at academic studies was to blame for these outcomes. He asked the epidemiologists to separate the student data into high and low stress responses about parental pressure in order to evaluate his hypothesis.

	NUMBER OF CONFIRMED AND SUSPECTED SUICIDES	PERSON-MONTHS OF OBSERVATION
High Stress (Upper Quintile)	9	34,400
Low Stress (Lower Quintile)	2	58,980

   Help Dr. Now by using the results of TEEN HELP to answer the following questions about parental stress:
   a. What are the average monthly incidence (density) rates of suicide per 10,000 students for those in the high and low stress groups?
   b. What is the relative risk of suicide among students with high stress compared to those with low stress? Interpret this finding. Is it a strong one?
   c. What is the risk of suicide attributable to stress for those in the highest quintile compared with those in the lowest quintile? Interpret this finding.

2. Another risk factor examined in TEEN HELP was whether the student felt isolated from his/her peers. Overall, the incidence rate for suicide was 1.1 per 10,000

students per month. At the time of the sixth assessment, the average monthly incidence density of suicide for those not feeling socially isolated was 0.8 suicides per 10,000 students and, for those feeling socially isolated, 3.4 suicides per 10,000 students. The relative risk for social isolation was therefore 4.3 (= 3.4/0.8), suggestive of a strong association. The first survey of the prevalence of the different risk factors among the students in the district found that 8 percent of the students felt socially isolated.

  a. Estimate the risk of suicide attributable to social isolation in this study (excess risk).

  b. Estimate the attributable fraction.

  c. Estimate the population attributable fraction.

  d. Interpret these findings.

10 | Observational Studies
CASE-CONTROL STUDIES

The retrospective method can be particularly useful in the study of diseases of a very low incidence and in the tentative exploration of hypotheses when not much is known about etiology of a disease.[1-2]

Harold Fred Dorn (1959)

CASE-CONTROL (CASE-REFERENT) STUDIES ARE SIMILAR to cohort studies in that they are both observational designs. They differ insofar as cohort studies are prospective, and case-control studies are not. Case-control studies are not prospective because the epidemiologist already knows the disease status of each subject when the study begins. Knowing the outcome is eminently practical when a disease is rare or if only a small group of cases of a new disease has been reported (a *case series*). Since the epidemiologist does not have to wait for the outcome to manifest in order to estimate its association with a potential etiologic factor, results can be obtained in a timely fashion. The measure of association for the case-control study design is the *odds ratio*, an estimate of the relative risk or risk ratio that would have been obtained if cohort data for the same exposure(s) and outcome were analyzed.

To begin a case-control study, the epidemiologist enrolls subjects based on their disease status (*cases* have the outcome of interest, while *controls* do not). The next step is to reconstruct subjects' exposure histories and use that information to estimate the association between one or more exposures (potential etiologic factors) and disease status. For example, consider that Reye's syndrome is a rare, acute, and often fatal illness that can damage brain and liver tissues. Case studies suggested that aspirin (salicylate) given to children during a viral illness could be a possible etiologic factor for the disease. Because of the severity of Reye's syndrome, all cases are likely to be identified through hospital admission records. The population at risk, however, would be all children experiencing a viral illness during the same time period as the cases. Complete ascertainment of such children is unlikely, as not all children with viral illnesses seek medical care. Because the population at risk cannot be reliably estimated, incidence rates for viral illnesses in children cannot be determined. To deal with this data limitation, the epidemiologist may select a case-control design.

The degree of association between Reye's syndrome and prior aspirin use was evaluated using the case-control design in the Public Health Service Reye Syndrome study.[3] Between February and May 1984, investigators identified 30 hospitalized children in 11 states with a confirmed diagnosis of Reye's syndrome who had chicken pox or a viral respiratory or gastrointestinal illness shortly before admission. Controls (n = 145) were identified as children of the same age and race, who had experienced a similar viral illness during the same time period and were treated at the same hospital or emergency room, or were part of the same school or community as the cases. Preliminary results from this study reported that of the 30 children with Reye's syndrome, 28 had ingested salicylates during their viral illness (93%); of the 145 controls, 66 had done so (46%). After review, two cases and their controls were excluded from the study as they were identified as having other chronic illnesses. Their exclusion did not significantly change the results, and further analysis to determine the measures of association are discussed below.

Measuring Association in Case-Control Studies

The data from a case-control study is arranged in a 2 × 2 table, and the odds of exposure for the cases (a/c) and controls (b/d) are then compared through the use of the *odds ratio* (OR). The equation for calculating the odds ratio shows that it is mathematically equivalent to a cross products calculation. Thus, the odds ratio is sometimes called a *cross products* ratio.[4]

$$Odds\ ratio = \frac{a/c}{b/d} = \frac{ad}{bc}$$

If the odds of exposure are the same for both the case and control groups, there is no statistical association between exposure and outcome (OR = 1.0, the *null value* for the *null hypothesis* that there is no difference between groups). If the odds of exposure are greater among the cases than

TABLE 10.1 Association Between the Development of Reye's Syndrome and Salicylate Use in Children

EXPOSURE	CASES	CONTROLS	TOTAL
Salicylate use	26	63	89
No salicylate use	2	78	80
Total	28	141	169

$$Odds\ ratio = \frac{ad}{bc} = \frac{26 \times 78}{63 \times 2} = \frac{2028}{126} = 16.1$$

SOURCE: Data adapted from Hurwitz et al. (1987).[5]

among the controls, the odds ratio indicates a positive association between the disease and the exposure. Similarly, if the odds ratio is less than 1.0, the association may indicate that the exposure (such as a vaccine) confers a protective effect.

Table 10.1 shows the 2 × 2 tabular results of the Reye's syndrome study after removal of the two cases and their respective controls, as well as the calculation of the odds ratio.[5]

The odds ratio of 16.1 means that children with Reye's syndrome (the cases) were a little more than 16 times as likely to have had the exposure (have taken salicylates during an immediately preceding viral illness) than were controls (children who did not take salicylates for a similar viral illness during the same time period), suggesting a strong statistical relationship.

Because the odds ratio is calculated from a sample of cases and controls rather than from the total population, it is an estimate of the true odds ratio. As with other estimated measures of association, it should be assessed using a confidence interval. A large confidence interval suggests the estimated odds ratio has a low level of precision. Conversely, a small confidence interval indicates a high degree of precision. The confidence interval can also serve as a proxy for the p value. If the confidence interval does not overlap the null value (OR = 1.0), the odds ratio may be considered statistically significant. The epidemiologist is ever cognizant, however, that a statistical association is but one aspect of making a causal inference (Chapter 4).

The Reye's syndrome study investigators estimated the odds ratio as 16.1 (95% CI = 3.5, 102.2). As the lower bound of the 95% confidence limit exceeds the null value of 1.0, the odds ratio is considered statistically significant at $p < 0.05$. These results, along with those from previous case-control studies on Reye's syndrome,[6–8] convinced the US Federal Drug Administration (FDA) in 1986 to issue a requirement that all nonprescription products containing aspirin be labeled with a warning about Reye's syndrome. The ruling was amended in 2003 to inform consumers of the symptoms of Reye's syndrome and advise that aspirin and nonaspirin salicylate drug products not be given to children or teenagers who have or are recovering from chicken pox or flu-like symptoms.[9]

Population Attributable Fraction

In Chapter 9 we introduced the concept of the *population attributable fraction (population attributable risk)*, the degree to which the incidence of an outcome would change if an exposure changed for an entire population. The same measure can also be useful for evaluating risk factors identified through the case-control study design. For example, a case-control study was launched in Spain where sporadic cases of diarrhea due to antibiotic-resistant *Campylobacter* were on the rise.[10] Between February 2005 and 2006, 81 cases and 81 age-matched controls were identified from the northeastern part of Spain. All subjects were interviewed by telephone using a structured questionnaire to elicit potential exposures that may have led to *Campylobacter* infection. Risk factors identified as statistically significant were contact with farm animals or pets (OR = 2.8; 95% CI = 1.1, 7.3), consuming chicken at least three times (OR = 6.1; 95% CI = 2.0, 18.5), or consuming unhygienically handled deli meat from a retail outlet (OR = 4.1; 95% CI = 1.2, 13.2) within one week prior to diagnosis. The population attributable risks for these exposures were reported as 19, 36, and 25 percent, respectively. The investigators reported that these three exposures may have cumulatively been responsible for as many as four out of five (80%) sporadic cases of *Campylobacter* in northeastern Spain during this time period.

Campylobacter has a complex epidemiology with many animal reservoirs and modes of transmission. The researchers noted that totally eliminating animal contact or the consumption of chicken or deli meats in the total population would be unrealistic. Instead, they recommended a combination of measures that included reducing the infectious agent in the food chain (particularly in poultry production); initiating a health education campaign for consumers, food-handlers, and caregivers to understand food safety issues; and handwashing.[10]

Designing a Case-Control Study

Various methods have been developed to identify subjects for case-control studies. Sometimes investigators recruit cases from one source and controls from a variety of different types of sources. Consistency of results when using

TABLE 10.2 Some Sources of Cases and Controls in Case-Control Studies*

CASES	CONTROLS
All cases diagnosed in the general population, from a sample of the general population, or from a disease registry	• Non-cases in the general population or a sample of the general population
All cases diagnosed in a community (hospitals, clinics, and other medical facilities such as physicians offices)	• Probability sample of that community (general population) obtained by various methods
All cases diagnosed in one or more hospitals	• Sample of patients in those same hospitals who do not have the outcomes being studied
Cases selected by any method	• Non-cases who are residents in the same block or neighborhood of cases • Spouses, siblings, or associates (schoolmates or workmates) of the cases

* Various combinations are possible.

different control groups increases the validity of inferences derived from the findings. Table 10.2 provides some options for selecting cases and controls.

One design issue is how many controls should be recruited for a case-control study. The epidemiologist must consider several factors when deciding on that number. For instance, if the exposures of interest are behaviors that potential controls may not wish to reveal (such as the use of illegal substances or personal sexual behaviors), it may be difficult to enroll controls. In other instances, appropriate controls may be plentiful, as when studying normal as compared to adverse birth outcomes. As a rule of thumb, epidemiologists will design a case-control study with at least as many cases as controls. When the disease is a rare one, the epidemiologist may try to increase the statistical precision of the study by increasing the number of controls. Statisticians have found that four controls per case may be an optimal number, but other ratios are also used.[11] Time and budgetary costs for enrolling and interviewing study subjects may dictate the size of the case and control groups.

Matching

Cases are usually selected from a population defined by a place (hospital or geographic area), specific time period, or other common characteristic (e.g., employment, membership in a health maintenance organization, or inclusion in a disease registry). To ensure comparability of cases and controls, and to control for known confounding variables, the epidemiologist often restricts the selection of controls to the same age range, race, and gender (or other characteristic, such as vital status) as the cases. For example, cases may be placed into 10-year age groups and controls selected for each of the groups. This technique is called a *frequency match (group match)*. The cases and controls in each age stratum can then be compared for homogeneity using statistical significance tests.[12-13] A second technique is to match each case to its own control subject (*individual match, pair-match, or sometimes simply "matched"*). The matched pairs will then be alike on all matching characteristics except for the variable (exposure) under investigation.

Matching has a drawback in that if many groups are chosen, or if pair matches are based on a large number of characteristics, the epidemiologist may encounter difficulties in finding suitable controls. For this reason the epidemiologist may need to reduce the number of strata, or, for pair matching, reduce the number of matching variables. With age matching, for example, it may be impossible to form pairs using 1-year age intervals. Grouping the ages of cases and controls into 5- or 10-year age strata, however, may make matching feasible.

The number of matching variables should be limited to those known to be related to the outcome. This prevents *overmatching*, a condition that may reduce the precision of the analysis. For example, once a variable is matched, its influence on the outcome can no longer be studied. Thus it may be preferable to gather information on potential confounders and adjust for them during statistical analysis rather than matching for them in the study design.

Preventing Bias

Good case-control study design requires use of either a representative (e.g., random) sample of cases from a large population or all cases from a smaller population. The former is exemplified by a random sample of lung cancer cases drawn from all lung cancer cases in a large population-based cancer registry; the latter is exemplified by using all cases of diarrhea in a daycare center.

Many times, ascertaining all cases of a health outcome is difficult, even in smaller populations. Consider an epidemiologist investigating miscarriages during the first trimester of pregnancy. A proportion of these miscarriages may occur in women who are not yet aware of their pregnancy or who may have no access to a health care provider to document the miscarriage. For the epidemiologist, obtaining a representative sample of women in the general population with early miscarriages would be difficult at best. Alternatively, the epidemiologist might be able to identify miscarriages among a smaller, well-defined population–perhaps women under a physician's care seeking to become pregnant. The results of the study might be biased, however, if the controls were selected from the general population.

Two types of bias concern the epidemiologist in case-control studies: *selection bias* and *information bias*. The former may occur if cases and controls have different probabilities of being selected, the latter if information on exposures is elicited from the case and control groups differently. Both types of bias must be controlled during the study's design, as they cannot be controlled in the statistical analysis after the data have been gathered.

Selection Bias

As early as 1856, W. A. Guy suggested that a spurious association might arise because of the different probabilities of admission to a hospital depending upon the disease and the characteristics of the subject (such as ability to pay for treatment).[14] The implication was that drawing cases and controls from hospitalized patients could lead to biased results, a conclusion mathematically demonstrated in 1946 by Joseph Berkson.[15] Epidemiologists work to minimize what has come to be known as *Berkson's bias* (*Berkson's fallacy*). When an outcome of interest is acute and rare, cases might be found only among hospitalized patients. In these instances, selecting more than one control group and using each control group both separately and in the aggregate during data analysis is standard practice (as in the Public Health Service Reye's syndrome study). Separate analyses may identify associations otherwise concealed due to selection bias.

Selection bias may be present in any situation where persons with different diseases or characteristics (such as disease severity, the ability to pay, or residing too far from a health care provider) enter a study at different rates or probabilities. Even if selection bias is present, it need not necessarily invalidate the study findings, and the epidemiologist should consider each situation on its own merits. For instance, selection bias is probably not a concern if the association can be demonstrated when different control groups are used for the analysis, when a dose-response relationship is apparent (Chapter 4), or when the statistical association is strong (see Chapter 9, Table 9.3).[16]

Information Bias

Once cases and controls are selected, information about exposures is collected. Such information may be biased by the interviewer's knowledge of the subject's status as either a case or control (*interviewer bias*). The subject's response may be influenced by the interviewer's manner or the way they structure questions for cases and controls. It is important, therefore, that interviewers are unaware (*blinded* or *masked*) of the subject's status and that standardized (*scripted, structured*) interviews are used for collecting study data. Alternatively, hospital patients may be interviewed or given a comprehensive, general-purpose survey at the time of admission. Several studies exemplify this technique. For example, patients at the Roswell Park Memorial Institute in Buffalo, New York were given a general health survey at the time of admission, that is, before the patient was seen by a physician and given a diagnosis.[17–19] Similarly, from 1976 to 2009, the Slone Epidemiology Center at Boston University obtained information about drug histories from patients entering hospitals in the Boston region, as well as in other cities. Upon admission, nurses used a standardized questionnaire to obtain information on the patient's demographics, life style habits, past and present illnesses, and lifetime medication use.[20] These and other studies gathering unbiased information have been highly successful in producing extensive data on exposures.

Another type of information bias relates to differences in subjects' ability to recall or acknowledge exposures (*recall bias*). For instance, the mother of a low birth weight infant may be more likely to remember taking a sip of wine during her pregnancy than might the mother with a child of normal birth weight. Alternatively, both cases and controls may deny or suppress the memory of particular exposures. Examples include denying exposures or suppressing memories of illegal activities or traumatic events.

Exposure information can sometimes be evaluated for recall bias by comparing responses with medical, employment, or school records. Several case-control studies of the relationship between the use of oral contraceptives and various disease outcomes assumed that women recalled their use of oral contraceptives with reasonable accuracy.[21–24] In one of the many tests of this assumption, the oral contraceptive histories of 75 women attending family planning clinics were compared with information available in the clinic records. The study found that the type of information obtained in the case-control studies was likely to be remembered with reasonable accuracy.[25] This is not always the case. For instance, when circumcision of sexual partners was found to be associated with cervical cancer risk, some investigators asked how many men were aware of their circumcision status. A study of Mexican military men revealed that only 8 percent of those reporting they were circumcised actually were when examined by a physician.[26] Such studies show that calculating odds ratios based on self-reported information that has not been independently verified may lead to biased results.

Most investigators take great pains to prevent interviewer bias by rigorously training study personnel in proper interview methods, standardizing survey instruments, and testing the process with mock interviews before data collection begins. Each interviewer's technique can be evaluated through the use of videotaping and debriefing mock interviews, by cross-training interviewers for peer comments, and by other means of bias detection at early stages in the study when corrective measures are still possible.

Additional Analyses

Odds ratios are the primary measure of association for case-control studies. They are flexible in that they can be calculated for all subjects in a study or for various subsets of cases and controls. For instance, consider a study to determine the association between oral contraceptive use before first pregnancy and female breast cancer. The investigators reported an odds ratio of 1.75 for women 45 years of age or younger (Table 10.3). In other words, for subjects in the study who were 45 years of age and younger, cases (those with breast cancer) were 1.75 times more likely than controls to have taken oral contraceptives before their first pregnancy.[27]

Could the amount of time taking oral contraceptives be a confounding factor? Might there be an amount of time taking oral contraceptives before first pregnancy where there is no effect? To address these questions, the investigators stratified the data by duration of oral contraceptive use. Table 10.4 contains the *stratum-specific odds ratios* for the association between breast cancer and the duration of oral contraceptive use before first pregnancy.

Note that the stratum-specific odds ratios increase with the duration of oral contraceptive use. Use of oral contraceptives for any time period before first pregnancy was associated with increased occurrence of breast cancer. Otherwise stated, there does not appear to be a *threshold effect* demonstrated in this study (*minimum dose* of oral contraceptive use associated with the development of breast cancer). A thorough investigation, however, requires that the epidemiologist calculate confidence intervals for each of the

TABLE 10.3 Oral Contraceptive Use Before First Term Pregnancy Among Female Breast Cancer Patients and Hospital Controls 45 Years Old and Younger

ORAL CONTRACEPTIVE USE	CASES	CONTROLS	ODDS RATIO (ESTIMATED RELATIVE RISK)
Yes	116	77	$OR = \dfrac{ad}{bc} = \dfrac{116 \times 274}{77 \times 235} = 1.75$
No	235	274	
Total	351	351	

SOURCE: Data extracted from McPherson et al. (1987).[27]

TABLE 10.4 Duration of Oral Contraceptive Use Before First Term Pregnancy Among Female Breast Cancer Patients and Hospital Controls 45 Years Old and Younger

DURATION OF ORAL CONTRACEPTIVE USE	CASES	CONTROLS	ODDS RATIO (ESTIMATED RELATIVE RISK)
<1 year	27 (a)	26 (b)	$OR = \dfrac{ad}{bc} = \dfrac{27 \times 274}{26 \times 235} = 1.2$
1–4 years	43 (a)	29 (b)	$OR = \dfrac{ad}{bc} = \dfrac{43 \times 274}{29 \times 235} = 1.7$
>4 years	46 (a)	23 (b)	$OR = \dfrac{ad}{bc} = \dfrac{46 \times 274}{23 \times 235} = 2.3$
No use	235 (c)	274 (d)	1.0

SOURCE: Data from McPherson et al. (1987).[27]

stratum-specific odds ratios and compare them against the referent group in order to verify the findings.

Summarizing Stratum-Specific Odds Ratios

When all stratum-specific odds are associated with an outcome, the epidemiologist may calculate a summary measure called the *Cochran-Mantel-Haenszel odds ratio* (OR_{CMH}), the *Mantel-Haenszel odds ratio* (OR_{MH}), or simply the *adjusted odds ratio* (OR_{adj}).[12–13] The calculation for this summary measure of association is:

$$OR_{CMH} = \frac{\sum \dfrac{ad}{n}}{\sum \dfrac{bc}{n}}$$

In the above equation, the sum of the cross-products calculations for each level is divided by the numbers of subjects in their respective levels, thereby yielding an adjusted odds ratio. The calculation for the adjusted odds ratio allows the levels with more subjects to carry relatively more weight in the equation. Thus, it is sometimes called a *weighted* or *pooled* odds ratio.

Analyzing Matched Cases and Controls

When confounding variables are controlled by the process of group- or pair-matching cases and controls, the analysis can become complex. An example comes from a study of chlamydia and ectopic pregnancy.[28]

TABLE 10.5 Matched-Pair Data for Determining
the Association between *Chlamydia trachomatis* and
Ectopic Pregnancy

MATCHED PAIRS	CONTROL EXPOSED	CONTROL NOT EXPOSED
Case exposed		109(*b*)
Case not exposed	36(*c*)	

SOURCE: Data from Chow et al. (1990).[28]

Researchers recruited cases of ectopic pregnancy from hospital admissions and controls from prenatal clinics. All the women were 12 to 24 weeks pregnant, had not had a bilateral tubal ligation or previous ectopic pregnancy, and did not become pregnant while using an intrauterine device (IUD). Cases and controls were matched for age (±1 year), ethnicity, and location. A total of 257 matched pairs were assembled. Each subject's blood was then tested for past exposure to chlamydia by antibody titer, and the pairs were placed into one of four categories: both case and control exposed (n = 72), case exposed and control not exposed (n = 109), case not exposed and control exposed (n = 36), or both case and control not exposed (n = 40) (Table 10.5).

In instances where both the case and control have the same exposure status, there is no additional information to be gained. Thus, cells *a* and *d* in Table 10.5 are of no use in the calculation of the odds ratio. The *discordant pairs*, however, may provide useful information. The calculation for the odds ratio in a matched case-control study is:

$$OR = \frac{cases\,exposed,\,controls\,not\,exposed}{controls\,exposed,\,cases\,not\,exposed}\,or\,\frac{b}{c} = \frac{109}{36} = 3.0$$

The odds ratio for a matched case-control study is interpreted in the same way as for nonmatched data. The interpretation for the above study is that women in this study who had an ectopic pregnancy were 3 times as likely to have had a prior infection with chlamydia as were women in this study who had normal pregnancies. While the association is a strong one, it is still an estimate and should be further evaluated with a confidence interval or a *p*-value that uses only the discordant pairs (*McNemar's test*).[29]

Interrelationships Between Risk Factors

Odds ratios can also be used to determine whether interrelationships exist between various characteristics or risk factors. A case-control study of lung

TABLE 10.6 Case-Referent Results Estimating Risk Ratios for Developing Lung Cancer when Cigarette Smoking and Asbestos Exposures Are Combined

CIGARETTES SMOKED DAILY	ASBESTOS EXPOSURE			
	NONE	LITTLE	MODERATE	HEAVY
0 to 4	1.0	1.2	2.7	4.1
5 to 9	2.9	1.2	7.8	11.9
10 to 19	9.1	1.9	24.6	37.3
20 to 29	16.5	19.8	44.6	67.7
>30	90.3	108.4	243.8	370.2

SOURCE: Adapted from Kjuus et al. (1986).[30]

cancer, cigarette smoking, and asbestos exposure among workers exposed to multiple risk factors in southern Norway provides an example of this.[30] All cases of lung cancer in men during 1979 to 1983 were ascertained from two neighboring counties in that nation. Each case was matched to a similarly aged control from the same geographical area. All men with conditions that would have precluded possible employment in the industrial sector (not healthy enough for heavy work) were excluded from the study. The 176 cases and 176 controls were interviewed about their history of smoking and exposures to asbestos. The number of cigarettes smoked daily was categorized into five levels from none to more than 30 cigarettes per day. Asbestos exposure was coded into four categories from none to heavy. The estimated risk ratios for each category of asbestos exposure and smoking habit are shown in Table 10.6. The risk increases when either smoking or asbestos exposure rises. When the factors are considered together, the effect appears synergistic.

Effect of Misclassification

Misclassification of disease state, exposure, or both can occur in any type of epidemiologic study. In a case-control study, misclassification of a person's outcome status may alter their probability of entering the study, potentially leading to selection bias. Information bias may also occur because exposures in a case-control study often cannot be measured directly. School, employment, or other historical records may or may not be complete. The subject's recall for reporting employment, residential, pharmaceutical, or behavioral exposures may not be accurate. If the subject is deceased, information about exposures may have to be estimated by a spouse, close relative, or friend.

Misclassification of information can be non-differential or differential. *Non-differential misclassification* occurs when errors in information are randomly distributed among cases and controls. For instance, many persons will typically underreport their own abortion, drug abuse, or smoking histories, as well as their number of sexual partners. If the underreporting is randomly distributed among all subjects, the likelihood that an association between exposure and outcome will be found is generally reduced.[31] *Differential misclassification* occurs when the amount and direction of misclassification differs between cases and controls, thus increasing or decreasing the estimate of the odds ratio.[32] For example, the spouses of cirrhosis patients might overreport alcohol consumption (overestimating exposure in the cases will increase the OR), while the spouses of controls might underreport the same behavior (underestimating exposure in the controls will decrease the OR).

The epidemiologist minimizes the effects of misclassification by verifying all study information using every feasible means. Information on subjects' individual characteristics or previous exposures might be confirmed by obtaining records from independent sources (such as hospitals, physicians, schools, military services, or employment records). Disease outcomes should be verified by an independent review of medical records, diagnostic tests, disease registry entries, or death certificates. The degree to which the information can be verified will depend upon the outcomes and exposures of interest. For example, information gathered on an individual's past alcohol consumption or diet generally poses serious problems for verification. Using health insurance records of prior illness or drug prescriptions may reduce the possibility of disease or exposure misclassification. Biological markers, when available, may confirm exposures. For example, the presence of cotinine (a metabolite of nicotine) in the blood, urine, or saliva can serve as a biomarker indicating exposure to cigarette smoke.

Adjusting for Confounding Variables

The epidemiologist may be interested in evaluating multiple exposures as potential risk factors. For example, in a study of lung cancer, exposures of interest may include a history of cigarette smoking, exposure to asbestos, and use of alcohol. Statistical techniques are available that that allow the exposures to be evaluated separately and in various combinations, such as linear, multiple linear, log-linear, and multiple logistic regression.[33] Using these statistical methods, the epidemiologist can determine which variables have an independent association with the outcome and which interact with each other, and to quantify the relative contributions of the exposures to the risk of developing the outcome. Once again, it is important to remember that any identified statistical associations cannot, in and of themselves, lead to a causal inference (Chapter 4).

Variations on the Case-Control Design

The epidemiologist may implement a modified case-control design within a cohort study (see Chapter 9) to address the problem of expensive or difficult to obtain information about exposures for an entire cohort. When the outcome of interest is fairly common, the *case-cohort design* may be an option. In this design, the epidemiologist selects as the cases a group of subjects from the cohort who have developed the outcome; controls, however, are sampled from all remaining subjects in the cohort (not simply those that are disease-free) to represent the total at-risk population.[34–35]

An example of the case-cohort design comes from the Tobago Prostate Survey, a population-based prostate cancer screening program for men over 40 years of age living on that Caribbean island.[36] The screenings included a risk factor questionnaire, blood collection for various studies, and a digital rectal exam. The investigators were interested in determining whether previous exposure to human herpes virus 8 (HHV-8) was associated with developing prostate cancer. The case-cohort design included 96 incident cases of prostate cancer identified through the screening cohort and 415 randomly selected subjects from the remainder of the cohort to represent the at-risk group. The at-risk group included 25 incident prostate cancer cases. The investigators reported that HHV-8 exposure increased with age for all men in the study (40–49 years, 3.5%; 50–59 years, 13.6%; 60 + years, 22.9%) and that men with higher prostate specific antigen (PSA) values were more likely to have HHV-8 seropositivity than men with normal PSA values (OR = 3.96, 95% CI = 1.53,10.2). The study did not, however, find an association between HHV-8 seropositivity and prostate cancer.

When the outcome of interest is rare, the *nested case-control* design may be an appropriate alternative to a full cohort analysis. In the nested case-control design, the epidemiologist selects as the cases subjects in the cohort who have developed the rare outcome. Subjects without the outcome are selected from the same cohort as controls. The nested case-control design is efficient for a rare disease, and the odds ratio provides a reasonable estimate of the relative risk. The nested case-control design was used by Levin and colleagues to examine the relationship between exposure to Epstein-Barr virus (EBV) and the development of multiple sclerosis (MS) among a cohort of more than 3 million active and reserve US military personnel.[37] Beginning in 1988, all individuals inducted into the military gave blood samples upon entry and again at 2-year intervals. The blood samples were stored in a serum repository, but the cost of conducting analyses to determine viral exposures for all 3 million subjects would be cost prohibitive. Instead, the 83 subjects meeting the diagnostic criteria for MS and who had at least one blood sample were selected as the case group. Two controls were selected for each subject, matched by age, sex, race/ethnicity, and date of blood collection. The serum samples for all subjects in the nested-case control study were then tested for antibodies to EBV, and the results for the two groups were compared. Strong positive associations were found between the presence of antibodies and the development of MS.

As the subjects selected for the case-cohort and nested case-control designs come from the same cohort, selection bias is minimized. Since information about exposures is collected for these designs before any subject experiences the outcome, information bias is also minimized. As the case and control groups in these designs may be matched, confounding can also be controlled.

Summary

In a case-control study, the epidemiologist selects subjects with and without the outcome of interest, reconstructs each subject's history of past exposures, and compares the proportion of exposures among the cases with that among the controls. If these proportions are different, then a statistical association exists between the exposure and the outcome. Cases can be ascertained from hospitals, clinics, disease registries, or during a prevalence or incidence survey in a population. Controls can likewise be sampled from similar sources or by using a random sample of the population. To prevent selection bias that can lead to spurious associations, the epidemiologist may choose to match each case with one or more controls, either using a group or individual matching protocol. Matching provides a means of controlling for known confounders, but the ability to generalize the findings to the general population is diminished. Data collection should be done equally for both cases and controls and should be independently verified whenever possible.

The measure of the strength of an association in a case-control study is the odds ratio, an estimate of the relative risk that can be calculated for both matched and unmatched designs. Misclassification of either the presence or absence of disease, or of exposure status, can affect the estimate of the odds ratio. Confounding factors can also affect the estimate. Statistical techniques such as the Mantel-Haenszel test and logistic regression can be used to adjust for confounding factors in the data analysis. However, such statistical techniques cannot make up for errors in study design or data collection. Another measure of association is the population attributable fraction, the proportion of the outcome of interest that is associated with various exposures.

Case-control studies have advantages over cohort studies in that they are generally lower in cost, require a shorter time to complete, and provide the ability to examine the relationship between a known health outcome and multiple risk factors. The design is particularly well suited for the study of rare health outcomes that are linked to environmental, drug, or treatment exposures, as they may lead to prompt public health or medical interventions.

On the other hand, the case-control design may prove problematic for determining whether the exposure preceded the disease. These studies are also subject to selection, recall, and misclassification biases. Well-designed case-control studies can minimize the introduction of biases, but the potential for their effect on results must be considered for each study question.

References

1. This quotation uses archaic terminology. Case-control studies were historically considered retrospective, while cohort studies were considered prospective by design.
2. Harold Fred Dorn, "Some Problems Arising in Prospective and Retrospective Studies of the Etiology of Disease," *New England Journal of Medicine* 261, no. 12 (1959): 571–579.
3. Eugene S. Hurwitz et al., "Public Health Service Study on Reye's Syndrome and Medications. Report of the Pilot Phase," *New England Journal of Medicine* 313, no. 14 (1985): 849–857.
4. Jerome Cornfield, "A Method of Estimating Comparative Rates from Clinical Data; Applications to Cancer of the Lung, Breast, and Cervix," *Journal of the National Cancer Institute* 11, no. 6 (1951): 1269–1275.
5. Eugene S. Hurwitz et al., "Public Health Service Study of Reye's Syndrome and Medications: Report of the Main Study," *Journal of the American Medical Association*. 257, no. 14 (1987): 1905–1911.
6. Stolley P. D., Tonascia J. A., Sartwell P. E., et al. "Agreement Rates between Oral Contraceptive Users and Prescribers in Relation to Drug Use Histories," *American Journal of Epidemiology* 107, no. 3 (1978): 226–235.
7. Ronald J. Waldman et al., "Aspirin as a Risk Factor in Reye's Syndrome," *Journal of the American Medical Association* 247, no. 22 (1982): 3089–3094.
8. Thomas J. Halpin et al., "Reye's Syndrome and Medication Use," *Journal of the American Medical Association* 248, no. 6 (1982): 687–691.

9. Food and Drug Administration, "Labeling for Oral and Rectal Over-the-Counter Drug Products Containing Aspirin and Nonaspirin Salicylates; Reye's Syndrome Warning. Final Rule," *Federal Register* 68, no. 74 (2003): 18861.

10. Fajo-Pascual M, Godoy P, Ferrero-Cancer M, et al. "Case-Control Study of Risk Factors for Sporadic Campylobacter Infections in Northeastern Spain," *European Journal of Public Health* 20, no. 4 (2010): 443–448.

11. Gail M, Williams R, David P. Byar, et al. "How Many Controls?" *Journal of Chronic Diseases* 29, no. 11 (1976): 723–731.

12. Cochran W. G., "Some Methods for Strengthening the Common χ 2 Tests," *Biometrics* 10, no. 4 (1954): 417–451.

13. Nathan Mantel, William Haenszel. "Statistical Aspects of the Analysis of Data from Retrospective Studies of Disease," *Journal of the National Cancer Institute* 22, no. 4 (1959): 719–748.

14. W. A. Guy, "On the Nature and Extent of the Benefits Conferred by Hospitals on the Working Classes and the Poor," *Journal of the Statistical Society of London.* 1856; 19 no. 1): 12–27.

15. Joseph Berkson, "Limitations of the Application of Fourfold Table Analysis to Hospital Data," *Biometrics* (1946): 2 no. 3): 47–53.

16. R. R. Monson, *Occupational Epidemiology, 2nd Edition.* Boca Raton, Florida: CRC Press, 1990.

17. Irwin D. J. Bross, "Effect of Filter Cigarettes on the Risk of Lung Cancer," *National Cancer Institute Monograms* 28 (1968): 35–40.

18. Irwin D. J. Bross and John Tidings, "Another Look at Coffee Drinking and Cancer of the Urinary Bladder," *Preventive Medicine* 2, no. 3 (1973): 445–451.

19. Morton L. Levin, Hyman Goldstein, and Paul R. Gerhardt, "Cancer and Tobacco Smoking; A Preliminary Report," *Journal of the American Medical Association* 143, no. 4 (1950): 336–338.

20. Slone Epidemiology Center, "Research Studies," Boston University School of Medicine, Boston, Massachusetts. Available at http://www.bu.edu/slone/research/studies/.

21. Collaborative Group for the Study of Stroke in Young Women, "Oral Contraceptives and Increased Risk of Cerebral Ischemia or Thrombosis," *New England Journal of Medicine* 288, no. 17 (1973): 871–878.

22. J. I. Mann et al., "Myocardial Infarction in Young Women with Special Reference to Oral Contraceptive Practice," *British Medical Journal* 2, no. 5965 (1975): 241–245.

23. David B. Thomas, "Relationship of Oral Contraceptives to Cervical Carcinogenesis," *Obstetrics and Gynecology* 40, no. 4 (1972): 508–518.

24. M. P. Vessey and Richard Doll, "Investigation of Relation between Use of Oral Contraceptives and Thromboembolic Disease," *British Medical Journal* 2, no. 5599 (1968): 199–205.

25. Roger Glass R, Brenda Johnson, and Martin Vessey, "Accuracy of Recall of Histories of Oral Contraceptive Use," *British Journal of Preventive & Social Medicine* 28, no. 4 (1974): 273–275.

26. Martin Lajous et al., "Determinants of Prevalence, Acquisition, and Persistence of Human Papillomavirus in Healthy Mexican Military Men," *Cancer Epidemiology, Biomarkers & Prevention* 14, no. 7 (2005): 1710–1716.

27. K. McPherson et al., "Early Oral Contraceptive Use and Breast Cancer: Results of Another Case-Control Study," *British Journal of Cancer* 56, no. 5 (1987): 653–660.

28. Joan M. Chow et al., "The Association between *Chlamydia trachomatis* and Ectopic Pregnancy. A Matched-Pair, Case-Control Study," *Journal of the American Medical Association* 263, no. 23 (1990): 3164–3167.

29. Steve Selvin, *Statistical Analysis of Epidemiologic Data, 3rd Edition*. New York: Oxford University Press, 2005.

30. Helge Kjuus et al., "A Case-Referent Study of Lung Cancer, Occupational Exposures and Smoking. II. Role of Asbestos Exposure," *Scandinavian Journal of Work, Environment & Health* 12, no. 3 (1986): 203–209.

31. Mustafa Dosemeci, Sholom Wacholder, and Jay H. Lubin, "Does Nondifferential Misclassification of Exposure Always Bias a True Effect Toward the Null Value?" *American Journal of Epidemiology* 132, no. 4 (1990): 746–748.

32. James J. Schlesselman, *Case-Control Studies: Design, Conduct, Analysis (Monographs in Epidemiology and Biostatistics)*. New York: Oxford University Press, 1982.

33. David G. Kleinbaum, Lawrence L. Kupper, and Hal Morgenstern, *Epidemiologic Research: Principles and Quantitative Methods (Industrial Health & Safety)*. Wiley; 1982.

34. Sander Greenland, "Adjustment of Risk Ratios in Case-Base Studies (Hybrid Epidemiologic Designs)," *Statistics in Medicine* 5, no. 6 (1986): 579–584.

35. Tosiya Sato, "Risk Ratio Estimation in Case-Cohort Studies," *Environmental Health Perspectives* 102, Supplement 8 (1994): 53–56.

36. A. C. McDonald et al., "A Case-Cohort Study of Human Herpesvirus 8 Seropositivity and Incident Prostate Cancer in Tobago," *Infectious Agents and Cancer* 6, (2011): 25, doi:10.1186/1750-9378-6-25. Available at http://www.ncbi.nlm.nih.gov/pubmed/22151996.

37. L. I. Levin et al., "Multiple Sclerosis and Epstein-Barr Virus," *Journal of the American Medical Association* 289, no. 12 (2003): 1533–1536.

Problem Set: Chapter 10

1. During the conduct of TEEN HELP (See questions, Chapter 9), Dr. Now and Superintendent Kwiet regularly met with many of the parents of participating students. At one such meeting, the parent of a student athlete pulled Dr. Now aside and asked if the health department would be investigating sports injuries. "Why?" Dr. Now asked. "My son is a pitcher on the varsity baseball team and he's had a series of knee injuries. We all know about arm and elbow injuries, but no one seems to believe his knee injuries could have anything to do with baseball. Yet, seven or eight of his teammates have had knee injuries in the past year and three of them are pitchers. That sounds suspicious to me, and anything you could do to help investigate this would be appreciated."

   Dr. Now approached Superintendent Kwiet about the knee injuries among baseball players. The superintendent thought that the health department should investigate, but there was not enough time to do another TEEN HELP if they wanted to make any changes during the current baseball season. "I think," said

Dr. Now, "we could conduct a case-control study in the next 4 weeks. That would give us enough information to let the baseball coach know that something needs to be done differently."

The health department contacted the pediatricians, orthopedic surgeons, and radiologists in the town to identify all male adolescents with knee injuries. Controls were a random sample of all male adolescents in the same county. The results are shown below:

SCHOOL ATHLETIC ACTIVITY	KNEE INJURIES	CONTROLS
Baseball Pitchers	13	7
Non-pitching Baseball Players	17	13
Other School Athletic Activity	22	40
No School Athletic Activity	23	70
Total	75	130

"That's interesting," said the superintendent. "The incidence of knee injuries among the pitchers is 13 out of 20, but ..." Dr. Now cut off the superintendent: "This is a different type of study, and you can't calculate incidence rates or anything like them. We have two separate groups of students, and we can only compare what's happened in one group with the others. We need to look at the odds ratios to see what the associations might be."

a. Calculate the odds ratios using male adolescents having no school athletic activity as the comparison group.

b. What are the population attributable fractions (PAFs) for these different groups of school athletes? Interpret these findings.

"Wow," said the superintendent when presented with these findings. "We need to do something. Are those odds ratios like the relative risks in TEEN HELP?" "I'm not sure," said Dr. Now. "They may be if the incidence of knee injuries in the male adolescent population is rare enough. Even if they're not rare, those odds ratios are well above 3.0 for baseball-associated activities. We need to have a talk with all of the school baseball coaches and the principals to see if there's something we can do to protect those boys' knees."

11 | Experimental Studies

RANDOMIZED CONTROLLED TRIALS

> By the allocation of the patients to the two groups we want to
> ensure that these two groups are alike except in treatment . . .
> this might be done, with reasonably large numbers, by a random
> division of the patients.[1]
>
> *A. Bradford Hill (1937)*

IN EXPERIMENTAL STUDIES, THE EPIDEMIOLOGIST controls the assignment of subjects to the study groups either as controls or as exposed to one or more treatments or levels of treatment. Having control of the experiment allows the investigator to prospectively evaluate how the groups respond to different preventive or therapeutic treatments. This chapter covers *randomized controlled trials* in which each individual in the study is randomly assigned to a treatment group. Chapter 12 will deal with *community* or *cluster randomized trials* in which groups of individuals are assigned to various treatment groups. By convention, all participants in randomized controlled trials are referred to as *subjects* regardless of whether or not they are patients under the care of a health care provider.

Randomized controlled trials include *prevention* (*prophylactic*) trials, used to determine the safety and efficacy of an agent for preventing disease. They also encompass *intervention trials* that target individuals with characteristics that increase the risk of developing a particular health outcome, and *therapeutic trials* that evaluate whether an agent or procedure can cure a disease, relieve its symptoms, or prolong the survival of those suffering from it.

An example of a therapeutic trial comes from a study of the efficacy of human embryonic dopamine neurons for Parkinson's disease. Subjects with Parkinson's disease were randomized to receive either an implantation of this material or a sham procedure in which burr holes were drilled into the skull but no implantation was performed. The younger subjects in the treatment group for this small (n = 40) randomized trial experienced some benefit, but the older patients did not.[2] Another example of a therapeutic trial compared two procedures for subjects with diabetic retinopathy (damaged blood vessels in the retina).[3] Each of 3,711 subjects was subjected to laser treatments (photocoagulation therapy) in an experiment where their eyes were randomized, so that one eye received treatment early in the course of the disease and the other eye was treated later. Five years later there was a 29 percent decrease in the incidence of severe visual loss in the eye treated earlier in the course of the disease.[4]

It may be difficult to classify some types of randomized controlled trials as purely preventive, intervention, or therapeutic. Consider the Justification for the Use of Statins in Prevention: an Intervention Trial Evaluating Rosuvastatin (JUPITER) study. In this study subjects with high C-reactive protein levels (an independent risk factor for cardiovascular disease) who did not have hyperlipidemia were randomized to receive either the drug rosuvastatin or a placebo. Subjects who received the drug treatment experienced a 47 percent reduction in the occurrence of myocardial infarction, stroke, or death from cardiovascular causes compared to the placebo group.[5] The study results demonstrated the need for physicians to intervene to reduce high C-reactive protein levels among their patients, even those without elevated serum lipid levels. While labeled an intervention trial, it is also clearly a therapeutic one.

The randomized controlled trial design can be used to determine whether reducing or eliminating a behavior suspected as being of etiologic importance is effective. The Finnish Diabetes Prevention Study provides an excellent example of an intervention study that is also a cessation experiment.[6] To determine the effect of lifestyle intervention on the development of Type II diabetes mellitus, 523 subjects with impaired glucose tolerance (at high risk for developing diabetes) were randomly allocated into two groups. One group received individualized counseling aimed at reducing weight, total intake of fat, intake of saturated fat, and increasing intake of fiber and physical activity; the control group received no such advice. The intervention group experienced average weight loss of 4.2 kg compared with an average loss of 0.8 kg in the control group after one year, and 3.5 kg and 0.8 kg, respectively, at the end of two years. The study demonstrated that cessation of a relatively high fat diet and a sedentary lifestyle resulted in a 58 percent reduction in the occurrence of Type II diabetes mellitus in the intervention group (4-year incidence of 11 percent in the treatment group and 23 percent in the control group).

The Physicians' Health Study is a similar example of a randomized controlled prevention trial. It involved 22,071 physicians and was designed for the purposes of determining whether low-dose aspirin consumption reduces total cardiovascular mortality and whether beta-carotene decreases cancer incidence in a healthy population.[7] The trial found a 39 percent decline in nonfatal myocardial infarction rates in the group that took aspirin compared with the control group but no effect for the beta-carotene. The results led the US Preventive Services Task Force and American Heart Association to recommend low-dose aspirin for the primary prevention of cardiovascular disease and for the secondary prevention of myocardial infarction and occlusive stroke.[8] These recommendations were subsequently amended to reflect the risk of gastric bleeding from aspirin therapy in some individuals.[9]

Randomized Controlled Trial Designs

Several designs have evolved for conducting randomized controlled trials: *clinical trials* (*parallel trials*), *factorial trials,* and *crossover trials.*

Clinical Trials

Clinical trials are widely used in medicine to assess *efficacy*, in other words, whether a therapeutic agent or procedure produces a desired effect. Whether a randomized design is appropriate often depends upon the developmental stage of a new therapy. For instance, *Phase 0 trials* are exploratory trials with *investigational new drugs* (IND). Such trials serve as first-in-human studies, using only a few healthy individuals to determine how the biological effects of an untested drug can be assessed. As Phase 0 trials do not have control subjects, they cannot be randomized.[10]

Phase I trials usually enroll fewer than 100 healthy volunteers to determine the safety and mode of action of the new treatment. This phase allows the dosage of the new treatment to be determined and to identify potential side effects. Subjects in Phase I trials may or may not be randomized to include a control group consisting of patients who receive either a treatment considered standard-of-care or, if there is no known treatment, a placebo.

Phase II trials test the efficacy of a new treatment in 100 to 300 subjects and compare the results from the treatment group to a group receiving the existing standard of care. Again, if no standard of care exists then the design may use a placebo as the comparative treatment. Phase II trials are increasingly, but not always, randomized.[11] A treatment may not show a statistically significant benefit at the conclusion of a Phase II trial. Rather, the purpose of these trials is to suggest that a treatment benefit may be present and, if so, how large a randomized controlled trial would be needed to conclusively demonstrate that benefit.

Phase III trials usually involve large numbers of subjects who are randomly assigned to the treatment and control groups (*arms* of the study). Phase III trials are definitive randomized controlled trials designed to assess the efficacy and safety of the new treatment. When the treatment being tested is a pharmaceutical, a Phase III trial is sometimes referred to as a *pivotal trial* or a *registrational trial*. If the results of a Phase III trial support both safety and efficacy, the new treatment may be approved for use by regulatory authorities.

Finally, *Phase IV trials* provide a follow-up of subjects after the new treatment has been approved by regulators and is in real-world use. Phase IV trials allow for determining long-term effects of the treatment and may even suggest potential new uses for the therapy.[11]

Registries of randomized controlled trials have been created to enable potential subjects with particular diseases to more easily find and enroll in these studies. The results of clinical trials are sufficiently important that in 2005, the International Committee of Medical Journal Editors (ICMJE), an organization of editors of more than a dozen of the largest medical journals worldwide, announced it would no longer publish the results of clinical trials not listed in a public-access randomized controlled trial registry. The World Health Organization maintains a global registry of clinical trials,[12] and regional registries also exist. These include but are not limited to the Pan African Clinical Trials Registry[13] and the European Union Clinical Trials Database (EudraCT).[14] In the United States, the National Library of Medicine (NLM) began a clinical trials registry for AIDS treatments; the registry gradually expanded so that it now includes all randomized controlled trials.[15] A private not-for-profit organization also supports voluntary registration of all randomized controlled trials using an International Standard Randomised Controlled Trial Number (ISRCTN) Register.[16] A list of all clinical trial registries is maintained by a human rights organization, Citizens for Responsible Care and Research, Inc. (CIRCARE).[17]

Factorial Trials

In a factorial trial, each subject is randomly assigned to a group that receives a specified ordering or combination of treatments. The factorial design has the advantage of allowing the epidemiologist to investigate several hypotheses simultaneously and determine possible interactions between treatments.

A classic example of a 2 × 2 factorial design is the Age-Related Eye Disease Study (AREDS), which examined the effect of high doses of zinc and antioxidant vitamins (vitamins C and E, and beta-carotene) on the progression of age-related macular degeneration (AMD).[18] The 3,640 subjects enrolled in this double-blind, placebo-controlled clinical trial were randomly assigned to one of four arms of the study: (1) both zinc and antioxidant vitamins, (2) zinc only, (3) antioxidant vitamins only, and (4) neither zinc nor antioxidant vitamins. The study found that the combination of antioxidant vitamins and minerals demonstrated an approximately 25% reduction in risk of developing advanced AMD at 5 years. The trial was then stopped and the AREDS formulation recommended for persons at high risk for AMD.[19]

The factorial design was possible for the AREDS study because the number of available subjects was large and the incidence of expected outcomes high. It follows that when the number of potential subjects for a study is limited (such as for a rare disease or condition), the factorial design will fail to detect statistically significant differences between the groups.

Crossover Trials

In a crossover trial, each subject in the study receives both the treatment and the comparator in a random sequence, each subject serving as his/her own control. An example of a crossover trial comes from a study to determine patient preference for one of two drugs formulated to treat advanced renal cell carcinoma (RCC). Of 169 patients with RCC, 114 met the criteria for treatment with either drug. The subjects were randomized to receive either (a) a therapeutic course of pazopanib, followed by a two-week *washout period* (the time of no treatment), and then a therapeutic course of sunitinib; or (b) the same treatments but in reverse order. Outcomes were assessed using a health-related quality of life (HRQoL) questionnaire. Subjects preferred pazopanib over sunitinib (70% vs 22%, with 8% of the subjects expressing no preference; $p < 0.001$) because they claimed the former treatment led to less fatigue, less diarrhea, and a better overall quality of life.[20]

Conducting a Randomized Controlled Trial

Conducting a randomized controlled trial begins by drafting a formal *protocol* which contains the *objectives* and *specific procedures* to be used in the trial. The protocol must be written before the start of the trial and should contain information on the methods for selecting and allocating subjects to the study groups. It must specify how the data will be collected, details on

the performance of any laboratory or other tests, and details on the administration of the therapy, intervention, or preventive treatment. Several guides
to drafting a protocol exist, and the interested reader should consult them
directly.[21] Once the protocol is written, the epidemiologist compiles a *manual
of procedures* (MOP). If situations arise during the trial, the manual is ref-
erenced for what the investigator must do. The epidemiologist must also
draft a *statistical analysis plan*, in which all aspects of data analysis are specified before the first subject is recruited. In the United States, the European
Union, and Japan, randomized controlled trials with drugs in development
must be conducted in compliance with *Current Good Clinical Practices*
(cGCP) guidance.

Subject Recruitment

The protocol should define the characteristics of the population to be studied (*the reference population*), taking into account the purpose of the study and
any anticipated difficulties in subject recruitment. *Inclusion criteria* are those
characteristics that qualify individuals for participating in the study; *exclusion criteria* are those that preclude individuals from participating. Inclusion
and exclusion criteria are often related to age and gender, type and stage of a
disease, particular risk factors, and previous or existing medical conditions or
medications. For example, a Phase II trial tested a new drug treatment (imatinib) for patients with acute lymphoblastic leukemia (ALL) who had a recurrence of their disease after initial treatment or who did not have a response
to treatment (*refractory disease*).[22] The trial set inclusion criteria as male or
female patients at least 18 years of age with a diagnosis of relapsed or refractory ALL and who had adequate liver function. Exclusion criteria included
prior treatment within 21 days, incomplete recovery from stem cell therapy, or
a history of noncompliance. Trial results indicated that the drug had low tox-
icity and induced a pronounced but brief therapeutic response. The research
team suggested the drug could provide *palliative* (symptom relief) therapy but
not curative treatment for this difficult and rapidly fatal disease.

Sample Size and Statistical Power

How many subjects are needed to detect a difference between the groups
receiving the new treatment and the comparator (standard of care or placebo
group)? One approach to setting the sample size is to specify some *parameters*
or qualities of the trial that will not be changed once the trial begins.[11] These
include the minimum difference in the size of the effect expected between the
treatment and comparative groups (*delta*), the *power* of the study to demonstrate

an association if one exists $(1-\beta)$, and the epidemiologist's willingness to be wrong in drawing statistical conclusions (the *level of significance* or α).

Consider a proposed clinical trial for a new drug to treat an aggressive and fatal disease. The study protocol defines success as increasing survival from the disease by at least 50 percent for at least one calendar year after the treatment begins. At the beginning of the trial, the epidemiologist assumes there is no difference between the treatment groups (the *null hypothesis*). At the end of the trial, there will be four possible outcomes, two of which are correct and two of which are not (Figure 11.1). Specifically, if the null hypothesis is true and the trial demonstrated no difference, then the epidemiologist would be correct in concluding there is no difference between treatments. If the null hypothesis is false (there really is a difference) and the study found a 50 percent reduction in mortality between the treatment groups, the epidemiologist would be correct in rejecting the null hypothesis.

Now consider the two instances where the outcomes of the trial could be in error. If the data indicated a false positive result (suggesting an efficacious treatment that in reality is not), then a *Type I error* (α-error) would lead to an incorrect conclusion. Alternatively, if the data gave a false negative result (failing to find a treatment effect that truly exists), then a *Type II error* (β-error) occurred.

If the epidemiologist sets the probability of a Type I error (α, the level of statistical significance) at 5 percent, then the chance of drawing a correct inference when the null hypothesis is true is 95 percent. If the epidemiologist sets the probability of a Type II error at 20 percent, the chance of drawing a correct inference when the null hypothesis is false is 80 percent ($1-\beta$ or the *power* of the study to detect a difference). Although the epidemiologist may be satisfied with

NULL HYPOTHESIS

H_0 : TREATMENT A = TREATMENT B

Decision on H_0	True No Difference	False Difference
Fail to Reject	Correct $1-\alpha$	Type II Error β
Reject	Type I Error (Level of Significance) α	Correct (Power) $1-\beta$

FIGURE 11.1 Possible outcomes of an experimental epidemiologic study design.

the power of a trial being as low as 60 percent, typically clinical trials are powered at 80 percent or more, because the consequences of inadequate power to detect a true difference may be profound. In one instance, an outbreak of surgical wound infections was attributed to the use of an ineffective prophylactic antibiotic. The clinical trial suggesting the antibiotic was efficacious had a sample size that was simply too small to demonstrate such efficacy. The result of the trial led to surgical complications that could have been avoided.[23]

The chances of committing Type I and Type II errors are inversely linked (when the chance for one type of error is decreased, the other is increased). Two ways exist to decrease both types of errors simultaneously: (1) Increase the size of the minimum effect (*delta*) that the trial will detect, or (2) increase the sample size. Tables are available for calculating the number of subjects needed for a randomized controlled trial,[24] as are various proprietary computer programs and free Web-based software. Using these tools, the epidemiologist can adjust the parameters of the study during the drafting of the study protocol.

Once the parameters of the trials are set, plans for recruiting subjects to the trial must be followed from the protocol. If it is not possible to enroll a sufficient number of subjects from one location, a multicenter randomized controlled trial design may be required. When a multicenter approach is employed, the epidemiologist must be careful in assuring that randomization does not result in most or all of the controls being recruited from only a few centers while those subjects receiving the active treatment come from all centers. When possible, the epidemiologist may elect to consider each center as its own stratum, both for randomization and during study analysis.

A second approach to dealing with limited numbers of subjects is using historical controls for the comparative group. These may include subjects serving as controls in a previous randomized controlled trial or observational study, or they might be the same group of subjects serving as their own historical controls. The use of historical controls as the comparison group may be acceptable if the outcome is sufficiently rare, the number of subjects is limited, or if the previous standard of care or the lack of any treatment resulted in a high case-fatality rate. In most instances, however, the epidemiologist avoids using historical controls. Not only may the practice result in misleading inferences, it may convert the study design from an experimental to an observational one.

Informed Consent

The conduct of a randomized controlled trial requires obtaining the *informed consent* of the potential study subjects before they enroll. Each subject must be informed of the purpose of the trial, the risks of using the treatment or intervention, the possible benefits of the treatment or intervention, and that they will be randomly assigned to either a treatment or a control group. Subjects must also be informed that they may withdraw at any time without effect on their care, and they must be given the name and contact information of the appropriate investigator to contact with any questions. If, after being provided with this information, the subject elects to participate in the study, they are said to have given their informed consent.

Informed consent must be obtained in writing in accordance with government regulations and rules of the institution(s) where the trial is to be conducted. In the case of minors or those unable to give informed consent, the investigator may need to obtain informed consent from a parent or guardian as well as *assent* from the potential subject. This will be determined after consideration of the study protocol, subject recruitment procedures, and data collection instruments by *Institutional Review Boards* (governed by US Federal Regulations) or *Research Ethics Committees* (the accepted global term) where the investigators conduct the trial.

Understanding the need for protecting human subjects in experimental trials requires a bit of historical context. After World War II, Nazi biomedical researchers were prosecuted for their abuses against prisoners in concentration camps during the war. Those abuses led to the development of the Nuremberg Code, a statement of the core ethical principles underlying the use of human subjects in experimentation. These principles include:

- *Respect for persons.* Each individual subject must be considered autonomous, able to make decisions about whether or not to participate in the research based on an informed consent process. Those who cannot make autonomous decisions must be protected from activities that may harm them.
- *Beneficence.* Investigators and their institutions are obligated to maximize the benefits and minimize the risks (economic, legal, physical, psychological, and social) of their research to subjects, their families, and society at large.
- *Justice.* The risks and benefits of research should be balanced. Research is not considered just when only one group of persons are selected for research, or if benefits will only accrue to groups selectively favored. Vulnerable populations such as those institutionalized or incarcerated, minorities, or the very sick may need to be protected.

Among several early notorious clinical experiments, the Tuskegee study stands out. The study started in Alabama during the 1930s, enrolling 301 black sharecroppers with syphilis and 299 black sharecroppers without the infection. The syphilitic subjects were told they had "bad blood" and were followed to observe the natural history of the disease.[25] When a treatment for syphilis became available (i.e., penicillin), it was withheld to allow the disease to manifest through to death. A national uproar ensued when the study came to light in 1972, and the study was found to be unethical.[26] In response, Congress established the framework under which clinical research in the United States has since been conducted. That framework is provided in the 1978 Belmont Report; it requires obtaining informed consent for participation from subjects and obligates the investigator to provide at least the standard of care to subjects in a research study.[27] This requirement has been incorporated into the cGCP guidance.

Randomization

In a randomized controlled trial, the treatment and comparison groups should be comparable in all respects except for use of the treatment being studied. This is achieved by using inclusion and exclusion criteria to match subjects for known factors, and by the use of random assignment to address unknown factors. Randomization helps to ensure that the distribution of *all* factors—known and unknown, measurable and not measurable—is based on chance. It helps ensure that both conscious and subconscious biases are avoided in the allocation of individuals to the treatment or comparison groups.

Simple random assignment can be achieved by the use of shuffled envelopes or other means of randomly assigning subjects to treatment groups. The process can be refined by *block randomization* or *stratification*. When an individual falls within a certain block or stratum (usually defined by demographic characteristics such as sex or age group), they are randomly assigned to either the treatment or the comparison group reflecting that stratum. Participants may also be classified by severity of disease and then randomly assigned to treatment or comparison groups to ensure approximately equal numbers in each category of severity. One study group receives the new treatment, preventive agent, or whatever type of intervention is under investigation. The other, the comparison group, receives the standard of care (control) treatment. Since potential study subjects may hesitate to participate if they do not think they have a high enough chance of receiving the new treatment, it is not unusual to design a clinical trial so that several subjects will receive the intervention for every subject receiving the standard of care treatment.

Data Collection and Management

The randomized controlled trial design requires that observations be made for each individual subject. In some situations the subject serves as the observer (such as in assessing pain); in other situations a health care provider assesses whether the individual's health status has been altered or if the disease has been prevented. The observer's knowledge of the subject's group assignment may introduce either a conscious or unconscious bias in thee assessment of treatment effect. To remove this potential source of bias in the observations, the protocol may call for a *single, double,* or *triple blinding* (*masking*) strategy for data collection and review.[28]

In a single-blinded study the subjects do not know their group assignment, so they will not introduce bias into their own observations; this is often accomplished by means of a *placebo*. Placebos mimic the effect of treatment, perhaps as an inert pill, a saline injection, or even sham surgery (as described above). The *placebo effect* has been widely studied, particularly for showing that individuals' perception of pain and other symptoms is influenced by their beliefs about which treatment they may have received.[29]

Double blinding prevents both the subject and the observer from knowing the subject's group assignment. This strategy is designed to ensure both equal treatment and unbiased assessment. Triple blinding goes one step further, in that neither the subject, the observer, nor the person reviewing the data know each subject's group assignment. This ensures that data collection and management are unbiased, along with group assignment and care.

Once collected, maintaining the integrity of the data is a key aspect of clinical trial design.[28] As required by the cGCP, the epidemiologist must be certain that the data from the trial are accurately recorded and correctly transferred from one data storage medium to another. To aid in this effort, all research data collection forms should have clear instructions, and both data entry and transfer should only be done through established protocols. One way of assuring that the integrity of the data has not been violated is to have a group of epidemiologists or biostatisticians who are not involved in the trial conduct an audit of the data.

Data Monitoring Committees

Of particular note in the Belmont Report is the requirement of the investigator to assess *equipoise,* namely that the potential risks of a study are at least equal to if not outweighed by the potential benefit of the treatment. Properly conducted randomized controlled trials begin with equipoise because one treatment has not been established as better than another. As the study progresses, however, data may reveal that equipoise is no longer present, particularly if there are adverse events reported from the treatment or if the treatment shows a clear benefit relative to the standard of care. For this reason, cGCP requires that randomized controlled trials use a *Data Monitoring Committee* (DMC) or *Data Safety and Monitoring Board*—a group of experts with the job of reviewing data accumulating from one or more clinical trials—on a regular basis. The DMC operates under a charter, a document detailing its membership, operation, and responsibilities. If the DMC determines that equipoise is in jeopardy, it may require a change in protocol to ensure that equipoise remains present. If the DMC determines that equipoise is no longer present, it may declare that continuing the trial is unethical and impose a halt.

Maintaining Compliance (Reliability)

The epidemiologist cannot be certain that a treatment is or is not effective unless ensured that the treatment group is actually receiving the prescribed treatment. Thus, some clinical trials require that compliance with therapy be assessed throughout the trial.[30] Enrolling only subjects that meet minimum standards of reliability is one way to maximize compliance. Exclusion criteria can be used to keep out individuals unlikely or unable to be compliant with the treatment, such as homeless persons, alcoholics, or the mentally ill. In other instances such individuals do qualify as subjects for randomized controlled trials; however, their compliance needs to be closely monitored. *Directly observed therapy* (DOT), in which a health care provider or other designated individual (excluding a family member) provides the treatment (usually a medication) and verifies subject compliance (usually by watching the subject swallow every dose) is an example of such an approach. This strategy has been used in randomized controlled trials of treatments for hepatitis C in a prison population in Spain,[31] of depression among HIV positive homeless individuals in San Francisco,[32] and for multidrug-resistant tuberculosis among subjects in Ukraine.[33,34]

When patients are likely to be compliant, a common strategy for documenting their compliance is to rely on a *pill count*. Subjects may be given more pills than needed for a given time period, instructed to return the unused pills at their next visit, and then the unused pills are counted by the health care provider (such as for extended periods of travel where the medications may not be able to be refilled). This strategy should never be used with unreliable subjects, especially if the medications have a street value (such as opiates). In those instances it is important to ensure that the subject returns for evaluation by dispensing only a limited amount of the medication.

Sometimes the epidemiologist can assess compliance by measuring the metabolites of the treatment (or lack thereof) in a biologic (blood or urine) specimen. An example of metabolic assessment of compliance comes from the Bath Breakfast Project, where about 70 men and women were randomized to either a large breakfast or overnight fasting until noon each day in a free-living environment.[35] Each subject's energy intake was measured by a food diary, and their energy expenditure was measured by heart rate/accelerometry during the first and last weeks of a six-week trial. Continuous glucose monitors measured both glycemic response to the treatment and compliance. The study reported that eating a daily breakfast was causally linked to higher physical activity thermogenesis in lean adults but with no change in resting metabolism. Importantly, cardiovascular health was unaffected by either treatment.

Data Analysis

The epidemiologist begins data analysis for a randomized controlled trial by comparing the characteristics of the treatment groups at baseline. If the groups are reasonably balanced in terms of characteristics, the data should then be assessed for internal consistency and for any patterns that may help interpret or explain potential findings. The next step is often comparing information, obtained at the time of enrollment, on the group of dropouts and persons lost to follow-up with that for all subjects who remained until the end of the trial. All subjects should also be assessed for compliance with the treatment protocols.

The standard analysis for randomized controlled trials focuses on the *intent to treat* (ITT) study population, which includes all subjects randomized for the trial, even if they were noncompliant, dropped out, or crossed over to another treatment. ITT is considered a pragmatic approach to statistical analysis from clinical trials, as it assumes that people are autonomous, making decisions about their lives in the real world rather than as part of a controlled experiment. To determine the impact of excluding those who did not complete the trial on the overall trial result, a *sensitivity analysis* may be done, first by assuming that all those who did not complete the trial had the worst possible outcome and, then, by assuming they had the best possible outcome (creating a range of results).

Another approach used to assess the results of a randomized controlled trial is the *number needed to treat* (NNT), the reciprocal of the difference in treatment effect. NNT may be explained as the average number of persons needed to be treated with the new treatment rather than the standard treatment to prevent one bad outcome. It provides the health care provider or insurer with an easily understood result, since a low NNT (in the absence of side effects) means a high treatment benefit. Treatments with a high NNT may be precluded from insurance coverage, as the costs may outweigh the benefits.

When analyzing for treatment effects, the epidemiologist may choose to conduct *time-to-event* (*survival*) analyses. These methods take into account *censored* data (information on subjects available only for an interval of time during the study) as well as information on those who complete the entire trial. Time-to-event analyses often use the *Kaplan-Meier approach* and their results shown as *survival curves* (*plots*). The Kaplan-Meier approach is a nonparametric technique focusing on the *median survival times* of the treatment groups, differences that can be tested using a *log-rank test*. Survival times can also be assessed using *Cox proportional hazard models*. These semi-parametric regression models yield *hazard ratios* (conceptually similar to the relative risk) with confidence intervals. The epidemiologist uses these measures to statistically assess the differences in survival times while adjusting for covariates of interest. The intricacies of these statistical techniques are beyond the scope of this text, and interested readers should seek additional resources to learn more about them.[36-37]

Reporting the Results

While randomized controlled trials are purported to be the gold standard in epidemiology, some investigators lack the ability to clearly explain the design, methods, and analysis of their trials when publishing their results. In 1996 a group of 30 medical journal editors, epidemiologists, and leaders in the conduct of such trials developed the *Consolidated Standards of Reporting Trials* (CONSORT) statement, which included a checklist and flow diagram (*CONSORT figure*) to aid authors in clearly reporting the enrollment, allocation, and follow-up methods used in the trial, along with the details of the statistical analysis and results. The CONSORT statement has been updated several times, most recently in 2010, and is now accepted globally as the standard for reporting clinical trials in scientific journals.

Publication bias is the tendency for scientific journals to selectively publish interesting and positive results for their readers. For the purposes of transparency and the spread of scientific knowledge, it is important that the results of all clinical trials be made available to both researchers and the general public. The 2007 Food and Drug Act Authorization Amendments requires the registration and reporting of results of clinical trials of drugs, biological products, and devices, conducted wholly or in part in the United States, regardless of funding source. The reporting system is Web-based, and many of the results must be presented in tabular form with no commentary. Because the reporting requirement is mandatory and time sensitive, scientific journals allow authors to submit their results for publication without a pre-publication penalty.

Limitations of Randomized Controlled Trials

Inferences derived from randomized controlled trials only reflect the experience of those subjects who consented to enroll (volunteers) and it is widely known that volunteers for such studies can differ from nonparticipants in notable ways. For instance, the National Diet-Heart Study, an early intervention trial regarding dietary fat intake, made it possible to compare the characteristics of those who volunteered and those who did not.[38-39] Volunteers were more likely than nonparticipants to be nonsmokers, concerned about health, members of community organizations, active in community affairs, employed in professional and skilled positions, and with more formal education. They were also more likely to be Protestants or Jews and to live in households with children. If any of these characteristics were related to the outcome being measured, the investigator would have to limit the inferences from the study's results and generalize cautiously.

The example above demonstrates the importance of gathering information on all potential subjects for a trial at the time of recruitment, not simply on those who agree to continue with the informed consent process. Gathering data on those who refuse to participate allows the epidemiologist to compare nonparticipants with the volunteers for the study, information that may be valuable for determining the extent to which the results of the trial can be generalized.

Randomized controlled trials are relatively expensive to conduct, and they may not always be practical for evaluating how treatment decisions impact outcomes for a broad expanse of patients. In some instances, the epidemiologist may opt to use a *large simple trial* (LST) for this purpose. Where randomized controlled trials assess efficacy, LSTs assess effectiveness, that is, the real-world effect of the intervention. They are useful for evaluating treatments for common conditions such as cardiovascular diseases, when a large study population is available and small effects may be detected that may have potentially large population impacts. The design is often used by large health care providers and third-party payers with access to big data from electronic medical records that allow for simplified collection of information on individuals.[40]

An example of the use of the LST design comes from the Ziprasidone Observational Study of Cardiac Outcomes (ZODIAC). Ziprasidone was developed as an antipsychotic medication with a better safety profile than existing treatments. However, some data suggested that it increased the risk of cardiac arrhythmia. The ZODIAC study was organized to investigate this issue, enrolling 18,154 schizophrenic subjects in 18 countries in North America, South America, Europe, and Asia. The study followed the subjects for one year with typical clinical care. In an analysis of nonsuicidal deaths (since schizophrenics experience an elevated risk of suicide),[41] no increased mortality was found among those using ziprasidone compared with an existing treatment (RR = 1.02, 95% CI = 0.76–1.39). The investigators concluded, "the findings of this study failed to show that ziprasidone is associated with an elevated risk of non-suicidal mortality relative to olanzapine [the comparator] in real-world use."[42]

Summary

A randomized controlled trial is an epidemiologic experiment in which all subjects are randomly assigned to either a treatment or comparison group. The process of randomization, if carried out properly, provides comparable groups for most factors so that differences in outcomes at the end of the trial can be attributed to the treatment(s).

There are three types of randomized controlled trials: therapeutic trials (in which the treatment of a disease is evaluated), intervention trials (in which an intervention is evaluated in persons at elevated risk of developing a disease before it manifests), and prevention trials (in which the efficacy of a preventive agent is evaluated). Regardless of the type of trial, three different designs may be employed: the clinical trial, the factorial trial, and the crossover trial. The factorial design is effective for testing more than one hypothesis if sufficient numbers of subjects are available and the outcome of interest is likely to develop. The crossover trial uses subjects as their own controls and randomizes the sequence of the treatment.

Randomized controlled trials are conducted according to a protocol, which describes in detail the design and rationale for the study. The study population is usually recruited until a predetermined sample size has been met, a size large enough to ensure that the study has adequate statistical power to determine whether the treatment is efficacious. After giving informed consent, subjects are randomly assigned to either the treatment or the comparison group. The effect of an intervention may be biased if either the subject or the assessor is aware of an individual's group allocation. It may be prudent to build masking into the study design to avoid this bias. During the course of the trial, subjects may be noncompliant with the study protocol, withdraw, or be lost to follow-up. Various methods (behavioral, biological, and statistical) are available to assess the degree of compliance. Methods should be built into the study design to minimize the number of subjects who either drop out or are lost to follow-up. It is important to know why subjects withdraw from a study and whether their loss introduced an important bias.

The nature of a randomized controlled trial necessitates concern with the ethical basis for its conduct. Institutional Review Boards and Data Monitoring Committees aid in holding trials to the highest standards of ethics and conduct, assuring that equipoise is always present. Such trials must be registered and the results reported in a timely fashion to guarantee transparency with the public and to ensure that scientific knowledge is shared.

To reiterate, the investigator specifies all aspects of a randomized controlled trial in the protocol and then follows that protocol rigidly. When this is done, subject enrollment, randomization, data collection, management, and analysis are carefully prescribed and the results should be reliable.

References

1. Austin Bradford Hill, "Principles of Medical Statistics," *Lancet* 229, no. 5915 (1937): 99–101.
2. C. R. Freed et al., "Transplantation of Embryonic Dopamine Neurons for Severe Parkinson's Disease," *New England Journal of Medicine* 344, no. 10 (2001): 710–719.
3. Early Treatment Diabetic Retinopathy Study Research Group, "Early Photocoagulation for Diabetic Retinopathy: ETDRS Report Number 9," *Ophthalmology* 98, no. 5, Supplement (1991): 766–785.
4. Frederick L. Ferris III, "Photocoagulation for Diabetic Retinopathy," *Journal of the American Medical Association* 266, no. 9 (1991): 1263–1265.
5. P. M. Ridker et al., "Cardiovascular Benefits and Diabetes Risks of Statin Therapy in Primary Prevention: An Analysis from the JUPITER Trial," *Lancet* 380, no. 9841 (2012): 565–571.
6. I. Hjermann et al., "Effect of Diet and Smoking Intervention on the Incidence of Coronary Heart Disease. Report From the Oslo Study Group of a Randomised Trial in Healthy Men," *Lancet* 2, no. 8259 (1981): 1303–1310.
7. Charles H. Hennekens and Kimberley Eberlein, "A Randomized Trial of Aspirin and Beta-Carotene among U.S. Physicians," *Preventive Medicine* 14, no. 2 (1985): 165–168.

8. Charles H. Hennekens, "Update on Aspirin in the Treatment and Prevention of Cardiovascular Disease," *American Journal of Managed Care* 8, no. 22, Supplement (2002): S691–S700.

9. U.S. Preventive Services Task Force, "Aspirin for the Prevention of Cardiovascular Disease: U.S. Preventive Services Task Force Recommendation Statement," *Annals of Internal Medicine* 150, no. 6 (2009): 396–404.

10. L. V. Rubinstein et al., "The Statistics of Phase 0 Trials," *Statistics in Medicine* 29, no. 10 (2010): 1072–1076.

11. Miquel Porta, ed., *A Dictionary of Epidemiology, 6th Edition*. New York: Oxford University Press, 2014.

12. World Health Organization, *International Clinical Trials Registry Platform*. Available at http://apps.who.int/trialsearch/.

13. Pan African Clinical Trials Registry (PACTR). Available at http://www.pactr.org.

14. European Medicines Agency, EU Clinical Trials Database. Available at https://www.clinicaltrialsregister.eu/about.html 15. US National Institutes of Health, National Library of Medicine, ClinicalTrials.gov. Available at http://clinicaltrials.gov/.

16. BioMed Central, "International Standard Randomised Controlled Trial (ISRCTN) Register." Available at http://www.controlled-trials.com/.

17. Citizens for Responsible Care and Research (ICIRCARE), Clinical Trial Registries. Available at http://www.circare.org/registries.htm.

18. "The Age-Related Eye Disease Study (AREDS): Design Implications, AREDS Report No. 1," *Controlled Clinical Trials* 20, no. 6 (1999): 573–600.

19. Emily Y. Chew et al., "Long-Term Effects of Vitamins C and E, Beta-Carotene, and Zinc on Age-Related Macular Degeneration: AREDS Report No. 35," *Ophthalmology* 120, no. 8 (2013): 1604–11.e4.

20. Bernard Escudier et al., "Randomized, Controlled, Double-Blind, Cross-Over Trial Assessing Treatment Preference for Pazopanib Versus Sunitinib in Patients with Metastatic Renal Cell Carcinoma: PISCES Study," *Journal of Clinical Oncology* 32, no. 14 (2014): 1412–1418.

21. International Conference on Harmonization (ICH) Working Group, *ICH Harmonized Tripartite Guideline: Guideline for Good Clinical Practice, E6(R1)*. Geneva, 1996. Available at http://www.ich.org/fileadmin/Public_Web_Site/ICH_Products/Guidelines/Efficacy/E6_R1/Step4/E6_R1__Guideline.pdf.

22. O. G. Ottmann et al., "A Phase 2 Study of Imatinib in Patients with Relapsed or Refractory Philadelphia Chromosome-Positive Acute Lymphoid Leukemias," *Blood* 100, no. 6 (2002): 1965–1971.

23. David E. Lilienfeld et al., "On Antibiotic Prophylaxis in Cardiac Surgery: A Risk Factor for Wound Infection," *Annals of Thoracic Surgery* 42, no. 6 (1986): 670–674.

24. Edmund A. Gehan, "Clinical Trials in Cancer Research," *Environmental Health Perspectives* 32 (October 1979): 31–48.

25. James H. Jones, *Bad Blood: The Tuskegee Syphilis Experiment*. New York: Simon & Schuster, 1993.

26. R. H. Brown et al., "Tuskegee Syphilis Study Ad Hoc Advisory Panel, Acknowledgements, Charge I," 1973. Available at http://biotech.law.lsu.edu/cphl/history/reports/tuskegee/report1.pdf.

27. National Commission for the Protection of Human Subjects of Biomedical and Behavioral Research, *The Belmont report: Ethical principles and guidelines for the protection of human subjects of research*. Bethesda, MD: ERIC Clearinghouse, 1978. Available at http://www.hhs.gov/ohrp/humansubjects/guidance/belmont.html.

28. Curtis L. Meinert, *Clinical Trials: Design, Conduct and Analysis*. New York: Oxford University Press, 2012.

29. Henry K. Beecher, "The Powerful Placebo," *Journal of the American Medical Association* 159, no. 17 (1955): 1602–1606.

30. R. Brian Haynes, *Compliance in Health Care*. Baltimore: Johns Hopkins University Press, 1979.

31. Pablo Saiz de la Hoya et al., "Directly Observed Therapy for Chronic Hepatitis C: A Randomized Clinical Trial in the Prison Setting," *Gastroenterology and Hepatology* (April 2014): S0210-5705(14)00081-8. doi:10.1016/j.gastrohep.2014.03.004.

32. A. C. Tsai et al., "Directly Observed Antidepressant Medication Treatment and HIV Outcomes among Homeless and Marginally Housed HIV-Positive Adults: A Randomized Controlled Trial," *American Journal of Public Health* 103, no. 2 (2013): 308–315.

33. Y. V. Efremenko et al., "Randomized, Placebo-Controlled Phase II Trial of Heat-Killed Mycobacterium Vaccae (Longcom Batch) Formulated as an Oral Pill (V7)," *Human Vaccines & Immunotherapeutics* 9, no. 9 (2013): 1852–1856.

34. Dmytro A. Butov et al., "Adjunct Immune Therapy of First-Diagnosed TB, Relapsed TB, Treatment-Failed TB, Multidrug-Resistant TB and TB/HIV," *Immunotherapy* 4, no. 7 (2012): 687–695.

35. J. A. Betts et al., "Bath Breakfast Project (BBP)—Examining the Role of Extended Daily Fasting in Human Energy Balance and Associated Health Outcomes: Study Protocol for a Randomised Controlled Trial [ISRCTN31521726]," *Trials* 12 (2011): 172, doi:10.1186/1745-6215-12-172.

36. David W. Hosmer, Stanley Lemeshow, and Susanne May, *Applied Survival Analysis: Regression Modeling of Time to Event Data*. Hoboken, NJ: Wiley-Interscience, 2008.

37. David G. Kleinbaum, *Survival Analysis: A Self-Learning Text, 3rd Edition (Statistics for Biology and Health)*. New York, NY: Springer, 2011.

38. National Diet-Heart Study Research Group Executive Committee on Diet and Heart Disease, "The National Diet-Heart Study: Final Report," *Circulation* 37 (1968), 3 Suppl: I1–428.

39. A. F. Crocetti, "An Interview Study of Volunteers and Non-Volunteers in a Medical Research Project," unpublished thesis, Johns Hopkins University, Baltimore, 1970.

40. B. Roehr, "The Appeal of Large Simple Trials," *British Medical Journal* 346 (February 29, 2013): f1317.

41. C. Bjorkenstam et al., "Suicide in First Episode Psychosis: A Nationwide Cohort Study," *Schizophrenia Research* 157, no. 1–3 (2014): 1–7.

42. B. L. Strom et al., "Comparative Mortality Associated with Ziprasidone and Olanzapine in Real-World Use among 18,154 Patients with Schizophrenia: The Ziprasidone Observational Study of Cardiac Outcomes (ZODIAC)," *American Journal of Psychiatry* 168, no. 2 (2011): 193–201.

12 | Experimental Studies

COMMUNITY AND CLUSTER

RANDOMIZED TRIALS

Studies in human populations can rarely approach the simplicity
and precision of physical experiments or those that can be
formulated as a purely mathematical concept. It is, nevertheless,
toward this ideal the studies should reach once the attempt is
made to establish a controlled experiment.[1]

Thomas Francis, Jr. (1957)

W HEN THE RISK FACTORS WITHIN a population are so prevalent
that a group of high-risk individuals cannot be identified, a
community-based intervention may be appropriate.[2–3] For example, a community-based intervention comparing the dental caries experience
of two communities, one with and the other without fluoride added to the
town's supply of drinking water, was discussed in Chapter 1. Preventive,
therapeutic, or social epidemiologic experiments in which whole communities (rather than individuals) serve as the units of analysis are called *community trials (lifestyle intervention trials, field trials).*[4]

In a community trial, the epidemiologist selects two or more communities that are as similar as possible. Assent for participation in a community
trial must be obtained through negotiation with local community and political leaders, or by using other means of community engagement.[5] For each
community at the study baseline, the epidemiologist collects information on
the prevalence of risk factors, as well as the incidence or prevalence of the
disease(s) of interest. Such data may be elicited directly though community
surveys or indirectly through a review of vital statistics or other administrative
records (for example, insurance forms and village health or school records).

Once baseline information (Time 1) has been established, one or more of the communities is designated for the intervention; the others serve as controls. Interventions might include a preventive agent such as fluoride for preventing dental caries,[6] a therapeutic agent such as vitamin A to treat night blindness,[7] or a social intervention to reducing the prevalence of smoking.[8] When the intervention stops (Time 2), the prevalence of the suspected risk factor(s) and the incidence or prevalence of the outcome(s) of interest are again determined for each community. The differences between the measures for the control and intervention communities are then compared, and the net differences are associated with the intervention.

By 1978, Cornfield and others began noting problems with the community trial design, including lack of randomization and low statistical power.[9–10] To address these issues, analytic methods were developed that allowed intact groups (*clusters*) to be studied in *cluster randomized trial* (*group randomized trial*) interventions.[11] Cluster randomized trials deliver interventions to entire communities, schools, workplaces, clinics, or households, and outcomes are measured on the individual subjects in the cluster. The design is often less expensive than a randomized controlled trial, easier to administer, and it may more accurately portray the way some interventions are delivered (i.e., changing the diet for a household rather than one individual in a household). Because the clusters are randomized to various treatment arms of the study, selection bias is minimized. As select individuals within the cluster may be placed at risk, the proposed intervention should undergo review by a research ethics committee before the trial begins. If the ethics committee deems there may be a risk to subjects within the clusters, assent for participation may be required from each subject as well as from the leaders of the cluster as a whole.[12]

Conducting a Community Trial

A community trial has six stages, each building upon the successful completion of its predecessor (Box 12.1). As in a randomized controlled trial, the first stage is developing the formalized protocol that includes the rationale, procedures, and organization of the trial. The protocol details all methods used for data collection, how effects and outcomes will be measured, the times when community surveillance data will be collected, and the methods of analyzing the study data. The protocol must also address how contingencies will be handled, such as adverse events related to the intervention.

BOX 12.1 STAGES IN A COMMUNITY TRIAL

1. Develop a protocol.
2. Recruit communities.
3. Establish baseline information, community surveillance.
4. Select the intervention and assign communities.
5. Maintain oversight of data monitoring.
6. Evaluate results.

Once the protocol is complete, the next stage addresses how communities will be selected, recruited, and assigned to the intervention or control group. The epidemiologist can determine the number and size of the communities needed for the trial using standard statistical formulas.[9,13-15] In a randomized controlled trial, sufficient statistical power to detect the desired effect is essential. Intervention trials may be expensive to implement, thus the number of communities studied may be small. For example, the Minnesota Heart Health Program studied only three pairs of communities in Minnesota and North and South Dakota (about 430,000 subjects in all). While the number of pairs was small, the study populations were sufficiently large to evaluate meaningful endpoints (able to detect a 14 percent decline in cardiovascular disease mortality with a Type I error of 5 percent and a statistical power of 85 percent) and to evaluate the effectiveness of specific educational programs.[16]

Ideally, the communities selected for study have self-contained health care systems and minimal migration.[17] They might be selected because of their high prevalence of the suspected risk factor(s) and/or disease(s), or because information on community demographics is easily obtained. Sometimes specific populations are selected for administrative convenience and favorable community relations. Regardless of why they are selected, the communities should be similar in as many respects as possible. Their population demographics, economies, and political cultures should be comparable in order to allay concerns that any differences in outcomes resulted from community differences rather than the intervention. In the Minnesota Heart Health Program, for example, three different community sizes were selected for study. Two communities were matched as towns, two as cities, and two as suburbs.[16]

Once communities are selected, they must be recruited for participation. In a randomized controlled trial, the investigator recruits individual subjects and enrolls them after obtaining their informed consent. In a community trial, the epidemiologist obtains assent for participation from local and regional elected officials, community leaders, and the local medical community.[18–19] Not only would it be unethical to proceed with the trial without community assent, it would probably be impossible without the cooperation of local leaders who can facilitate the local logistics of the trial. After obtaining community assent, the epidemiologist must inform community members that they will be participating in a study. Examples of so doing include notification by tribal leader decree, through notices posted throughout the community or in local newspapers, by snail mail, or through diverse types of electronic media.

The next step is to establish baseline data and, if none exists, set up a data collection (surveillance) system. Information on risk factors and outcomes must be collected and assessed similarly before and at the end of the intervention. In most cases the epidemiologist assesses the data at regular intervals during the intervention to at least monitor for adverse effects. Data monitoring of risk factors may be assessed through community-wide surveys or by estimating risk through the use of administrative data such as tax revenues collected from the sale of cigarettes or alcohol.

Outcomes may be measured using community-wide surveys or through administrative data such as hospital records or insurance claims. Vital statistics or disease registry data, for instance, provide useful information on mortality or the incidence of disease. In some instances, data monitoring for deaths may require reviewing the records of local political or religious organizations. Information about adverse birth outcomes might require obtaining information from local midwives. Whatever surveillance systems are used, they should be sensitive to the outcomes of interest.[20]

Community surveillance requires a protocol for data acquisition and for methods used in community outreach.[21] Community support can be developed using endorsements from local political, social, and medical leaders. Local leaders may also be able to facilitate access to information gathered by systems outside of official channels. Outcomes must be clearly defined (with diagnostic criteria), and the means of validating reported outcomes must be specified. Finally, any data collected on risk factors and outcomes requires proper management and protection.

In community trials, the intervention is often a health education initiative (for example, use of condoms to reduce the risk of HIV infection).[22–23] In such a case, the community designated for intervention might receive an educational program designed to increase the rate of condom use. If the trial is not randomized, the epidemiologist selects the community designated for the intervention. Otherwise, a coin might be flipped or another method of randomization may determine which community is assigned to the intervention. For instance, the Community Intervention Trial for Smoking Cessation (COMMIT) study selected 11 pairs of communities. Each pair was randomly assigned by roulette (spinning a wheel containing two possible outcomes) either to an intensive smoking cessation program (the intervention) or to no intervention (the comparison).[24]

During the course of a community trial, the surveillance data are analyzed at regular intervals to promptly identify any adverse effects of the intervention. A committee of experts not otherwise associated with the trial (a Data Monitoring Committee) might meet regularly to review the data and decide whether the trial should continue. If adverse effects of the intervention are detected, the trial must be stopped for ethical reasons.[20]

At the trial's conclusion, the data are analyzed to determine if the intervention was effective. In the first stage of the analysis, no adjustment is made for any potential confounding factors. It is important, however, to also analyze the data with such adjustments and to report both sets of results.

Examples of Community Trials

Two nonrandomized community trials, both started in 1972, provide classic examples of this type of experimental design. Epidemiologists developed the North Karelia Project in response to a community's desire to reduce its high cardiovascular disease rates. The project focused on community health education, training of health care providers, increased availability of healthier foods, and the development of community-based health behavior support networks. In contrast, the Stanford Five-City Project focused solely on community-based health education efforts as the means to reduce cardiovascular morbidity.

The North Karelia Project

Around 1970, the province of North Karelia, Finland, had the highest frequency of cardiovascular disease in the world.[3] Representatives of the province demanded governmental action to reduce the prevalence of the disease. Local authorities, in collaboration with the World Health Organization, developed a protocol for a community intervention to reduce cigarette smoking, serum cholesterol levels, and hypertension, all cardiovascular disease risk factors prevalent within North Karelia. A similar province, Kuopio, was selected as the comparison community.

TABLE 12.1 Average Annual Age-Adjusted Ischemic Heart Disease Death Rates per 100,000 Persons in North Karelia and the Rest of Finland from 1969 to 1986, by Gender

DATES	MEN		WOMEN	
	NORTH KARELIA	REST OF FINLAND	NORTH KARELIA	REST OF FINLAND
1969–1971	715	491	132	90
1972–1974	637	470	96	87
1975–1977	592	469	89	80
1978–1980	538	417	82	71
1981–1982	501	383	75	63
1983	541	343	56	58
1984	509	343	81	57
1985	526	342	75	58
1986	439	317	93	54

SOURCE: Tuomilehto et al. (1989).[26]

Epidemiologists conducted surveys in both provinces to provide baseline data for the three risk factors. Myocardial infarction and stroke registries were also established in both areas to monitor cardiovascular disease. The intervention in North Karelia was launched in 1972 and included health education among influential citizens, training for health care providers, community health education, screening for hypertension, and building needed health care facilities.[25] The program was evaluated every five years. After the first evaluation, the Finnish government launched national efforts to reduce the cardiovascular disease risk factors throughout the country.[3] Thus, comparisons between the intervention and control provinces after the first evaluation had to consider the impact of the national effort.

Table 12.1 shows the results of the North Karelia Project by 1986, with notable declines in the death rates from ischemic heart disease for both males and females in the intervention province.[26] However, ischemic heart disease mortality also declined from the early 1970s through the 1980s for both males and females in the rest of Finland. Thus, the investigators attributed to declines in the mortality rates to the overall decline in the prevalence of cardiovascular disease risk factors in the entire population rather than solely to the intervention.[27]

The Stanford Projects

The Stanford Three-Community Study examined the impact of a community health education campaign in California communities on the prevalence of cigarette smoking, elevated serum cholesterol levels, and high blood pressure.[22] In two communities, mass-media campaigns were conducted over a period of two years. In one of them, face-to-face counseling was also provided for a subgroup of high-risk individuals. A third community did not receive the intervention and served as the control. In all three communities, people were interviewed and examined before the educational campaign began. The baseline values for the risk factors were remarkably uniform. At follow up, each subject's knowledge and behavior with respect to diet and smoking were assessed and their blood pressure, weight, and plasma cholesterol were measured. The intervention had positive effects on all risk factors except weight; the risk of developing cardiovascular disease in the intervention communities was reduced by approximately 25 percent.[28]

The Stanford Five-City Multifactor Risk Reduction Project expanded upon the Three-Communities project, including two intervention cities (Monterey and Salinas) and three control ones (Modesto, San Luis Obispo, and Santa Maria).[29] All of the cities were located in northern California and selected for size, distance from Stanford, and access to media markets. Random assignment of the cities was not possible due to the range of local broadcast media coverage. The intervention cities would have broadcast messages, but the messages would not be broadcast to the cities serving as controls.

Community health education began in the intervention cities in 1980 and ended in 1986; monitoring for cardiovascular morbidity and mortality continued in all the cities until 1992. The investigators reported that cardiovascular morbidity and mortality began to decline in the intervention cities around the time the educational efforts ended; similar declines were noted in the control cities. The report suggested that external influence(s) might be responsible for the declines in cardiovascular diseases in all the communities—perhaps innovations in medical management had improved cardiovascular disease outcomes, or perhaps social pressures led individuals in all the communities to reduce their risk factors for developing the disease.[30]

Both the North Karelia Project and the two Stanford trials developed in response to local concerns about elevated cardiovascular disease mortality rates. The use of randomization to assign the intervention either to North Karelia or Kuopio would not have been practical or ethical. Randomization in the Stanford Five-City Project also would have been problematic, since two of the three communities shared a common television station used as part of the intervention.

Cluster Randomized Trials

When the opportunity presents itself to use a randomized approach, the epidemiologist uses randomized treatment assignment for communities or clusters of individuals. Random assignment helps to ensure that the distribution of *all* factors—known and unknown, measured and not measurable—except for the intervention being studied—is based on chance. It helps ensure that a factor (e.g., investigator preference and geographic convenience) that may lead to a biased outcome is controlled. The community focus of cluster randomized trials lends itself to assessing the utility of public health interventions, but the design has also been found useful for assessing the effectiveness of clinical interventions. In these instances the outcome of interest may be related to the delivery of care rather than the efficacy of a specific treatment of a disease.

The epidemiologist follows the exact same six steps in conducting a cluster randomized trial as for a (nonrandomized) community trial, with the exception that during the fourth stage the assignment is made randomly. It is the use of randomization that affords the epidemiologist the ability to ensure that all factors other than placement in the treatment or control groups are equally distributed between the clusters.

Examples of Cluster Randomized Trials

An example of a cluster randomized trial using the workplace as the cluster unit is the WHO Collaborative Trial in the Multifactorial Prevention of Coronary Heart Disease (CHD).[31] Between 1971 and 1977, workers in 80 factories in four countries (Belgium, Italy, Poland, and the United Kingdom) were screened for cigarette smoking, blood pressure, weight, and serum cholesterol level. The 80 factories were arranged into 40 pairs of facilities of approximately comparable size, location, and type of industry. Within each pair, one factory was randomly assigned to receive the intervention (a health education program for smoking cessation, cholesterol-lowering dietary advice, exercise, weight reduction, and control of hypertension); the other served as the control. The random allocation of factories to the intervention group reduced the possibility for selection bias, and the outcome measures of interest were the incidence of and mortality from CHD. Preliminary results indicated that reducing exposure to risk factors could reduce CHD in middle-aged men up to 25 percent and that a community health education intervention could be beneficial for this purpose.[32]

The Aceh Study

The Aceh Study was a cluster randomized trial using the village as the cluster unit to determine whether vitamin A supplementation would reduce childhood mortality. Previous epidemiologic observations established that Indonesian children with ophthalmologic signs of mild vitamin A deficiency (*xerophthalmia*) experienced elevated death rates.[7] Sommer and his colleagues hypothesized that vitamin A could reduce mortality among these children. Aceh Province had 2,048 villages with no existing or planned vitamin supplementation program. Of these, 450 villages were selected and randomly assigned to either the intervention (n = 229) or control (n = 221) groups. Eighteen villages started vitamin A supplementation programs before the baseline surveys began and were excluded from the trial; they were replaced with adjacent villages lacking vitamin supplementation programs. Assent for community participation was obtained from village leaders.

A baseline survey of each of the 450 villages was undertaken. All children up to five years of age were examined for xerophthalmia. To maintain the ethics of the trial, any child found to have the condition during the baseline survey was referred for immediate treatment and excluded from further participation. About one to three months after the baseline survey was complete, volunteers gave a single capsule containing 200,000 IU of vitamin A and 40 IU of vitamin E to children one to five years old in the intervention communities.

At baseline, 29,236 children were enrolled; follow-up was completed on 89 percent of the children treated and 88 percent of the children serving as controls. During the six-month follow-up period, 101 children in the intervention villages and 130 children in the control villages died. The difference in the mortality rates between the intervention and control villages was 36 percent. The relative risk of dying for boys was 69 percent higher in the control villages; for girls, the risk was less pronounced at 9 percent. Xerophthalmia declined by 85 percent in the intervention villages. The investigators concluded that vitamin A supplementation would likely reduce mortality in areas where vitamin A deficiency is common.[7] Capsules were distributed during the follow-up examination at the end of the study in both intervention and control communities.

The Prevention Trial in the Cherokee Nation

Community-based participatory research (CBPR) brings academic and community partners together to address community problems. In response to a high prevalence of underage drinking among Native American and other high-risk rural youth, the CBPR approach brought together a University of Florida research team with partners from Cherokee Nation Behavioral Health. The partners shared the goal of finding effective interventions that could reduce alcohol use among youth. The Prevention Trial in the Cherokee

Nation was designed as a cluster randomized trial using isolated towns as the cluster unit.

The Cherokee Nation consists of approximately 300,000 citizens, with about half living in a 14-county nonreservation area of northeastern Oklahoma. This region contains many rural towns with populations containing large proportions of Native Americans, whites, and persons of mixed race. The CBPR team designed a cluster randomized trial to compare two complex environmental and behavioral interventions as implemented in isolated towns (separated by at least 30 miles from the nearest neighboring town) that each had 400 to 700 high schools students.[33] Twelve towns fit the criteria, and they were randomly assigned to the various arms of the study: CONNECT intervention only, CMCA intervention only, both interventions, and no intervention (a factorial design).

The CONNECT intervention included (1) one-on-one screening and group motivational sessions for high school students; (2) high school staff and community training in risk identification, communication, and support; and (3) family and community media campaigns to shift family and social norms relative to underage alcohol use. The CMCA intervention placed direct-action teams into the community, charging them with three tasks: (1) reduce the number of outlets that illegally sell alcohol to minors; (2) reduce youth access to alcohol through family and friends; and (3) reduce community tolerance of youth alcohol consumption (Table 12.2).

After the towns were randomized, several high schools (the clusters) were recruited for participation. Assent for participation was obtained from school superintendents and each high school principal. Passive consent for student participation was obtained from parents. Archival data was found on

TABLE 12.2 Study Design for the Prevention Trial in the Cherokee Nation

CLUSTER	TREATMENT
A. Treatment town $n \approx 250$ youth	CONNECT only
B. Treatment town $n \approx 250$ youth	CMCA only
C. Treatment towns ($n = 2$) $n \approx 500$ youth	CONNECT and CMCA
D. Control towns ($n = 2$) $n \approx 500$ youth	None
E. Control towns ($n = 6$, archival) $n \approx 250$ youth per town	None

SOURCE: Data from Komro et al. (2014).[33]

each town for items such as juvenile justice system reports, alcohol-related car crashes, juvenile substance abuse admissions, graduation rates, and more. Baseline data for each town was then collected in two ways. First, to assess adherence with legally mandated age checks for purchasing alcohol, an underage youth (accompanied by a young-looking adult team member) attempted to purchase alcohol at the sales outlets in each town. The attempts were repeated monthly over a four-year period to monitor the effectiveness of the CMCA intervention. A survey of student behaviors was also implemented quarterly over the four-year period to monitor the CONNECT intervention. While the results of this complex behavioral intervention are still pending, the Prevention Trial in the Cherokee Nation provides an excellent example of how time-series data monitoring with two distinct interventions and multiple comparison groups can be woven together using the randomized cluster trial design and community-based participation.

The Quality Initiative in Rectal Cancer Trial

Cluster randomized trials may be used to assess different approaches designed to encourage clinicians to change their health care delivery practices. An example of using this study design is the Quality Initiative in Rectal Cancer Trial.[34] The investigators sought to reduce the occurrence of two adverse health outcomes following rectal cancer surgery (local recurrence and permanent colostomy) by using a quality-improvement strategy to change surgical practices. In this instance the hospitals define the cluster, and the patients of the participating surgeons at each hospital populate the cluster. The intervention included attending workshops, having one of the study team surgeons demonstrate optimal surgical technique, using postoperative questionnaires, and auditing results.

Some 56 surgeons in the intervention group (558 patients) and 49 surgeons in the control group (457 patients) participated in the study. The rates of permanent colostomy were 39 percent in the intervention group and 41 percent in the control group; for local recurrence, the corresponding rates were 7 percent and 6 percent. The investigators concluded that this particular quality initiative failed to reduce the frequency of the two adverse outcomes.

Loss to Follow-Up

A major concern for any community or cluster randomized trial is that some individuals will be lost to follow-up, and that the composition of the groups may have consequently changed during the course of the trial.[13] Individuals who leave the trial may be different from those who remain, thus creating problems for the epidemiologist in interpreting trial results. For instance, persons who move into the community after an intervention has been administered may not be exposed to it (e.g., vaccine administration), yet their health outcomes are included along with other members of the community at the end of the trial.[21] If more persons are lost to follow-up in the intervention group than in the control group, the effectiveness of the intervention may also be obscured.[35] Thus, communities or clusters of individuals identified for participation in these trials should be selected for stability whenever possible.

Comparing Experimental Designs

In randomized controlled trials, subjects are assigned individually to the treatment groups (at its simplest, treatment and placebo) and the unit of statistical analysis is the subject (Chapter 11). In community or cluster randomized trials, entire communities or clusters are assigned to the various arms of the study, and the unit of analysis is the cluster.[23]

The choice between a randomized clinical trial and a community or cluster randomized trial essentially depends on the prevalence of the disease in the population, the complexity of the intervention, and the resources available to conduct the trial. The larger the population to be studied, the more desirable a community or cluster randomized trial becomes.[2] For instance, hypercholesterolemia is prevalent in many communities in the United States. Screening and intervention for all persons with elevated serum cholesterol levels in these communities would consume large amounts of health care resources. An educational program developed to lower dietary cholesterol intake, if effective, would likely consume fewer resources than screening and treating the entire population. The effectiveness of that intervention could only be demonstrated through a community or cluster randomized trial.

Summary

A community trial is an experimental epidemiologic study design in which entire communities are assigned to either treatment or control groups. It is an alternative to a randomized controlled trial and useful when the outcome of interest is so common that it may be difficult to identify a high-risk group.

Cluster randomized trials use intact groups (households, schools, clinics, workplaces) as the clusters and randomizes them to the various arms of the study. Outcomes are measured on the individual subjects in the cluster.

The first step in conducting a community or cluster randomized trial is to develop a protocol that includes all of the procedures, definitions, and justifications for the conduct of the trial. The next step is the identification and recruitment of the communities or clusters to be studied. Baselines for the factors targeted for intervention or treatment and the outcomes of interest are then established. Surveillance procedures to monitor changes in the factors and the outcomes are also put into place at this time. The intervention is then implemented. Data monitoring continues throughout the conduct of the trial. At the trial's conclusion, the data are analyzed to determine if the intervention had the desired effect. These designs are useful when the risk factor(s) or outcome(s) of interest are so prevalent in the population that a high-risk group may be difficult to identify, when the intervention is more appropriately delivered at the group rather than the individual level (e.g., community efforts to encourage condom use or prevent transmission of HIV), or when the interventions are complex and require large numbers of subjects for analytical purposes.

References

1. Thomas Francis, Jr., "Symposium on Controlled Vaccine Field Trials: Poliomyelitis," *American Journal of Public Health and the Nation's Health* 47, no. 3 (1957): 283–287.
2. T. E. Kottke et al., "Projected Effects of High-Risk Versus Population-Based Prevention Strategies in Coronary Heart Disease," *American Journal of Epidemiology* 121, no. 5 (1985): 697–704.
3. Pekka Puska, Aulikki Nissinen, and Jaakko Tuomilehto, "The Community-Based Strategy to Prevent Coronary Heart Disease: Conclusions from the Ten Years of the North Karelia Project," *Annual Review of Public Health* 6, no. 1 (1985): 147–193.
4. Miquel Porta, ed., *A Dictionary of Epidemiology, 6th Edition*. New York: Oxford University Press, 2014.
5. George Okello et al., "Challenges for Consent and Community Engagement in the Conduct of Cluster Randomized Trial among School Children in Low Income Settings: Experiences from Kenya," *Trials* 14 (May 16, 2013): 142, doi:10.1186/1745-6215-14-142.
6. David B. Ast and Edward R. Schlesinger, "The Conclusion of a Ten-Year Study of Water Fluoridation," *American Journal of Public Health & the Nation's Health* 46, no. 3 (1956): 265–271.
7. Alfred Sommer et al., "Impact of Vitamin A Supplementation on Childhood Mortality. A Randomised Controlled Community Trial," *Lancet* 1, no. 8491 (1986): 1169–1173.

8. M. H Gail et al., "Aspects of Statistical Design for the Community Intervention Trial for Smoking Cessation (COMMIT)," *Controlled Clinical Trials* 13, no. 1 (1992): 6–21.

9. Jerome Cornfield, Randomization by Group: A Formal Analysis. *American Journal of Epidemiology* 108, no. 2 (1978): 100–102.

10. David M. Murray, *Design and Analysis of Group-Randomized Trials*. New York: Oxford University Press, 1998.

11. Alan Donner and Neil Klar, *Design and Analysis of Cluster Randomization Trials in Health Research*. Hoboken: Wiley, 2010.

12. Charles Weijer et al., "The Ottawa Statement on the Ethical Design and Conduct of Cluster Randomized Trials," *PLoS Medicine* 9, no. 11 (2012): e1001346.

13. Carol Buck and Allan Donner, "The Design of Controlled Experiments in the Evaluation of Non-Therapeutic Interventions," *Journal of Chronic Diseases* 35, no. 7 (1982): 531–538.

14. Allan Donner, Nicholas Birkett, and Carol Buck, "Randomization by Cluster: Sample Size Requirements and Analysis," *American Journal of Epidemiology* 114, no. 6 (1981): 906–914.

15. Allan Donner, "Statistical Methodology for Paired Cluster Designs," *American Journal of Epidemiology* 126, no. 5 (1987): 972–979.

16. David R. Jacobs, Jr., et al., "Community-Wide Prevention Strategies: Evaluation Design of the Minnesota Heart Health Program," *Journal of Chronic Diseases* 39, no. 10 (1986): 775–788.

17. Irving I. Kessler and Morton L. Levin, *The Community as an Epidemiologic Laboratory: A Casebook of Community Studies*. Baltimore: Johns Hopkins University Press, 1970, 1–22.

18. J. P. Elder et al., "Organizational and Community Approaches to Community-Wide Prevention of Heart Disease: The First Two Years of the Pawtucket Heart Health Program," *Preventive Medicine* 15, no. 2 (1986): 107–117.

19. Roger Sherwin, "Controlled Trials of the Diet-Heart Hypothesis: Some Comments on the Experimental Unit," *American Journal of Epidemiology* 108, no. 2 (1978): 92–99.

20. Pekka Puska, "Intervention and Experimental Studies," in *Oxford Textbook of Public Health, 2nd Edition*, eds. W. W. Holland, R. Detels, and G. E. Knox. Oxford and New York: Oxford University Press, 1991, 113–122.

21. Richard F. Gillum, Paul T. Williams, and Edward Sondik, "Some Considerations for the Planning of Total-Community Prevention Trials—When Is Sample Size Adequate?" *Journal of Community Health* 5, no. 4 (1980): 270–278.

22. John W. Farquhar et al., "Community Education for Cardiovascular Health," *Lancet* 309, no. 8023 (1977): 1192–1195.

23. John W. Farquhar, "Symposium on CHD Prevention Trials: Design Issues in Testing Life Style Intervention: The Community-Based Model of Life Style Intervention Trials," *American Journal of Epidemiology* 108, no. 2 (1978): 103–111.

24. COMMIT Research Group, "Community Intervention Trial for Smoking Cessation (COMMIT): Summary of Design and Intervention," *Journal of the National Cancer Institute* 83, no. 22 (1991): 1620–1628.

25. Erkki Vartiainen et al., "Fifteen-Year Trends in Coronary Risk Factors in Finland, with Special Reference to North Karelia," *International Journal of Epidemiology* 20, no. 3 (1991): 651–662.

26. Jaakko Tuomilehto et al., "Trends and Determinants of Ischaemic Heart Disease Mortality in Finland: With Special Reference to a Possible Levelling Off in the Early 1980s," *International Journal of Epidemiology* 18, Supplement 1 (1989): S109–S117.

27. J. T. Salonen et al., "Contribution of Risk Factor Changes to the Decline in Coronary Incidence during the North Karelia Project: A Within-Community Analysis," *International Journal of Epidemiology* 18, no. 3 (1989): 595–601.

28. Nathan Maccoby et al., "Reducing the Risk of Cardiovascular Disease," *Journal of Community Health* 3, no. 2 (1977): 100–114.

29. Stephen P. Fortmann et al., "Community Surveillance of Cardiovascular Diseases in the Stanford Five-City Project: Methods and Initial Experience," *American Journal of Epidemiology* 123, no. 4 (1986): 656–669.

30. Stephen P. Fortmann and Ann N. Varady, "Effects of a Community-Wide Health Education Program on Cardiovascular Disease Morbidity and Mortality: The Stanford Five-City Project. *American Journal of Epidemiology* 152, no. 4 (2000): 316–323.

31. World Health Organization European Collaborative Group, "Multifactorial Trial in the Prevention of Coronary Heart Disease: I. Recruitment and Initial Findings," *European Heart Journal* 1 no., 1 (1980): 73–80.

32. World Health Organization European Collaborative Group, Multifactorial Trial in the Prevention of Coronary Heart Disease: III. Incidence and Mortality Results. *European Heart Journal* 4, no. 3 (1983): 141–47.

33. Kelli A. Komro et al., "Prevention Trial in the Cherokee Nation: Design of a Randomized Community Trial," *Prevention Science* 16, no. 2, (2014): 291–300, doi: 10.1007/s11121-014-0478-y.

34. Marko Simunovic et al., "The Cluster-Randomized Quality Initiative in Rectal Cancer Trial: Evaluating a Quality-Improvement Strategy in Surgery," *Canadian Medical Association Journal* 182, no. 12 (2010): 1301–1306.

35. John W. Farquhar et al., "Effects of Communitywide Education on Cardiovascular Disease Risk Factors," *Journal of the American Medical Association* 264, no. 3 (1990): 359–365.

36. S. Leonard Syme, "Life Style Intervention in Clinic-Based Trials," *American Journal of Epidemiology* 108, no. 2 (1978): 87–91.

IV | Using Epidemiologic Information

> . . . one-to-one provider–patient relationships, so advantageous for the clinician, can actually be a disadvantageous distortion for the community [public health] practitioner committed to the broader target of equitable programming for a total population.[1]
>
> *William H. McBeath (1981)*

EPIDEMIOLOGIC METHODS ARE OFTEN applied in a wide variety of disciplines and sub-disciplines. Some epidemiology textbooks on the market are dedicated entirely to cancer, chronic disease, environmental, genetic, health promotion, infectious disease, managerial, medical, nursing, nutritional, obesity, occupational, oral health, perinatal, pharmaceutical, physical activity, social, and spatial epidemiology, as well as epidemiology for the plant and veterinary sciences. Part IV covers two broad areas of epidemiology straddling multiple (though not all) disciplines—clinical and field applications. In addition, it addresses how epidemiology aids both clinical and public health practitioners in developing evidence-based practices.

Clinicians use epidemiology when screening for and diagnosing disease. They also use it when selecting tests and treatments for their patients, and when evaluating patient outcomes. Chapter 13 introduces some additional methods epidemiologists have developed to evaluate patient outcomes (such as quality of life) and the costs related to the health care provided. Comparative effectiveness research (CER) addresses the question of which of two or more treatments is better for the individual patient or population, as appropriate. The chapter covers only the very basics of CER, as this is a vast and rapidly expanding area of epidemiology.

Public health professionals utilize epidemiologic methods for investigating disease outbreaks, bioterrorism events, and natural disasters in real time and place. These field methods are discussed in Chapter 14, including the data gathering and statistical tools that allow the epidemiologist to evaluate the status of public health problems on site and immediately communicate their findings. Geographic information systems (GIS) may be used to document existing or potential public health problems and can be used to engage communities in participatory research. The capabilities and limitations of GIS, as well as social media, are described so that the epidemiologist may use them effectively. Lastly, the chapter closes with consideration of surveillance techniques used in the field, building on the discussion of surveillance introduced in Chapter 7.

Chapter 15 addresses the development of evidence-based practices for both clinical and public health purposes. The results of many epidemiologic studies are now widely available via electronic searches, but the precision afforded by the results requires an understanding of the hierarchy of data. The results of various studies may be synthesized using meta-analysis, a means of summarizing results so they may inform decisions by public health officials, health policy makers, or clinicians.

Reference

1. William H. McBeath, Testimony before the Subcommittee on Health and the Environment, Committee in Energy and Commerce, US House of Representatives. April 3, 1981.

13 | Clinical Applications

The practice of medicine is an art, based on science.[1]
Medicine is a science of uncertainty and an art of probability.[2]

William Osler (1849–1919)

C LINICIANS APPLY THE PRINCIPLES OF epidemiology to everyday practice in two ways: clinical decision making and contributing to the understanding of how the health services they provide are linked with various types of patient outcomes. The first category, clinical decision making, includes recommending a preventive practice, ordering screening or diagnostic tests and procedures, assigning diagnoses, and recommending treatments. The second category uses reported clinical, administrative, and other data to evaluate how patients respond to the health services they receive, in other words, *outcomes research.*

Screening for Disease

Several epidemiologic study designs can be used to evaluate the efficacy of screening tests. Population-based studies provide a great deal of information about screening tests, but they often cannot adjust for potential confounders. Case-control and cohort studies may be able to control for some confounding factors, but they cannot control for several types of bias, some of which may make screening programs appear more effective than they really are. Two major types of bias of concern to the epidemiologist evaluating screening programs are length bias and lead time/overdiagnosis bias.

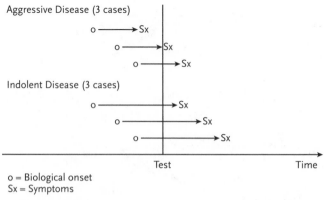

FIGURE 13.1 Graphical explanation of length bias.

Length Bias

Length bias occurs when one group in a study has cases of disease that are more aggressive than the comparator. Consider that aggressive tumors have shorter asymptomatic periods than do indolent (slow to progress) ones. It follows that the probability of picking up an aggressive tumor during the window of opportunity for early detection (the sojourn period; see Figure 3.1, p. 42) is shorter. Thus, screening programs are more likely to pick up cases with less aggressive tumors, and screened cases will be overrepresented in the diagnosed cohort. As individuals with less aggressive disease are more likely to have more favorable outcomes compared to those with more aggressive forms of the same disease, the screening program will appear to be more effective than it really is (Figure 13.1).

For instance, a review of cases reported to the Finnish Cancer Registry found that women with screening-detected cancer have a longer time to disease recurrence and live longer than women with cancers detected clinically.[3] Shen and colleagues confirmed this finding via analysis of three large breast cancer screening trials—the Health Insurance Plan (HIP) of New York and two Canadian National Breast Cancer Screening Studies.[4] The investigators noted that clinicians should be made aware that women with tumors detected on screening mammograms were more likely to have nonmetastatic disease compared to those who were diagnosed clinically. In other words, the method of detection was clearly prognostic.

Lead Time and Overdiagnosis Bias

Lead time is the amount of time gained in treating a disease because it is detected by screening before symptoms appear. *Lead time bias (zero time shift*

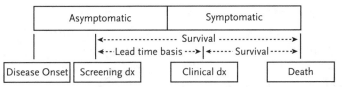

FIGURE 13.2 Graphical explanation of lead time bias.

or *stage shift*) occurs in a study when a group of individuals who had their disease detected early because of screening appear to have increased survival times compared to those whose disease was detected when the disease later became symptomatic.[5] In other words, early detection through screening may not have improved survival, even though it appeared to do so because of lead time bias (Figure 13.2).

As an example, the development of the prostate-specific antigen (PSA) test to screen for prostate cancer caused a rapid spike in the reported number of cases of the disease, as well as downward shifts in age at diagnosis and stage of the tumor.[6] The researchers concluded that the PSA test was an effective screening tool, bringing new cases to light at an earlier stage. A decade later, Telesca and colleagues calculated that PSA screening produced an average lead time of approximately 4.59 years for whites and 6.78 years for blacks, in effect picking up indolent cases.[7] They also found that the initial increase in prostate cancer reporting after the advent of the PSA test had leveled off, yet 22.7 and 34.4 percent of white and black cases, respectively, were overdiagnosed.

Overdiagnosis bias occurs when cases detected through screening include individuals who would likely have died of other causes before their disease had become symptomatic or progressed to a life-threatening stage. Overdiagnosis may also lead to overtreatment, sometimes with significant sequelae that reduce the patient's quality of life or that may even shorten life. Long-term evaluation of PSA screening showed more cases diagnosed, but little to no change in mortality from prostate cancer. Thus, in May 2012 the US Preventive Services Task Force suggested that providers discourage PSA screening. The task force concluded with moderate certainty that the benefits of PSA screening for prostate cancer do not outweigh the harms associated with overdiagnosis.[8]

Screen Patients, Not Populations

Length and lead time biases, as well as the limitations of screening tests, pose significant problems when screening entire populations. For instance, South Korea has high age-standardized cancer incidence and mortality rates compared to other industrialized countries.[9] To address public concerns and the costs associated with cancer treatments, the government instituted the National Cancer Screening Program (NCSP) in 1999. The early detection of breast, cervical, colorectal, liver, and stomach cancers was expected to reduce the overall burden of these diseases on society. Women over 30 years of age were offered free Pap smears, and women over 40 were offered free mammograms and clinical breast exams every two years. All South Koreans over the age of 40 years were offered free endoscopy or upper gastrointestinography every two years to screen for stomach cancer. Those over 40 years of age or who were in a high risk group were offered free sonography or alpha fetoprotein screenings for liver cancer every six months. All South Koreans over the age of 50 years were offered free fecal occult blood screenings for colorectal cancer every two years.

In 2010, the effectiveness of the NCSP was evaluated. The sensitivity of the screening programs (the proportion of disease correctly identified through screenings; see Chapter 7, p. 130) ranged from a low of 35 percent for breast cancers to a high of 77 percent for cervical cancers. More than half of all stomach and liver cancers were missed, as were almost two-thirds of all breast cancers. The *positive predictive values* (the proportion of true positives out of all positive tests; see Chapter 7, p. 131) of the screening programs ranged from 0.6 to 5.7 percent. In other words, even for the best of the NCSP population-based cancer screening programs, more than 94 percent of positive tests were inaccurate (false positives). The researchers reported that biases were also likely present in the screening programs. Patients with indolent tumors were more likely to have been picked up by periodic screening programs (*length bias*, Figure 13.1), and they may have appeared to survive longer because their tumors were identified in the presymptomatic phase (*lead time bias*, Figure 13.2). This means the NCSP was less effective than expected for reducing cancer mortality and increasing survival times for the South Korean population as a whole. In essence, the NCSO massive screening effort had been poorly designed, with customized cancer communication suggested as a good alternative.[9]

While population-based screening for cancer has limitations, the clinician has the responsibility of using judgment to determine which patients or groups of patients would best benefit from screening. Not only do patient characteristics matter, but so do time and place factors. Consider the utility of a rapid HIV screening test for asymptomatic pregnant women in labor. In clinical practice, a positive result from a standard HIV screening test requires Western blot confirmation, the results of which will not be available in time to inform interventions during labor and delivery. Could a rapid HIV test replace standard testing practices in this situation? As false positive tests cause serious anxiety for both mother and the delivery team, what might be the positive predictive value of the rapid test?

To address these questions, the Mother-Infant Rapid Intervention at Delivery (MIRIAD) study evaluated 7,753 laboring women whose HIV status was unknown at the time of admission.[10] Each woman had the rapid HIV test and the standard HIV test, and both results were compared with the Western blot as the reference test. HIV prevalence in the women enrolled in the study was 0.7 percent (52 of 7,753). Sensitivity was 100 percent for both tests (all cases were correctly identified). Sensitivity was 99.9 and 99.8 percent, respectively (those who tested negative were almost all negative). The positive predictive value, however, was 90 percent for the rapid test (52/58) and 74 percent for the standard test (52/70).[11] In other words, the rapid test identified six false positives, two fewer than the standard test, which identified eight. The benefit of the rapid test was not only earlier treatment but also 16 percent fewer false positives.

Epidemiologists use the metrics of *accuracy, sensitivity, specificity*, and *positive* and *negative predictive values* to assess the efficacy of screening tests. The clinician, however, makes decisions about whether or not to screen based on a patient's individual risks, not the risk of the population as a whole. Consider that about 8 percent of screening mammograms in US women are reported as being abnormal, but only 10 percent of women identified as having an abnormal mammogram end up with a breast cancer diagnosis. As a result, women who get 10 annual screening mammograms have about a 50 percent chance of at least one of them being a false positive.[12] False positives suffer anxiety, additional radiation exposure with repeat mammograms, and many unnecessary procedures. While these statistics show that screening mammograms at the population level pose a large burden on society, the clinician knows that if there is a family history of breast cancer, the risks of not having an annual mammogram far outweigh the risks of a false-positive scare.

The clinician also has to take into account the acceptability (cultural and physical discomfort) of a screening test for the patient. For example, some women with high-risk pregnancies may refuse prenatal testing because of cultural or religious beliefs. Those who welcome such testing may still feel that the risk of miscarriage following amniocentesis outweighs the benefit of knowing fetal status. Only a frank discussion between the clinician and patient can sort out these complex issues and contribute to informed clinical decision making.

Clinical Decision Making

In all aspects of medical practice, the health care provider (for example, the dentist, nurse, physician, veterinarian, or allied health professional) faces a series of choices—choices that are made in a specific context for a particular patient. Despite the intention to provide well-reasoned care, patterns of diagnosis and treatment have sometimes been less than optimal. For example, a well-intentioned intervention that has since gone out of favor is tonsillectomy and adenoidectomy for children who present with tonsillitis. A 1945 study evaluated this practice by asking three groups of pediatricians to screen a group of children for tonsillitis.[13] The first group examined 389 children and referred 174 (45 percent) for tonsillectomy. The 215 "healthy" children who were not referred for tonsillectomy were then screened by a second group of physicians. The second group of physicians recommended tonsillectomy for 99 (46 percent) of the "healthy" children. The process was repeated, and a third group of physicians examined the 116 remaining "healthy" children, referring 51 (44 percent) of them for tonsillectomy. Perhaps surprisingly, all three groups of pediatricians referred between 44 and 46 percent of the children they evaluated for tonsillectomy. Was this due to physician expectation that almost half of all children benefit from the procedure? Or was it perhaps due to the lack of objective and validated criteria for the surgery?

The subjective nature of clinical decision making poses challenges for the clinician seeking to diagnose and create an optimal treatment plan that meets each patient's needs. Health care providers must take into account the patient's diagnosis, but they must also consider each patient's biomedical, cultural, economic, social, or other circumstances. Epidemiologic research contributes to clinical decision making in that it provides information about the different options available for diagnosing and treating various diseases. Still, clinicians must sort through patient factors and epidemiologic research findings to present options for treatment plans to the patients for consideration. In some instances, clinicians trying to sort out various options can be aided by the formal process of decision analysis.

Decision Analysis

Health care providers make probabilistic decisions that are informed by their training, the current literature in their field, and their personal experiences. When a provider orders a test, he/she has some sense of the probability that the results will be positive. If that probability is close to zero, there would be little point in ordering the test. Similarly, if the provider is already sure of the

TABLE 13.1 Steps in Clinical Decision Analysis

STEPS	EXPLANATION
1. Frame the question	Consider all treatments, no treatment, and, if appropriate, the possibility of combined treatments.
2. Create a decision tree	Diagram the problem, showing the clinical options and the possible outcomes of each. Outcomes can include loss of life, complete recovery, and the risks of side effects.
3. Assign probabilities to the outcomes	Use the literature or experience to estimate probabilities for branches and points of the decision tree.
4. Assign utilities to the outcomes	Utilities are the relative values assigned to any scale (e.g., years of survival, dollars spent, or an arbitrary scale of 0 to 100).
5. Calculate the expected utility	The probability of an outcome is multiplied by the utility value. These are averaged with for all outcomes in the same decision tree branch.
6. Perform sensitivity analysis	Repeat the analysis under different assumptions. This helps clarify the contribution of different factors to the ultimate decision.

diagnosis, the test is uninformative. In other situations, though, a formalized structure for making a treatment decision can assist the health care provider in formulating a treatment plan. Decision analysis is an approach that weighs the probabilities of various outcomes. It is one way to develop a protocol or checklist, such as those now increasingly used by health care providers, and it can inform health policy makers about resource needs in the community. The steps to performing a formalized decision analysis appear in Table 13.1.

An example of decision analysis comes from a study to determine the best surgical treatment of coronal angular deformity of the lower limb in children, a condition that can lead to osteoarthritis of the knee.[14] The question was framed (Step 1) so as to determine the best intervention to temporarily fuse the growth plate: staples, percutaneous screws, or a tension band plate. A literature review identified 34 studies addressing the three procedures and served as the basis for developing a decision tree (Step 2). Each treatment had two outcomes (complication or no complication), and branching indicted two types of complication (metal failure or incomplete correction) with the latter having two results: further observation or another surgical procedure (osteotomy). Probabilities for each outcome were based on reports in the literature (Step 3), and all of the data were entered into the decision tree. Figure 13.3 shows the results for one of the treatment groups in the decision tree, the tension band plate intervention.

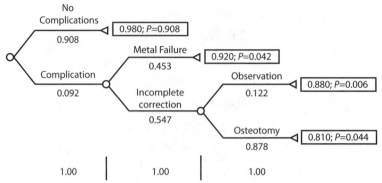

SURGICAL INTERVENTION
Tension Band Plate

No
Complications
0.908   0.980; P=0.908

Metal Failure
0.453   0.920; P=0.042

Complication
0.092   Observation
               0.122   0.880; P=0.006
Incomplete
correction
0.547   Osteotomy
               0.878   0.810; P=0.044

1.00   1.00   1.00

FIGURE 13.3 Example of outcomes from one arm of a decision tree.
SOURCE: Sung et al. (2014).[14]

The literature reported that 90.8 percent of children undergoing the tension band plate intervention experienced no complications (probability = 0.908). Of the 9.2 percent that did experience complications, 54.7 percent were from incomplete correction and 45.3 percent were from metal failure. Of those with incomplete correction, 87.8 percent required osteotomy and 12.2 percent were followed with observation. Note that sum of the outcomes for each subset of branches in Figure 13.3 sums to 100 percent (1.00). Thus, a child undergoing the tension band plate intervention had a 4.4 percent chance of having a complication ending in osteotomy ($0.092 \times 0.547 \times 0.878$ = 0.044).

Utility scores, measures that quantify health-related quality of life (Step 4), were developed by having 25 pediatric orthopedic surgeons respond to a questionnaire asking them to score each scenario depicted in the decision tree on a scale from 0 (death) to 100 (perfect health). The mean score of having no complications from a treatment was 98; an outcome requiring osteotomy was scored as 81 or 82. The mean scores were then converted to probabilities (0–1.0), and each was entered into the decision tree at the end of its respective branch, along with the calculated probability of having that outcome.

Statistical analysis software was used to calculate the expected utility of each of the interventions (Step 5), along with sensitivity analyses that varied the probabilities of each outcome (Step 6). The investigators reported that the tension band plate may provide a slightly better quality of life (0.969) than the staples and the percutaneous screws interventions (0.962 and 0.957, respectively). The analysis was not without some limitations. For one, the utilities were surgeon-derived rather than patient-derived. For another, the probabilities were calculated from the evidence reported in the literature rather than from randomized controlled trials. Publication of these types of results may aid clinicians in advising their patients about the possible outcomes of each of several treatment options, and can provide realistic expectations that can aid in patients' decision making.

Outcomes Research

Outcomes research is "the study of the end results of health services that takes patients' experiences, preferences, and values into account ... intended to provide scientific evidence relating to decisions made by all who participate in health care."[15] It includes convenience, cost, geographical accessibility, and patient preferences for procedures and treatments. The results of outcomes research are used by governments, employers, and insurers who seek to minimize costs while providing acceptable levels of care. Providers may also implement outcomes research in their practices.

In England and Wales, the National Institute for Health and Care Excellence (NICE) assesses health technologies and clinical practices for the National Health Service (NHS). From an outcomes research perspective, NICE recommends the adoption of new technologies (including pharmaceuticals) when that technology appears to be cost-effective. The first pharmaceutical reviewed by NICE was zanamivir (a drug developed for the treatment influenza) in 1999. That evaluation concluded that the drug should not be made available to the NHS. Since that first evaluation, NICE has established itself as one of the pioneer users of outcomes research data for developing health policy, and its methods are now studied globally as an exemplar for assessing the value of new pharmaceuticals and other health care technologies.

Quality of Care

One of the areas that concerns outcomes researchers (or outcomes epidemiologists) is the quality of care provided to patients. Chapter 7 discussed the development of DALYs and QALYs, measures of the burden of disease at the population level. Measuring outcomes at the individual level, however, requires evaluating the health services available to individuals and the quality of care that begins with patient–physician interactions. Put forth by Donabedian in 1966, one model considers quality of care in terms of structure, process, and outcomes. *Structure* refers to the physical location, equipment, staff, and financing where the health care service of interest is provided. For example, is the facility conveniently located? Is it accessible to patients with disabilities? Is the equipment used in the facility state of the art? *Process* covers all interactions between patients and providers, including clinical evaluation; tests, procedures, and treatments; and patient compliance and satisfaction with the interactions that occur at that location. *Outcomes* include the effects of the health care service provided on the health status of both the individual patient and the entire population served.

As an example, Blayney applied the Donabedian model to an academic medical center.[16] The author recommended evaluating the structure where patient care was delivered as well as the infrastructure (including informatics, a concept not yet applicable when the original model was put forth) of the facility. With regard to process, he also recommended measuring both patient satisfaction and patient adherence to treatments. Finally, he noted that while the gold standard for outcomes usually focuses on total recovery and long-term survival, it is important to include quality of life measures, as these are especially important for patients with chronic illnesses. In areas that were identified as needing improvement at the medical center being evaluated, systematic quality improvement (QI) measures were implemented. Blayney suggested that continuing the evaluative process on an ongoing basis using the Donabedian model should result in lean management, established metrics for success, waste reduction, and the addition of value for both patients and providers at the medical center.

Comparative Effectiveness Research

Comparative effectiveness research (CER) reviews and compares available evidence on the effectiveness, costs, and benefits of various treatments. Wennberg pioneered the use of population-level data for evaluating variations in treatments using 1969 information from a health data system in Vermont.[17] The results of his study demonstrated that the availability of health care in an area, not clinical need, drove the utilization of services. For example, the two areas with the lowest number of providers in Vermont had 13 tonsillectomies per 10,000 people. In contrast, the two areas with the highest number of providers had 151 tonsillectomies per 10,000 people. Other surgical procedures, the number of days of hospital stay, and the number of nursing home beds showed the same pattern. Wennberg concluded that too much medical care and the likelihood of *iatrogenic illness* (one inadvertently caused by a medical treatment or diagnostic procedure) was as important as not having enough medical care available for communities.

As clinical practices move towards implementing electronic medical records and as ever larger data bases become available for evaluation, CER is likely to become an increasingly important tool for outcomes research. Physician-recorded outcomes as well as patient-recorded outcomes will also become more widely available for large epidemiologic and health economic studies.[18] These large studies should allow finding the best treatment option for the average patient, but they do not take into account the needs of individual patients. One type of CER that does take the individual patient into account, however, is *patient-centered outcomes research* (PCOR).

PCOR seeks to improve patient care and outcomes through research guided by patients, caregivers, and the health care community. It informs patient-centered medicine in which the clinician and patient form a partnership to make therapeutic decisions together. The partners must consider the diagnosis as well as the cultural, psychological, and social factors that may influence the patient's prognosis. PCOR provides information regarding treatment alternatives and the likely outcomes for a heterogeneous group of patients, not just the average one. Such information allows for more informed discussions about the potential for individualized courses of therapy. Snyder and colleagues note that because PCOR incorporates the patient perspective, methods that measure patient-reported outcomes (PROs) are critical.[19]

Patient-Reported Outcomes

Patient-reported outcomes (PROs) are patients' direct reports of their health status—what they are able to do and how they feel—without these responses being filtered or interpreted by anyone else. PROs can be measured using survey tools that measure *health-related quality of life* (HRQoL) in various ways. Hundreds of HRQoL instruments have been developed for use with specific diseases, but seven have been designed to be applicable for the general population. These appear in Table 13.2.

Derived from the Medical Outcomes Study (MOS), the SF-36 health survey is the most commonly used of the instruments in Table 13.2.[20] The MOS examined (1) clinical end points; (2) physical, social, and role functioning in everyday living; (3) patients' perceptions of their general health and well-being; and (4) satisfaction with their treatment. In a cross-sectional design, the MOS evaluated 22,462 patients of 523 randomly selected clinicians from different health care settings in three US cities (Boston, Chicago, and Los Angeles). A subsample of 2,349 patients with chronic illnesses (diabetes, hypertension, coronary heart disease, and/or depression) became subjects for a longitudinal

TABLE 13.2 Quality of Life Instruments Designed for General Use

QUALITY OF LIFE INSTRUMENT	MEASURES	USED FOR
Medical Outcomes Study 36-Item Short Form (SF-36)	✓ Vitality ✓ Physical functioning ✓ Bodily pain ✓ General health perceptions ✓ Physical role functioning ✓ Emotional role functioning ✓ Social role functioning ✓ Mental health	✓ Evaluating individual health status. ✓ Researching the cost-effectiveness of a treatment. ✓ Monitoring and comparing disease burden.
Nottingham Health Profile (NHP)	✓ Sleep ✓ Mobility ✓ Energy ✓ Pain ✓ Emotional reactions ✓ Social isolation	✓ Reflecting patient rather than professional perceptions of health.
Sickness Impact Profile (SIP)	✓ Physical dimensions o Somatic autonomy o Mobility control ✓ Psychological dimensions o Psychological autonomy and communication o Emotional stability ✓ Social dimensions o Mobility range o Social behavior	✓ Constructing a measure of sickness in relation to impact on behavior.

Instrument	Dimensions	Purpose
Dartmouth Primary Care Cooperative Information Project (COOP) Charts	✓ Physical fitness ✓ Feelings ✓ Daily activities ✓ Social activities ✓ Pain ✓ Change in health ✓ Overall health ✓ Social support ✓ Quality of life	✓ Providing clinicians with immediate about the health status of their patients.
Quality of Well-Being (QWB) Scale	✓ Mobility ✓ Physical activity ✓ Social activity ✓ Symptoms/problem complexes	✓ Summarizing HRQoL in a single measure (0 to 1).
Health Utilities Index (HUI) (in more than one version)	✓ Sensation (vision, hearing, speech) ✓ Mobility (ambulation, dexterity) ✓ Emotion ✓ Cognitive ✓ Self-care ✓ Pain ✓ Fertility	✓ Summarizing HRQoL in a single measure (0 to 1).
EuroQol Instrument (EQ-5D)	• Mobility • Self-care • Usual activities • Pain/discomfort • Anxiety/depression	• Summarizing HRQoL in a single measure (0 to 1).

study to monitor treatments, hospitalizations, and the outcomes of care. Various survey instruments were tested on 1,440 patients in the subsample, and the investigators reported that the SF-36 was reliable for measuring both physical and mental health from the patient's point of view.[21]

Summary

Clinicians apply the principles and practices of epidemiology as they order screening and diagnostic tests, make treatment decisions, and evaluate the effectiveness of those treatments on the health outcomes of their patients. Some may even have utilized decision analysis to inform them of the probabilities of complex treatment options. Clinicians understand the purpose and worth of patient-centered outcomes research for their practices and appreciate the importance of measuring patient outcomes that include quality of life measures.

Many clinical practitioners may already be participating in epidemiologic research in ways they may not perceive. Every birth or death certificate they file builds a database for descriptive epidemiologic studies. Every case reported to a disease registry helps build a database for epidemiologic research. Some physicians refer their patients for clinical trials. Many clinicians obtain HRQoL surveys on their patients to evaluate whether treatments are working. Those who run health care facilities may evaluate their institution's structures and processes, as well as patient outcomes, and perhaps even include patient satisfaction surveys as part of their quality improvement efforts. What is clear is that as medical informatics continues to advance, clinicians and their patients will be providing increasing amounts of information that should yield rich databases for epidemiologic, health services, and health outcomes research.

References

1. Sir William Osler, *Teacher and Student. Aequanimitas, with Other Addresses to Medical Students, Nurses and Practitioners of Medicine.* Philadelphia: Blakiston, 1904.
2. Sir William Osler, R. B. Bean, compiler, W. B. Bean, editor, *Sir William Osler: Aphorisms from his Bedside Teachings and Writings.* New York: H. Schuman, 1950.
3. Heikki Joensuu et al., "Risk for Distant Recurrence of Breast Cancer Detected by Mammography Screening or Other Methods," *Journal of the American Medical Association* 292, no. 9 (2004): 1064–1073.
4. Yu Shen et al., "Role of Detection Method in Predicting Breast Cancer Survival: Analysis of Randomized Screening Trials," *Journal of the National Cancer Institute* 97 no. 16 (2005): 1195–1203.

5. Miquel Porta, ed., *A Dictionary of Epidemiology, 6th Edition*. New York: Oxford University Press, 2014.

6. A. Farkas et al., "National Trends in the Epidemiology of Prostate Cancer, 1973 To 1994: Evidence for the effectiveness of Prostate-Specific Antigen Screening," *Urology* 52, no. 3 (1998): 444–8; discussion 448–9.

7. Donatello Telesca, Ruth Etzioni, and Roman Gulati, "Estimating Lead Time and Overdiagnosis Associated with PSA Screening from Prostate Cancer Incidence Trends," *Biometrics* 64, no. 1 (2008): 10–19.

8. US Preventive Services Task Force, "Screening for Prostate Cancer," May 2012. Available at http://www.uspreventiveservicestaskforce.org/Page/Document/RecommendationStatementFinal/prostate-cancer-screening.

9. M. Jung, "National Cancer Screening Programs and Evidence-Based Health Care Policy in South Korea," *Health Policy* 119, no. 1 (2015): 26–32, doi:10.1016/j.healthpol.2014.08.012.

10. Marc Bulterys et al., "Rapid HIV-1 Testing During Labor: A Multicenter Study," *Journal of the American Medical Association* 292, no. 2 (2004): 219–223.

11. D. J. Jamieson et al., "Rapid Human Immunodeficiency Virus-1 Testing on Labor and Delivery in 17 US hospitals: The MIRIAD Experience," *American Journal of Obstetrics and Gynecology*. 197, no. 3, Supplement (2007): S72–S82.

12. Donald Berry, "Commentary: Screening Mammography: A Decision Analysis," *International Journal of Epidemiology* 33, no. 1 (2004): 68–68.

13. Harry Bakwin, "Pseudodoxia Pediatrica," *New England Journal of Medicine* 232, no. 24 (1945): 691–697.

14. Ki Hyuk Sung et al., "Determining the Best Treatment for Coronal Angular Deformity of the Knee Joint in Growing Children: A Decision Analysis," *Biomed Research International Vol. 2014* (2014): article ID 603432, doi:10.1155/2014/603432.

15. Carolyn M. Clancy and John M. Eisenberg, "Outcomes Research: Measuring the End Results of Health Care," *Science* 282, no. 5387 (1998): 245–246.

16. Douglas W. Blayney, "Measuring and Improving Quality of Care in an Academic Medical Center," *Journal of Oncology Practice* 9, no. 3 (2013): 138–141.

17. John Wennberg and Alan Gittelsohn, "Small Area Variations in Health Care Delivery," *Science* 182, no. 4117 (1973): 1102–1108.

18. Albert W. Wu et al., "Measure once, Cut Twice—Adding Patient-Reported Outcome Measures to the Electronic Health Record for Comparative Effectiveness Research," *Journal of Clinical Epidemiology* 66, no. 8, Supplement (2013): S12–S20.

19. C. F. Snyder et al., "Patient-Reported Outcomes (Pros): Putting the Patient Perspective in Patient-Centered Outcomes Research," *Medical Care* 51, no. 8, Supplement 3 (2013): S73–S79.

20. Alvin R. Tarlov et al., "The Medical Outcomes Study: An Application of Methods for Monitoring the Results of Medical Care," *Journal of the American Medical Association* 262, no. 7 (1989): 925–930.

21. John E. Ware et al., "Comparison of Methods for the Scoring and Statistical Analysis of SF-36 Health Profile and Summary Measures: Summary of Results from the Medical Outcomes Study," *Medical Care* 33, no. 4, Supplement (1995): AS264–AS279.

14 | Field Epidemiology

... the committee defines the substance of public health
as: organized community efforts aimed at the prevention of disease
and promotion of health. It links many disciplines and rests upon
the scientific core of epidemiology.[1]

Committee for the Study of the Future of Public Health (1988)

Field Epidemiology Defined

Field epidemiology (applied epidemiology, hospital epidemiology, intervention epidemiology, or shoe leather epidemiology) is "the practice of [epidemiology] in real time and real place, which in turn involves both science and art."[2] Definitions of field epidemiology[3-4] generally agree that:

- A health-related problem arises unexpectedly
- A timely response is demanded
- The epidemiologist goes to the field to investigate the problem
- The investigation is limited because of time or other situational constraints

Field epidemiologists do more than respond to health-related events after they occur. They also apply scientific methods to generate new knowledge and evidence for both current and future decision making. For example, field epidemiologists work as part of multidisciplinary teams to design and implement new surveillance and public health preparedness programs. They also participate in public health research and train the next generation of field epidemiologists.

The Rise of Field Epidemiology

Field epidemiology has a longstanding history dating back to the epidemiologist John Simon and the English Privy Council in Victorian England. As the role of the state in public health evolved, so did field epidemiology activities in the United Kingdom. In the United States, such activities were under the purview of the state and local health departments, with the Public Health Service supporting those activities when requested. Following the Second World War, the US Communicable Disease Center (CDC) was established with a primary mission of malaria control in the American south. The agency's founder, Assistant Surgeon General Joseph Mountin, advocated for the agency taking on other communicable diseases, and in 1947 the CDC began operations in a headquarters in Georgia. Four years later, Alex Langmuir was recruited to the CDC to establish an epidemiology training program, the Epidemic Intelligence Service (EIS). Since the agency's creation the CDC has responded to approximately 5,000 requests for *Epi-Aids* (epidemiologic field investigations), including more than 550 international requests ranging from elevated radiation exposure following cardiac imaging scans to events of mass hysteria.[5-6]

Similar to the EIS program in the United States, the European Programme for Intervention Epidemiology Training (EPIET), created in 1995, began establishing a network of field epidemiologists to strengthen the epidemiology workforce throughout the European Union. In 2007 EPIET was merged with the newly created European Centre for Disease Prevention and Control (ECDC) headquartered in Stockholm, Sweden.[8] These agencies work together with the World Health Organization and various regional agencies to identify and rapidly respond to global health threats.

Field Investigations

The investigation of a foodborne outbreak, a common occurrence in many local communities, was presented in Chapter 1. It is also possible to investigate outbreaks at a regional or even global level. Indeed, some of these large-scale efforts have yielded impressive results. For example, smallpox has been globally eradicated, polio and Guinea worm are on the edge of eradication, and several other infectious diseases have been targeted for eradication (e.g., cysticercosis or tapeworm, lymphatic filariasis, measles, mumps, and rubella) or control (onchoceriasis or river blindness, schistosomiasis, and trachoma). Outbreaks of persistent (cholera), new (SARS), and reemerging (tuberculosis) diseases require rapid response in order to arrest their spread. Outbreaks may occur due to bioterrorist events, in the aftermath of war or natural hazards, or from everyday environmental and occupational exposures. How do epidemiologists respond when called upon for aid in the field? The simple answer is that it depends upon the situation, but the pathway to a field investigation is clear.

Fieldwork is undertaken in a series of steps (Box 14.1). First, the epidemiologist must establish the purpose of the project. Is the purpose of the fieldwork to help control the spread of a disease, or to identify possible etiologic factors for the outbreak? Perhaps aid has been requested to train additional public health workers, follow up on previous cases, or assess the burden of disease in an endemic area.

Once the purpose of the fieldwork is determined, the epidemiologist considers logistics. Will the epidemiologist lead the investigation, serve as advisor to other public health personnel, or function as part of a multidisciplinary team? Is the project site so remote as to preclude the use of telephones or computers? Is protective clothing required? How will environmental or biological samples be handled and transported? How will the epidemiologist communicate findings, to whom, and with what intended effect? These questions, and more, should be carefully considered before embarking on fieldwork.

For an infectious disease outbreak with a known etiological agent, some of the steps in Box 14.1 may happen contemporaneously because of the speed

---

BOX 14.1 STEPS IN AN OUTBREAK INVESTIGATION

1 Prepare for fieldwork
2 Establish the existence of an outbreak
3 Verify the diagnosis
4 Construct a working case definition
5 Find cases systematically and record information
6 Perform descriptive epidemiology (time, place, persons)
7 Develop hypotheses
8 Evaluate hypotheses epidemiologically
9 As necessary, reconsider, refine, and reevaluate hypotheses
10 Compare and reconcile with laboratory and/or environmental studies
11 Implement control and prevention measures
12 Initiate or maintain surveillance
13 Communicate findings

SOURCE: *Principles of Epidemiology in Public Health Practice*, 3rd Edition (CDC, updated 2011). http://www.cdc.gov/ophss/csels/dsepd/SS1978/SS1978.pdf

required for response. For example, the Ministry of Health in Guinea (West Africa) reported an outbreak of Ebola hemorrhagic fever (86 cases with 59 deaths, case fatality ratio = 68.5%) to the World Health Organization in March 2014 (Step 2).[9] Biologic samples from the cases sent to the Pasteur Institute in Lyon, France, suggested *Zaire ebolavirus* as the causative agent (Step 3). Field agents followed up on reports of suspected cases, including those in neighboring countries (Steps 4 and 5). *Médecins sans Frontières* (Doctors without Borders) went into the epicenter of the outbreak to establish treatment centers to isolate suspected cases and treat confirmed cases in an effort to help stem the spread of the disease and to attempt to reduce case fatality (Step 11). Field efforts required strict adherence to biosafety guidelines in laboratories, barrier nursing procedures, use of personal protective equipment by all health care workers, disinfection of contaminated objects and areas, and safe burials (Step 11). Community education efforts were instituted to reduce human-to-human transmission and to encourage community identification of additional cases (Step 11). Case-finding expanded to neighboring countries (Step 4), confirmed and suspected cases were isolated, contacts of cases were followed up and monitored (Step 11), and surveillance was aggressively maintained (Step 12). On August 8, the World Health Organization (WHO) declared the epidemic to be a Public Health Emergency of International Concern,[9] and many countries instituted public health education efforts (Step 13) along with screening international travelers and isolating potential cases.

Efforts to find the origin of the 2014 Ebola outbreak happened contemporaneously (Steps 6–10). Finding the cause of the outbreak would allow epidemiologists to stop further infections from the source, better understand the disease, and, hopefully, to prevent future outbreaks. At the time of the investigation Ebola was known to be a *zoonotic disease*, transmissible from vertebrate animals to man. *Primary* cases were known to result from an individual being exposed to an infected living or dead animal. *Secondary cases* (human-to-human) were known to arise from exposure to the bodily fluids of infected individuals.[10] The *reservoir* (natural habitat) of the virus was not known.

The epidemiologic investigation gathered data on possible sources of transmission from hospital records as well as from interviews with patients, their contacts, neighbors, family members, and others. Case tracing, a line listing of cases, and an epidemic curve (see Chapter 3) identified the *index case* (the first case) as a 2-year-old child who died in Meliandou, in Guéckédou prefecture, on December 6, 2013 (Figure 14.1).

The investigative team reported that the virus was likely transmitted from an infected animal to the index case and then spread among close contacts

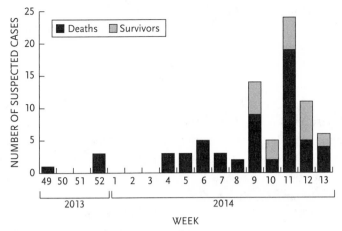

FIGURE 14.1 Number of suspected cases of Ebola virus disease, Guéckédou (80 suspected cases with 59 deaths).

SOURCE: Baize et al. (2014).[11] Used with permission.

for months before a *cluster* of cases appeared in local hospitals and the outbreak was reported.[11] The cluster of cases grew to become the largest Ebola epidemic in history, with secondary cases reaching Europe and the United States by the end of 2014.

Clusters

A *cluster* is a greater than expected number of cases of disease occurring within a group of people in a geographic area over a defined period of time. It is not unusual for physicians, parents, neighbors, or co-workers of the cases to report a cluster to local authorities in the hope that a field investigation will find and eliminate the cause(s). When the cluster has an infectious etiology,[12] or if the disease of concern is rare,[13] a field investigation may be quite effective. However, when the etiologic agent(s) are noninfectious or the outcome of concern is fairly common (such as cancer), the results have historically been limited.[14]

Increasing public demand for field investigations of noninfectious disease clusters led to the National Conference on Clustering of Health Events in Atlanta, Georgia in 1989. The *cluster busters* at the conference reported that noninfectious cluster investigations rarely produced important findings. Rather, cluster investigations had become efforts in managing public expectations.[15] Following the conference, CDC published guidelines for investigating noninfectious disease clusters, injuries, birth defects, and previously unrecognized syndromes or illnesses.[16] The guidelines were revised for cancer clusters in particular in 2013 to reflect improved data sources, new investigative techniques and analytical methods, and lessons learned.[17] CDC recommended a four-step response to an initial report of a cancer cluster:

1. *Initial contact and response*: The responder (most likely a local health department) should be empathetic, collect information from the inquirer, and refer them to the relevant unit as quickly as possible.
2. *Assessment*: The responder should consider the evidence as presented by the inquirer and the biologic plausibility that the cancers could share a common etiology.
3. *Determining the feasibility of conducting an epidemiologic study*: The responder must develop a study hypothesis, conduct a literature review, consider population health and risk factors, confirm cases, and verify whether there are data on the environmental contaminants of concern.
4. *Conducting an epidemiologic study to assess the association between cancers and environmental causes*: If the conditions for an epidemiologic investigation are met, implementation may proceed. The study should be designed to add both to epidemiologic and public health knowledge, if possible.

Because reports of cancer clusters usually involve few cases, the ability of an epidemiologic investigation to statistically detect a causal association is often low. Failure to provide a satisfactory response to public concerns, however, erodes public trust. Public health agencies must therefore respond to reports of cancer clusters with timely and effective communication. Agencies must be transparent about the progress of a cancer cluster investigation and the likelihood that it will be able to identify potential etiologic factors.

Terrorism

When events are potentially linked to terrorism (anthrax, dirty bombs, explosions, plague, smallpox, and more), epidemiologic field investigations need to be coordinated with those of law enforcement. The epidemiologist must help identify and isolate known cases, interview potential cases and their contacts, take environmental or biological samples to identify exposures, and set up surveillance. At the same time, law enforcement needs to preserve the crime scene, take suspects into custody, interview witnesses, and guarantee the *chain of custody* for any evidence that may be used at trial. Field and law enforcement investigators need to collaborate and respect the protocols of their concurrent investigations, as both efforts are designed to ensure the health and safety of the public as well as meet the need for justice.

For example, infection with *Bacillus anthracis* is rare in the United States, with no case of inhalation anthrax reported between 1976 and 2001. In October 2001 a media worker in Florida was diagnosed with inhalation anthrax, and a multistate team of investigators from public health and law enforcement (federal, state, and local) was formed. Coordinated through CDC's Emergency Operations Center, the group worked collaboratively to identify additional cases of anthrax, describe case and exposure characteristics, and prevent further cases through public health interventions (limiting exposure to contaminated sites, providing vaccines, etc.).[18] By November 20 of that year, 22 cases of either cutaneous or inhalational anthrax were identified. Five of the cases died (*case-fatality rate* = 45%). Twenty of the 22 cases had been either mail handlers or had worked at facilities where contaminated mail was processed. The epidemic curve showed that the contaminated letters were mailed in two waves, with the letters passing through a postal facility in Trenton, New Jersey. Further environmental sampling traced the mailing to a specific mail drop box in Princeton, New Jersey. Although the perpetrator was not apprehended, the rapid response to the public health emergency was swift and effective. Persons deemed at risk for inhalational anthrax were identified, and antimicrobials for postexposure prophylaxis were recommended. While the collaborative team had to refine their study methods and recommendations, they were able to respect the protocols needed for both the public health and criminal investigations.

Disasters

Disasters originate from natural, man-made, or complex causes. *Natural disasters* are catastrophic events not caused by human actions. These include but are not limited to acute events such as earthquakes, floods, tornados, and volcanic eruptions. Natural disasters may also develop slowly, such as drought or other climate change. *Man-made disasters* are caused by human actions, whether purposeful or not. Examples include environmental contamination (biological or toxic), industrial accidents or explosions, structure failures (bridges, tunnels, etc.), human error, and purposeful decisions that result in social and political violence.[19] Sometimes natural and man-made disasters overlap to create *complex emergencies*. Complex emergencies happen because the infrastructure to provide relief has been disrupted or may never have existed, or because governing structures are weak or uncooperative.[20]

Regardless of whether the disaster is natural, man-made, or complex in nature, the epidemiologist may serve a part of an initial response team, doing a "walk through" to directly observe and estimate the number of deaths, the number remaining to be rescued, or the number of victims requiring emergency medical attention. "Quick and dirty" surveys may need to be developed to set baseline quantitative information. Rapid health screenings may need to be instituted to determine the need for nutritional supplementation or the need for vaccine programs. Surveillance systems may need to be created to detect disease outbreaks or monitor the long-term health effects on both disaster victims and first responders.[21] The field epidemiologist needs to be flexible and ready to respond as circumstances may require.

For example, while the events of September 11, 2001 needed to be investigated as acts of terrorism, they also needed to be handled as a complex emergency. Deaths and injuries had to be estimated and systems put into place to identify victims and notify their families. Safety measures needed to be implemented for first responders and cleanup workers dealing with structurally unstable and environmentally contaminated environments. Surveillance systems needed to be put into place to determine the immediate and long-terms effects of the attacks on the surviving victims, the first responders, and the communities affected.

Epidemiologic data show that 2,823 persons died in the attacks of September 11, both in the planes used as weapons and on the ground. Cross-sectional surveys of 3,271 civilian survivors of the twin tower collapse found that 1 in 6 suffered symptoms of posttraumatic stress disorder two to three years after the event.[22] Ten-year surveillance of a cohort of 50,000 rescue, recovery, and cleanup workers, and 400,000 additional persons living in the areas surrounding the lower Manhattan site, showed lasting health effects from the event. Fully 20 percent suffered from mental health disorders (four times the prevalence in the general population), along with increased incidence of respiratory illnesses and heart disease.[23] Studies to determine the effects of September 11 on cancer incidence and overall mortality continue.

The epidemiologist occupies a central role in dealing with both disease outbreaks and other adverse health events in the field. They may provide key information for public health and law enforcement authorities and for political leaders who have to respond to events in real time. Their findings may also influence health planning and policy initiatives after the investigation is over. To aid in their ability to provide key information, the field epidemiologist has several tools at his/her disposal.

Tools for Field Investigations

One of the most useful tools to the field epidemiologist is *Epi Info*™—free, widely used software that is available in several languages.[24] Using Epi Info, the epidemiologist can draft questionnaires, enter data, and create line listings of the cases, their demographic characteristics, and their potential exposures. The software generates descriptive and epidemiologic statistics such as relative risks, along with graphs that include options for epidemic curves. Epi Info has been used in innumerable field investigations, in situations as disparate as rapidly assessing the water, sanitation, and hygiene situation in a relief camp in Uganda,[25] evaluating the association between malaria and population growth in Brazil,[26] and investigating an outbreak of pertussis in rural Texas.[27] The software also provides the epidemiologist with simple mapping capabilities, another tool widely used in field investigations.

Maps are powerful visualization tools. *Spot maps* aid the epidemiologist in identifying clusters of disease and can target potential sources of exposure. Spot maps are often created by placing colored pins or stick-on spots on street maps to identify where pedestrian accidents have happened, rabid animals have been found, or wells have been contaminated. Spot maps allow the identification and monitoring of potential "hot spots" where public health interventions might be needed. The field epidemiologist may also create a spot map as a visual aid for communicating findings to local residents. Because spot maps are low-tech, they remain a vital tool for many field investigations.

Epi Info includes access to *shapefiles* (geospatial information) that allow the epidemiologist to generate *choropleth* maps depicting the value of a variable (such as the occurrence of disease) among non-overlapping geographic units (e.g., states, counties, municipalities, census tracks, villages, or postal codes). While choropleth maps have the ability to portray differences in outcomes or exposures spatially, they also have serious limitations. Consider the likelihood that an outbreak of disease will be evenly distributed across the unit of geographic analysis. A spot map is able to show hot spots, but a choropleth map will show the entire geographic unit at risk. Which is more useful? Now consider that diseases rarely respect political boundaries (state lines, town limits), particularly when populations are mobile. It is entirely possible that a choropleth map will miss identifying an outbreak if cases occur across the units of analysis so that the incidence of disease in any given unit is not elevated. To evaluate whether this is a problem, the epidemiologist should examine the data at varying *geographic scales* (the size of the geographic unit) so as not to miss an effect.[28]

Geographic information systems (GIS) provide powerful analytic tools that consider multiple map layers and examine the relationships among the variables represented on those layers at varying geographic scales. GIS is useful for evaluating whether patterns are random, clustered, or dispersed—information of importance to the field epidemiologist. It is widely used to produce spatial optimization models, to identify where and how emergency services are best located, or to model the movement of pollutants through air and water so that populations can be evacuated if needed.

Using *remote sensing* (obtained without making physical contact for measurement) and *satellite imagery* data, a GIS specialist can help the epidemiologist demonstrate environmental changes that have or may impact the biological health of plants, animals, and humans. Properly used, GIS can identify areas where disease vectors are likely to present the greatest risk, where toxic exposures are the highest, or where crop failures are likely to result in famine. What GIS technology cannot do, however, is provide the epidemiologist with a tool for hypothesis testing. Spatial data are limited for use with inferential statistics because each geographic unit represents a population rather than a sample. Indeed, places are not randomly located nor are they independent of the places next to them. Despite these data limitations, the use of GIS in epidemiology is expanding.

One way that GIS is expanding for use by the epidemiologist is through public participation. *Public Participatory GIS* (PPGIS) is a technique that enlists the help of community members in data collection, mapping, analysis, and decision making. The field epidemiologist may ask community members to review local maps for accuracy, to help locate areas for search and rescue, or to identify community assets that can be mobilized during or after an emergency. For instance, the Coastal Services Center in the National Oceanic and Atmospheric Administration (NOAA) now recommends that PPGIS be used to aid coastal communities in planning for resilience after disasters. The agency learned the value of PPGIS when it was implemented in affected communities after the Indian Ocean tsunami in 2004.[29]

PPGIS is useful for *community asset mapping*, the production of maps of various types of resources with input from community members.[30] Community asset maps reflect the social structure and culture of each individual community, information that can be invaluable to the field epidemiologist assigned to a new location. The field epidemiologist may also ask community members to use cell phones or portable global positioning system (GPS) units to mark the locations of informal gathering places, as well as the locations of environmental contaminants or known disease vectors. For example, PPGIS informed decisions regarding placement of primary health care services for nomadic tribes in Chad,[31] identification of areas of arsenic contamination of ground water in rural Texas,[32] and location of areas where vector suppression was needed for malaria control in Tanzania.[33]

Surveillance

The field epidemiologist may need to implement various types of surveillance to monitor environmental exposures; identify, potentially isolate, and treat known cases; or find potential cases through contact tracing. Sentinel surveillance (see Chapter 7) may be instituted to provide early warning of potential outbreaks. As an example, caged chickens have been used as sentinel animals to identify when West Nile virus risks are elevated in places as disparate as the Senegal River Delta[34] and the Los Angeles area in California.[35] Knowing the presence of the vector may allow the field epidemiologist to suggest approaches that limit the transmission of the disease to humans. Similarly, companion animals have been used as sentinels to monitor zoonotic parasites among indigenous populations in Canada. Identifying the parasites in animal companions allows the field epidemiologist to suggest interventions that reduce worm infestations, diarrheal and cystic diseases, and diseases such as ocular and visceral larva migrans.[36] Diagnoses of Lyme disease in pets also signal the danger of increased risk to humans residing in an area,[37] and this allows the field epidemiologist to suggest implementing health education programs that include preventive measures such as using repellents and protective clothing, and doing tick checks.

Reports of infectious diseases from centralized systems may also help the field epidemiologist to estimate the scope of an outbreak. For instance, the *National Outbreak Reporting System* (NORS) for identifying outbreaks of enteric diseases in the United States was presented in Chapter 1. Similarly, *PulseNet International* is a global network of laboratories that evaluate the molecular footprints of foodborne disease agents, helping the field epidemiologist link similar cases so that common exposures can be identified and evaluated.[38] For example, PulseNet International aided in linking cases of *Shigella sonei* reported from multiple countries. The cases were traced to a common exposure—air travel from Hawaii to various global destinations in 2004.[39] Overall, 204 cases were confirmed, and 300 to 1,500 additional individuals were estimated to have been infected, with the source identified as contaminated meals served on outbound flights that were provided by a single caterer.[40]

Being able to identify cases of infectious disease as early as possible is of primary importance for preventing outbreaks from becoming pandemics.

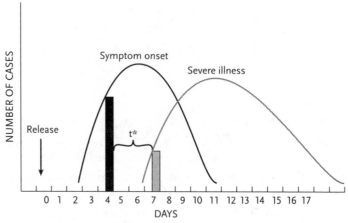

FIGURE 14.2 Syndromic surveillance—rationale for early detection.
SOURCE: Henning (2004).[41]

Syndromic surveillance, for instance, detects early cases of illness before health authorities confirm them (see Chapter 7). Consider that an increase in calls to a poison control center, a rush on over-the-counter sales of anti-diarrheal medications, or a sudden rash of animal deaths might not necessarily command attention as an outbreak in traditional surveillance systems. If these events are reported to a centralized system and monitored in real time, as-yet-undiagnosed outbreaks might be detected. In other words, the epidemic curve is shifted to the left through syndromic surveillance, detecting outbreaks in their prediagnostic phase (Figure 14.2).[41]

Crowdsourcing is the process of obtaining information from large groups of people via digital media, a process made possible by the development of highly efficient search engines. For instance, the *Global Public Health Intelligence Network* (GPHIN) was developed by Health Canada in 2000. GPHIN monitors digital media sources around the world, scanning the media for health events. GPHIN then disseminates that information to public health authorities in real time. This system was able to identify the SARS outbreak in 2003, months before it was reported to the World Health Organization (WHO).[42] By creating awareness among global public health authorities, the outbreak was contained before it could become a pandemic.

HealthMap, another real-time global health monitoring system, was developed at the Boston Children's Hospital. This system scans various reporting systems for cases of infectious diseases and displays them on interactive maps by time and disease agent. The maps are accessible to the public on both an interactive website and a smartphone application. Other surveillance systems based on crowdsourcing include *Sickweather.com*, which scans social media sites such as Facebook and Twitter for symptoms of select diseases, and *Google Flu Trends*, which aggregates information from Google searches about the flu. Aggregates of flu-related queries identified by Google Flu Trends cannot be matched to the number of reported cases of the flu, but they may suggest early flu activity in various regions.[43]

Participatory surveillance allows individuals to report their own symptoms to an online database. An example of participatory surveillance system is *Flu Near You*, a website linked to HealthMap that allows any individual in Canada or the United States who is at least 13 years old to register to participate. Flu Near You contacts each registrant by email weekly, eliciting information about whether they developed flu symptoms or were immunized against the flu during the past week. The results of the data collection are portrayed on HealthMap.[44]

The widespread use of social media provides additional tools for surveillance. For example, the New York City Department of Health and Mental Hygiene used online reviews of restaurants by their patrons on Yelp, a business review website, to identify unreported cases of foodborne illness.[45] The Chicago Department of Health monitored Twitter, a microblogging service, to identify tweets suggesting symptoms of food poisoning. Over 10 months the project identified and responded to 270 tweets. Individuals with symptoms were referred to a reporting website where netizens could enter information on where and what they ate. Those reports resulted in 133 restaurant inspections (16 percent of the restaurants reported failed inspection, 25 percent passed but with critical or serious violations).[46] Being able to correct inspection violations quickly is important for preventing additional foodborne outbreaks.

Crowdsourcing and *infoveillance* (a digital, or real time epidemiologic study) can also be used to identify and potentially counter misinformation about outbreaks. For instance, in 2013 an outbreak of an avian virus (H7H9) previously unreported in humans appeared in southeast China. The outbreak totaled 108 confirmed cases with 23 deaths within the first month, with sporadic cases appearing for the remainder of the year. Most cases were traced to an exposure to infected birds at a live poultry market. No person-to-person transmission could be documented.

The H7H9 flu outbreak received widespread media attention in China, along with a great deal of misinformation circulated via various types of electronic media. To evaluate the problem, an infoveillance study was launched to determine the speed and extent of the misinformation.[47] The investigators obtained crowdsourcing data through China's most popular search engine (Baidu) and microblog site (Sina) and identified 32 different rumors that circulated rapidly throughout 19 provinces. One rumor of a case in a local school was started by a student and eventually forwarded by 34,000 people. Another rumor, that "eating chicken feet with pickled peppers" caused the infection, was found to have spread through five provinces within a few weeks of the first confirmed case of H7H9. The investigation found that a single case in a new area causes more public attention and viral spread of the information (accurate or not) than do additional cases in the same geographic area affected by the original outbreak. The investigators concluded that the first three days of an outbreak are critical for releasing timely information that is transparent, and the first week may be the critical period for health education. Failure to counter rumors with transparent reporting can be detrimental to effective public health interventions.

Summary

Field epidemiology takes place in real time and in real places at risk for developing or having already developed significant health problems. The field epidemiologist may be asked to estimate the scope of a problem, implement case findings, identify potential causal factors, work with law enforcement or first responders in emergency situations, set up surveillance in the field, or train additional field epidemiologists in their "science and art." Whether responding to the report of a foodborne outbreak, disease cluster, bioterrorist event, or disaster, fieldwork is undertaken in a series of steps designed to provide the effort with the greatest chance of success.

The field epidemiologist has a variety of tools that he/she may employ in preparation for going to the field (*crowdsourcing*, various types of *surveillance, GIS*), for use during a field investigation (*spot maps, Epi Info*), for use with the community once in the field (*PPGIS, community asset mapping*), and for evaluating the results of their efforts once the request for assistance has been completed (*observational studies, infoveillance*). Field epidemiologists go where they are needed, work to prevent outbreaks from becoming epidemics, and use the tools of their trade in creative ways. They are the test pilots of epidemiology.

References

1. Committee for the Study of the Future of Public Health, *The Future of Public Health*. Washington, DC: National Academies Press, 1988.
2. R. C. Dicker, "A Brief Review of the Basic Principles of Epidemiology," in *Field Epidemiology*, ed. M. B. Gregg. New York: Oxford University Press; 2008, 16–37.

3. R. A. Goodman and J. W. Buehler, "Field Epidemiology Defined," in *Field Epidemiology*, ed. M. B. Gregg. New York: Oxford University Press, 2008, 3–15.

4. Miquel Porta, ed., *A Dictionary of Epidemiology, 6th Edition*. New York: Oxford University Press, 2014.

5. P. S. Brachman and S. B. Thacker, "Evolution of Epidemic Investigations and Field Epidemiology During the *MMWR* Era at CDC—1961-2011." *MMWR Surveillance Summaries* 60, Supplement 4 (2011): 22–26.

6. Centers for Disease Control and Prevention, Epidemic Intelligence Service at NCEH/ATSDR, "Epi-AID Investigations." Available at http://www.cdc.gov/nceh/eis/epi_aid.html.

7. Louis Wolfe, *Disease Detectives*. New York: Franklin Watts, 1979.

8. European Programme for Intervention Epidemiology Training (EPIET). Available at http://ecdc.europa.eu/en/epiet/Pages/HomeEpiet.aspx.

9. Sylvie Briand et al., "The International Ebola Emergency," *New England Journal of Medicine* 371, no. 13 (2014): 1180–1183.

10. David L. Heymann, *Control of Communicable Diseases Manual, 20th Edition*. Washington, DC: Association American Public Health, 2014.

11. Sylvaine Baize et al., "Emergence of Zaire Ebola Virus Disease in Guinea," *New England Journal of Medicine* 371, no. 15 (2014): 1418–1425.

12. Denise Koo and Stephen B. Thacker, "In Snow's Footsteps: Commentary on Shoe-Leather and Applied Epidemiology," *American Journal of Epidemiology* 172, no. 6 (2010): 737–739.

13. Cristina Bosetti et al., "Occupational Exposure to Vinyl Chloride and Cancer Risk: A Review of the Epidemiologic Literature," *European Journal of Cancer Prevention* 12, no. 5 (2003): 427–430.

14. Michael Goodman et al., "Cancer Clusters in the USA: What Do the Last Twenty Years of State and Federal Investigations Tell Us?" *Critical Reviews in Toxicology* 42 no. 6 (2012): 474–490.

15. Kenneth J. Rothman, "A Sobering Start for the Cluster Busters' Conference," *American Journal of Epidemiology* 132, no. 1 Supplement (1990): S6–S13.

16. Guidelines for Investigating Clusters of Health Events. *MMWR – Recommendations and Reports* 39, RR-11 (1990): 1–23.

17. Investigating Suspected Cancer Clusters and Responding to Community Concerns: Guidelines from CDC and the Council of State and Territorial Epidemiologists. *MMWR – Recommendations and Reports* 62, RR-08 (2013): 1–24.

18. C. M. Greene et al., "Epidemiologic Investigations of Bioterrorism-Related Anthrax, New Jersey, 2001," *Emerging Infectious Diseases* 8, no. 10 (2002): 1048–1055.

19. Dona Schneider and Meredeth Turshen, "Social Moderators of Environmental Health: Political and Social Violence," in *Encyclopedia of Environmental Health*, eds. J Nriagu et al. Oxford, UK: Elsevier, 2011, 623–630.

20. P. B. Spiegel et al., "Occurrence and Overlap of Natural Disasters, Complex Emergencies and Epidemics During the Past Decade (1995-2004)," *Conflict and Health* 1 (2007): 2.

21. R. Waldman and E. K. Noji, "Field Investigations of Natural Disasters and Complex Emergencies," in *Field Epidemiology, 3rd edition*, 459–478, ed. M. Gregg. New York: Oxford University Press, 2008.

22. Laura DiGrande et al., "Long-Term Posttraumatic Stress Symptoms among 3,271 Civilian Survivors of the September 11, 2001, Terrorist Attacks on the World Trade Center," *American Journal of Epidemiology* 173, no. 3 (2011): 271–281.

23. New York City Department of Health, "What We Know about the Health Effects of 9/11." Available at http://www.nyc.gov/html/doh/wtc/html/home/home.shtml.

24. Centers for Disease Control and Prevention, Epi Info ™ 7.1.5. Available at http://wwwn.cdc.gov/epiinfo/index.htm.

25. Lynn M. Atuyambe et al., "Land Slide Disaster in Eastern Uganda: Rapid Assessment of Water, Sanitation and Hygiene Situation in Bulucheke Camp, Bududa District," *Environmental Health* 10 (2011): 38.

26. Éldi Vendrame Parise et al., "Epidemiological Profile of Malaria in the State of Tocantins, Brazil, from 2003 to 2008," *Revista do Instituto de Medicina Tropical de São Paulo* 53, no. 3 (2011): 141–147.

27. Anthony O. Eshofonie et al., "An Outbreak of Pertussis in Rural Texas: An Example of the Resurgence of the Disease in the United States," *Journal of Community Health* 40, no. 1 (June 2014): doi: 10.1007/s10900-014-9902-2.

28. Dona Schneider et al., "Cancer Clusters: The Importance of Monitoring Multiple Geographic Scales," *Social Science & Medicine* 37, no. 6 (1993): 753–759.

29. National Oceanographic and Atmospheric Administration, *Stakeholder Engagement Strategies for Participatory Mapping* (2009). Accessed March 30, 2015. http:/coast.noaa.gov/digitalcoast/_/pdf/participatory-mapping.pdf.

30. Janice C. Burns, Dagmar Pudrzynska Paul, and Silvia R. Paz, *Participatory Asset Mapping*. Los Angeles: Advancement Project—Health City, 2012. Available at http://communityscience.com/knowledge4equity/AssetMappingToolkit.pdf.

31. M. Wiese, I. Yosko, and M. Donnat, "Participatory Mapping as a Tool for Public Health Decision-Making in Nomadic Settings. A Case Study among Dazagada Pastoralists of the Bahr-el-Ghazal Region in Chad," *Medecine Tropicale: Revue du Corps de Sante Colonial* 64, no. 5 (2003): 452–463.

32. S. E. O'Bryant et al., "Long-Term Low-Level Arsenic Exposure Is Associated with Poorer Neuropsychological Functioning: A Project FRONTIER Study," *International Journal of Environmental Research and Public Health* 8, no. 3 (2011): 861–874.

33. Stefan Dongus et al., "Participatory Mapping of Target Areas to Enable Operational Larval Source Management to Suppress Malaria Vector Mosquitoes in Dar es Salaam, Tanzania," *International Journal of Health Geographics* 6, no. 1 (2007): 37.

34. Assane Gueye Fall et al., "West Nile Virus Transmission in Sentinel Chickens and Potential Mosquito Vectors, Senegal River Delta, 2008-2009," *International Journal of Environmental Research and Public Health* 10, no. 10 (2013): 4718–4727.

35. Jennifer L. Kwan et al., "Sentinel Chicken Seroconversions Track Tangential Transmission of West Nile Virus to Humans in the Greater Los Angeles area of California," *American Journal of Tropical Medicine and Hygiene* 83, no. 5 (2010): 1137–1145.

36. Janna M. Schurer, Janet E. Hill, and Champika Fernando, "Sentinel Surveillance for Zoonotic Parasites in Companion Animals in Indigenous Communities

of Saskatchewan," *American Journal of Tropical Medicine and Hygiene* 87, no. 3 (2012): 495–498.

37. Janna M. Schurer et al., "People, Pets, and Parasites: One Health Surveillance in Southeastern Saskatchewan," *American Journal of Tropical Medicine and Hygiene* 90, no. 6 (2014): 1184–1190.

38. Bala Swaminathan et al., "Building PulseNet International: An Interconnected System of Laboratory Networks to Facilitate Timely Public Health Recognition and Response to Foodborne Disease Outbreaks and Emerging Foodborne Diseases," *Foodborne Pathogens & Disease* 3, no. 1 (2006): 36–50.

39. Centers for Disease Control and Prevention, "PulseNet International: Tracking foodborne disease outbreaks throughout the world." Available at http://www.cdc.gov/ncezid/dfwed/stories/pulsenet-international.html.

40. K. Gaynor et al., "International Foodborne Outbreak of *Shigella sonnei* Infection in Airline Passengers," *Epidemiology & Infection* 137, no. 03 (2009): 335–341.

41. Kelly J. Henning, "What is Syndromic Surveillance?" *Morbidity and Mortality Weekly Report* 53, Supplement (2004): 5–11.

42. John S. Brownstein, Clark C. Freifeld, Lawrence C. Madoff, "Digital Disease Detection—Harnessing the Web for Public Health Surveillance," *New England Journal of Medicine* 360, no. 21 (2009): 2153–2157.

43. Jeremy Ginsberg et al., "Detecting Influenza Epidemics Using Search Engine Query Data," *Nature* 457, no. 7232 (2008): 1012–1014.

44. Rumi Chunara et al., "Flu Near You: An Online Self-Reported Influenza Surveillance System in the USA," *Online Journal of Public Health Informatics* 5 (2013): 1. http://www.ncbi.nlm.nih.gov/pmc/articles/PMC3692780/

45. Cassandra Harrison et al., "Using Online Reviews by Restaurant Patrons to Identify Unreported Cases of Foodborne Illness—New York City, 2012-2013," *Morbidity and Mortality Weekly Report* 63, no. 20 (2014): 441–445.

46. Jenine K. Harris et al., "Health Department Use of Social Media to Identify Foodborne Illness—Chicago, Illinois, 2013-2014," *Morbidity and Mortality Weekly Report* 63, no. 32 (2014): 681–685.

47. Hua Gu et al., "Importance of Internet Surveillance in Public Health Emergency Control and Prevention: Evidence from a Digital Epidemiologic Study During Avian Influenza A H7N9 Outbreaks," *Journal of Medical Internet Research* 16, no. 1 (2014): e20.

15 | Evidence-Based Practices

It is surely a great criticism of our profession that we have not
organized a critical summary, by specialty or subspecialty, adapted
periodically, of all relevant randomized control trials.[1]

Archibald Cochrane (1979)

HE EPIDEMIOLOGIST NEEDS TO ASSESS all of the available data to discern if a statistical relationship exists between a potential etiological
factor and a given health outcome. Similarly, health care providers
need to be able to assess all of the available data on the efficacy and/or
effectiveness of a given therapy in order to provide the best care for their
patients. During the latter quarter of the twentieth century, online search
engines and electronic access to journal articles allowed for more access
than at any time in history to the published results of scientific studies.
This vast and growing amount of literature required a systematic approach
to reading it (see Appendix 1) and, for those conducting studies, required
that they report their results in a standardized fashion so that others could
replicate their work (see Appendix 2). The ability to systematically read and
review the literature allowed for the development of *evidence-based practices*
for both public health and medicine—practices that support decisions being
made rationally and with consistency. Evidence-based practices are those
that are supported by scientific evidence. In public health these practices
are termed *evidence-based public health;* in the clinical fields they are termed
evidence-based medicine.

Evidence-Based Public Health

Because of the nature of public health and its focus on populations, evidence-based public health (EBPH) relies on various types of evidence, not only the results of epidemiologic studies. This has perhaps impeded agreement on what constitutes EBPH as, despite more than a decade of debate, there is still no consensus. Brownstein and colleagues[2] summarized the characteristics of EBPH as follows:

- Making decisions using the best available peer-reviewed evidence (both quantitative and qualitative research)
- Using data and information systems systematically
- Applying program-planning frameworks (that often have a foundation in behavioral science theory)
- Engaging the community in assessment and decision making
- Conducting sound evaluation
- Disseminating what is learned to key stakeholders and decision makers

These characteristics not only require the skills of the epidemiologist to synthesize evidence that can be used to formulate EBPH practices, but also the skills, willingness, cooperation, and support of the entire public health workforce in order for the practices to be implemented.

As practicality is the watchword of public health, using an evidence-based approach to optimize the impact of limited resources makes imminent sense. Many organizations can assist practitioners in the development of EBPH practices. In the United States these include, among others, the Prevention Research Center at Washington University, founded in 1997; the National Network of Public Health Institutes (NNPHI), formed in 2001; and the Council for Training in Evidence-Based Behavioral Practice, established in 2006. At the global level, however, the situation for EBPH is more problematic.

Because populations are complex and their situations vary widely, the epidemiologist needs to know not just whether something works generally, but under which particular circumstances. Shelton reports that the World Health Organization and other global organizations rely on the results of randomized controlled trials for the development of their evidence-based practices.[3] This presents a mismatch in expectations for developing global EBPH practices as the results obtained from randomized controlled trials cannot be generalized to whole populations. To address global public health problems, multiple methodologies might be used to gather information that is applicable in diverse situations.[3] Only by being flexible will EBPH be able to address thorny global issues such as eliminating preventable child and maternal mortality.

Evidence-Based Medicine

Evidence-based medicine (EBM) differs from EBPH in that it focuses on the individual rather than on populations. While EBPH has a number of stakeholders, including public health practitioners and health policy makers, EBM is patient-centric. For this reason, the results of randomized controlled trials and their associated systematic reviews serve as the scientific basis for developing EBM practices.

The impact of EBM can be seen in the increasing development of treatment protocols, checklists, and similar tools for use by both the clinician and the clinical epidemiologist. With regard to prevention, for more than three decades the US Preventive Services Task Force (USPSTF) has provided recommendations regarding preventive medical practices based on the available evidence (see Chapter 13 for a discussion of PSA screening). The concept of EBM received an endorsement in a 1991 article by the editor of the *British Medical Journal*,[4] and shortly thereafter the *Journal of the American Medical Association* (JAMA) began publishing a series of articles called "Users' Guides to the Medical Literature."[5] The spark was ignited for a paradigm shift in medical education—away from emphasizing clinical experience and intuition, toward training residents in EBM.[6]

EBM has not only been integrated into medical education but also into medical practice globally. Specifically, a conference was held in Sicily for evidence-based health care teachers and developers in 2003. The educators came to a consensus that:

> . . . decisions about health care should be based on the best available, current, valid and relevant evidence. The decisions should be made by those receiving care, informed by the tacit and explicit knowledge of those providing care, within the context of available resources.[7]

The consensus document also noted that all health care professionals should understand and implement evidence-based practices and that teaching these skills should be integrated into medical education. To achieve the goal of implementing evidence-based practices, the starting point should be a systematic review of all available epidemiologic study results.

TABLE 15.1 Hierarchy of the Evidence from
Epidemiological Studies

RANK	STUDY DESIGN
1	Meta-analyses
2	Experimental designs Randomized controlled trials Large simple trials Randomized cluster trials
3	Observational designs Cohort studies Case-control studies
4	Descriptive studies Prevalence studies Cross-sectional studies Ecological studies Case series Case reports

Evaluating the Evidence

To understand how systematic reviews of the literature are used for formulating evidence-based practices, it is important to understand how the results of epidemiologic studies are ranked for their scientific merit. The epidemiologist uses a *hierarchy of evidence* to estimate the value of results generated by the various epidemiologic study designs (Table 15.1). At the top of the hierarchy is *meta-analysis*, a quantitative systematic review technique for incorporating the results from any number of epidemiologic studies into a summary measure that represents all of the studies selected.

Just below meta-analysis in the hierarchy are the experimental epidemiologic study designs, that is, the *randomized controlled trial*, the *large simple trial*, and the *randomized cluster trial*. The nature of experimental designs, with their ability to control for confounding variables (both identified and as yet unknown), provides confidence in the study results. In fact, some epidemiologists refer to randomized controlled trials as the "gold standard" of epidemiologic studies. If so, then meta-analysis, with its ability to summarize the results of multiple experimental studies, might be considered the "platinum standard."

Underneath experimental epidemiologic study designs are observational study designs, namely cohort and case-control studies. These designs do not always afford the control of confounding that experimental studies do. However, the presence of a comparison group provides a basis for assessing associations between potential etiological factors and health-related outcomes. The results of observational studies are useful both individually and particularly when combined in a meta-analysis.

Lastly, beneath all of the other levels in the hierarchy are the results of descriptive studies, including cross-sectional studies, case series, and anecdotal case reports. As the latter two have no comparison group, they provide little in the way of usable results except, perhaps, for generating hypotheses.

Using this informal hierarchy, the epidemiologist can assist in formulating evidence-based practice recommendations for both public health and the clinical fields. At its core, an evidence-based approach means that decision making is based on the results of studies using the best available data. How to evaluate those studies in the aggregate is the true challenge.

Collaborative Reviews

The sheer volume of scientific publications available for review has become burdensome for the individual practitioner and epidemiologist alike. To evaluate this ever-growing body of literature, collaborative work groups have been formed to systematically review publications in their areas of expertise. For example, the *Cochrane Collaboration* is a not-for-profit organization named for Archie Cochrane, a British epidemiologist whose work focused on assessing the efficacy and effectiveness of health care interventions. The Cochrane Collaboration hosts more than 50 collaborative groups with participants from around the globe, who work together to systematically review the literature on health care interventions (primarily randomized controlled trials) within their areas of expertise. The *Cochrane Reviews* created by these groups provide a key component of EBM, the evidence upon which clinical practices can be justified. The collaborative reviews are available online in the *Cochrane Library*, accessible to both health care professionals and patients making treatment decisions.[8]

The *Campbell Collaboration* (C2) is an organization that functions similarly to the Cochrane Collaboration but with a focus on social interventions. The organization is named for the American sociologist Donald Campbell, who advocated for the assessment of governmental interventions as the basis for rational policy formation. Like the Cochrane Collaboration, C2 is organized around specific areas of study.[9] The *Campbell Systematic Reviews* are available via the *Campbell Library*.[10]

An example of how collaborative reviews contribute to evidence-based practice comes from the Evidence, Expertise, Exchange (3e) Initiative. A panel of 78 multinational rheumatologists developed 10 clinical questions to be answered about the diagnosis and management of gout. A systematic review was undertaken of the literature from 14 countries in Europe, South America, and Australasia, and the data extracted, synthesized, and assessed for bias. The panel had multiple rounds of discussion about the data and held formal votes that resulted in 10 recommendations aimed at improving patient care.[11]

Collaborative reviews using the expert panel evaluative process are useful for developing best practices in both public health and the clinical fields. The summaries generated by collaborative reviews may also be useful for families and patients seeking to ensure that clinical recommendations are relevant and up-to-date. Expert panels are not the only means of evaluating literature reviews, however. The quantitative approach to summarizing the results in the literature, *meta-analysis*, may also be used.

Meta-Analysis

A meta-analysis identifies a research question, specifies the sources from which studies addressing that question will be identified, transforms the study findings to a common metric, and statistically analyzes the findings. An early proponent of this method, Thomas Chalmers, noted several purposes for meta-analyses: [12]

- To resolve conflicting conclusions by examining quality, subjects, and inventions
- To increase [statistical] power for major endpoints and subgroup analyses
- To sharpen boundaries of effect size in the case of positive studies
- To answer new questions

When a meta-analysis focuses on the results from randomized clinical trials, another purpose may be added to this list. A meta-analysis can purposefully generate the *number needed to treat* (NNT) to prevent an event from happening,[13] a clinically relevant measure that expresses the benefit of one intervention over another (see Chapter 11).

Meta-analyses are not restricted to evaluating clinical trials data. They can be employed across the hierarchy of epidemiologic evidence. To illustrate this, we will review the steps for conducting a meta-analysis using the example of Bahekar and colleagues who evaluated the relationship between periodontal disease (PD) and coronary heart disease (CHD).[14] This example is useful because more than one level in the hierarchy of evidence was used, and the results have implications for clinical and preventive medicine as well as for dentistry and public health.

Conducting a Meta-Analysis

The first step in a meta-analysis is to define the question or establish the aim or purpose of the analysis. As several studies reported conflicting results about the relationship between PD and CHD, Bahekar and colleagues wanted to evaluate whether PD posed an increased risk for the disease.[14] To do this, they had to find all completed epidemiologic studies addressing the question of interest, a task that can present a significant challenge.

Common sources for identifying *primary studies* (those that collect original data) are AMED (complementary and alternative medicine literature), CINAHL (nursing and allied health literature), Embase (biomedical literature with a focus on the pharmacological effects of drugs), MEDLINE (indexed academic biomedical, dental, healthcare, medical, nursing, and veterinary literature), PsycINFO (psychology literature), and PubMed (includes MEDLINE citations, plus ahead-of-print listings and citations from some additional life science journals). Open access publication and digital repositories such as PubMed Central are also searchable, and decisions about whether or not to use such resources must be made. Should material that has not been peer-reviewed be included in the meta-analysis? If not, might *publication bias* be a problem? Publication bias is a type of selection bias that occurs when the results of published studies are not representative of all of the research done in a particular area (e.g., studies conducted but not published in the peer-reviewed literature).[15] For instance, if researchers only submit their positive results to peer-reviewed journals fearing that negative results will not be published, then the literature that appears in those journals will be biased.

In our example, the investigators chose to search the PubMed computerized database (1966–2006), the Cochrane Controlled Trials Register (1970–2006), Embase (1980–2006), and CINAHL (1982–2006). They also completed a manual review of published articles and review papers, and chose not to include unpublished studies. Using a fixed set of search terms for PD (chronic periodontal infections, gingivitis, periodontal disease, tooth diseases) and CHD (atherosclerosis, cardiovascular disease, coronary artery disease, stroke), the researchers identified 320 articles.[14]

Before examining any of the articles identified through the search process, it is important to lay out the inclusion and exclusion criteria for which studies will be used in the meta-analysis. The criteria in our exemplar were studies using human subjects with a sample size of at least 80 persons. The outcome (CHD) was defined as the clinical presence or absence of coronary artery disease; exposure (PD) was defined as either clinically diagnosed or self-reported periodontal disease. Implementing the criteria reduced the number of articles from 320 to 20: 10 prospective cohort studies, 5 case-control studies, and 5 cross-sectional studies. When each study was reviewed for completeness of the data, the number of studies was further reduced to five for each study design.[14]

Once the studies to be included in any meta-analysis are finalized, the data must be extracted from them according to a preset protocol. In our example, two individuals independently extracted the data from each study to minimize information bias. A single database could not be assembled because the outcome measure (*relative risk, odds ratio, prevalence*) for each of the study designs was different. Thus, three separate databases were created and each database was analyzed separately.[14]

It can be useful to understand the results of the individual studies used in a meta-analysis by displaying them in a *forest plot*. Each study is shown as a "branch" (the outcome measure for that study along with its confidence interval) in the forest plot. The "trunk" represents the null value for that study design. For instance, Figure 15.1 shows the results of the cohort studies used in the PD and CHD example. Note the value for the trunk of the forest plot on the right side of the figure is 1 (RR = 1) and the two largest of the cohort studies have confidence intervals that include the null value.

Meta-analysis can derive various summary measures (*relative risk, hazard ratio, odds ratio*, or *risk difference*) through the use of statistical modeling. In the *fixed effects model* the epidemiologist assumes that the true effect (outcome) of the treatment (exposure) is constant, and any observed variations are due to sampling error. This allows the data to be weighted so that the treatment effects in larger studies are given preference in the analysis to those in smaller ones. Conversely, the *random effects model* uses the effect sizes from all of the studies, so that no study is discounted and no study can dominate the estimate of the effect. The result of the random effects model, then, is the mean of the distribution of effects.

In our example, the investigators selected the fixed effects model for their analyses.[14] The results of all three meta-analyses evaluating the association between PD and CHD were statistically significant at $p < 0.001$. The cohort studies (86,092 subjects) yielded a relative risk of 1.14, the case-control studies (1,423 subjects) yielded an odds ratio of 2.22, and the prevalence of CHD in the cross-sectional studies (17,724 subjects) was 59% higher risk among those with PD compared to those without PD.[14] The ability to show a statistically significant association between PD and CHD across the hierarchy

Model	Study name	Subjects	Risk ratio	Lower limit	Upper limit	p-Value
	Destefano (9)	N = 9760	1.250	1.058	1.477	0.009
	Howell (13)	N = 22037	1.010	0.884	1.155	0.884
	Joshipura (11)	N = 441199	1.040	0.863	1.254	0.681
	Mattila (10)	N = 214	1.210	1.078	1.358	0.001
	Wu (12)	N = 9962	1.170	1.042	1.313	0.008
Fixed	Overall	N = 86,092	1.141	1.074	1.213	0.000

FIGURE 15.1 The relative risk of CHD in periodontitis: prospective studies.

SOURCE: Bahekar et al. (2007).[14] Used with permission.

of the evidence using the platinum standard of meta-analysis strengthens confidence in the results. As CHD is a complex disease with multifactorial etiology, adding PD as a risk factor has important implications for biologic research, suggests interventions for clinicians and dentists who see patients with PD, and may provide a focus for public health prevention efforts.

Publishing the Results of Systematic Reviews

Prior to the past several decades there were no standards for how systematic reviews should be conducted or how the results of such reviews should be reported in the literature. The Cochrane Handbook[16] provided guidance on how to perform a systematic review, and it quickly became the unofficial standard. In 1996, the QUOROM Statement (QUality Of Reporting Of Meta-analyses) was developed, laying out reporting standards for the results of meta-analyses based on randomized controlled trials.[17] Standards for publishing the results of meta-analyses based upon observational studies were published in 2000—the Meta-analysis of Observational Studies in Epidemiology (MOOSE) guidelines.[18] MOOSE differs from QUOROM in that it requires that each observational study be rated for quality. In our example of PD and CHD, the cross-sectional studies were rated on their internal validity (good, fair, or poor) using criteria developed by the US Preventive Services Task Force.[14]

In 2009, the QUOROM Statement was updated and became known as the Preferred Reporting Items for Systematic Reviews and Meta-Analyses (PRISMA).[19] The PRISMA guidelines include 27 items that should be able to be easily found by anyone reading the results of a systematic review. Being able to readily find these key components means that the meta-analysis should be able to be replicated or updated to aid in the formulation of evidence-based practices.

Limitations of Systematic Reviews

It is important for those reporting study results, as well as those formulating guidelines for EBPH and EBM practices, to understand not only the strengths but also the limitations of systematic reviews. Whether the systematic review is qualitative or quantitative in nature, publication bias (discussed above) must be of concern. Publication bias should be considered when inclusion and exclusion criteria are formulated, and these should be reported when the results of the review are published (as per PRISMA guidelines).

The second limitation is *homogeneity*, the assumption that all of the studies selected for a meta-analysis are sufficiently similar so that their results can be pooled. If the way subjects are selected, the way exposures and outcomes are measured, or if the period of follow-up differs among the studies, the assumption of homogeneity may not hold. Remember that in the PD and CHD example, each study design required a separate meta-analysis because the outcome measures differed. Within each meta-analysis, however, the investigators still had concerns about homogeneity. They reported that the studies differed greatly in the way PD was assessed, how CHD was measured, and how adjustments were made for confounding.[14] Thus, reviewers should factor into their conclusions the degree to which the assumption of homogeneity is or is not supported in the analysis.

Summary

Evidence-based practices support rational and consistent decision making in both the public health and the clinical fields. Such practices are primarily developed from systematic reviews, either through the collaborative review process undertaken by a panel of experts or by the quantitative technique of meta-analysis. All systematic reviews pose concerns about publication bias, and meta-analysis poses an additional concern about the homogeneity of the studies being pooled for review.

Despite these limitations, developing and continually evaluating evidence-based practices is important. The effort adds to our understanding of treatments that provide the best outcomes, prevention programs that yield the best results, and the best ways to improve the health and well-being of society as a whole. Yet, evidence-based practices may face challenges—cultural, economic, and political—that will attempt to undermine their import. To address these challenges, clinical and public health professionals should gather and evaluate data used to develop evidence-based practices carefully and transparently, communicate the findings clearly, and engage patients and communities in the decision-making processes that affect them directly.

References

1. A. L. Cochrane *1931-1971: A Critical Review. Medicines for the Year 2000*, 1–11. London: Office of Health Economics, 1979.
2. John S. Brownstein, Clark C. Freifeld, Lawrence C. Madoff, "Digital Disease Detection—Harnessing the Web for Public Health Surveillance," *New England Journal of Medicine* 360, no. 21 (2009): 2153–2157.
3. J. D. Shelton, "Evidence-Based Public Health: Not Only Whether It Works, but How It Can Be Made to Work Practicably at Scale," *Global Health: Science and Practice* 2, no. 3 (2014): 253–258.
4. Richard J. Smith, "Where's the Wisdom? The Poverty of Medical Evidence," *British Medical Journal* 303 (1991): 798–799.
5. Gordon Guyatt et al., *Users' Guides to the Medical Literature: A Manual for Evidence-Based Clinical Practice, 2nd Edition*. Chicago: AMA Press, 2008.
6. Gordon Guyatt et al., "Evidence-Based Medicine: A New Approach To Teaching the Practice of Medicine," *Journal of the American Medical Association* 268, no. 17 (1992): 2420–2425.
7. Martin Dawes et al., "Sicily Statement on Evidence-Based Practice," *BMC Medical Education* 5, no. 1 (2005): 1.
8. The Cochrane Library. Available at http://www.cochrane.org/cochrane-reviews/about-cochrane-library.
9. J. Schuerman et al., "The Campbell Collaboration," *Research on Social Work Practice* 12, no. 2 (2002): 309–317.
10. The Campbell Collaboration Library. Available at http://www.campbellcollabora-tion.org/lib/.
11. Francisca Sivera et al., "Multinational Evidence-Based Recommendations for the Diagnosis and Management of Gout: Integrating Systematic Literature Review and Expert Opinion of a Broad Panel of rheumatologists in the 3e Initiative," *Annals of the Rheumatic Diseases* 73, no. 2 (2014): 328–335.
12. Thomas C. Chalmers, "Meta-Analysis in Clinical Medicine," *Transactions of the American Clinical and Climatological Association* 99 (1988): 144–150.
13. Miquel Porta, ed., *A Dictionary of Epidemiology, 6th Edition*. New York: Oxford University Press, 2014.
14. Amol Ashok Bahekar et al., "The Prevalence and Incidence of Coronary Heart Disease Is Significantly Increased In Periodontitis: A Meta-Analysis. *American Heart Journal* 154, no. 5 (2007): 830–837.
15. Drummond Rennie and Annette Flanagin, "Publication Bias. The Triumph of Hope Over Experience," *Journal of the American Medical Association* 267, no. 3 (1992): 411–412.

16. Julian P. T. Higgins and Sally Green eds., *Cochrane Handbook for Systematic Reviews of Interventions, Version 5.1.0.* The Cochrane Collaboration, 2011. Available at www.cochrane-handbook.org.

17. David Moher et al., "Improving the Quality of Reports of Meta-Analyses of Randomised Controlled Trials: The QUOROM Statement. Quality of Reporting of Meta-analyses," *Lancet* 354, no. 9193 (1999): 1896–1900.

18. D. F. Stroup et al., Meta-analysis of Observational Studies in Epidemiology (MOOSE) Group, "Meta-analysis of Observational Studies in Epidemiology: A Proposal for Reporting," *Journal of the American Medical Association* 283, no. 15 (2000): 2008–2012.

19. David Moher et al., "Preferred Reporting Items for Systematic Reviews and Meta-Analyses: The PRISMA Statement," *British Medical Journal* 339 (2009): b2535.

V | Conclusion

I N OUR DISCUSSION ABOUT THE fundamentals of epidemiology, we described how the epidemiologist's ultimate goal is to find and reduce or eliminate exposure to those factors causing diseases or other adverse health outcomes. Epidemiologic methods developed over time, with a focus on the *comparative* approach, to determine why diseases occur at different times, in different places, and among different populations. Of particular concern to the epidemiologist is how to show cause, that is, to identify a particular etiological factor rather than simply document the results of various disease processes (Part I). Patterns of death, disease, and other health outcomes can be identified using descriptive studies (Part II) and hypotheses about the causes of these patterns can be tested by employing well-designed analytic studies (Part III). Epidemiologic knowledge may be used to inform clinical decision making, to investigate health-related conditions in the field in real time and place, or to develop evidence-based practices to improve the health and well-being of society as a whole (Part IV).

While most of the examples used in this book come from clinical medicine and public health, they could just as easily come from plant science or veterinary medicine. The triads of *time, place, person* and *agent, host, environment* are applicable in all of these settings. The value of the epidemiologic characterization of disease lies in both the prevention of adverse health outcomes and in suggesting potential routes of treatment. At the same time, tools either pioneered or strongly advocated by epidemiologists, such as QALYs and DALYs, have themselves entered into the realms of health policy formulation and execution. Such efforts underscore the degree to which the epidemiologic perspective can impact the health of populations.

Finally, we would be remiss in not noting how adaptive and responsive epidemiology can be when addressing the myriad changes taking place in our global environment. That the epidemiologist can marshal resources to develop the knowledge base needed to contain and, ideally, eliminate a disease is testimony to the power of the field to advance the public's health. Concepts such as vital statistics; the incidence, prevalence, and virulence of diseases; the sensitivity, specificity, and predictive value of screening tests; and the results of randomized controlled trials and meta-analyses for developing evidence-based practices, among others, provide the *foundations of epidemiology*. These foundations inform individuals, researchers, health care providers, and health policy makers who make decisions that can enhance the health of not just individuals but also populations in the aggregate.

APPENDIX 1 | Guide to Reading the Epidemiologic Literature

Goal
- What was the underlying goal of the study? Was a hypothesis stated?

Design
- What was the study design? Was the design appropriate to the goal of the study?

Subjects
- Describe the sample (e.g., cross-sectional, random, matched, etc.).
- What sample size(s) were selected and why (e.g., convenience, sample size calculation)?
- Was the method of selection different for case and control subjects? If so, why?
- Were inclusion and exclusion criteria described?
- How successful was enrollment? Did the authors describe those that refused to participate?
- How successful was retention? Did the authors describe those who were lost to follow-up?

Exposure
- How was exposure defined?
- How was exposure measured (e.g., biological measurements, employment records, etc.)?
- Were the methods used to estimate exposure reliable and reproducible?

Outcome
- How was outcome defined?
- How was it measured (e.g., self-report, physician diagnosis, death certificate)?
- What means were used to avoid missing outcomes?

Data analysis
- What method of analysis was used (OR, RR, rate difference, hazard ratio, other)?
- How were confounders handled?
- What was the resulting statistical power of the study?

Results
- Are the results clearly presented and internally consistent?
- Was a statistical association found? How strong is it?
- Did the authors discuss possible sources of error in the study design (e.g., random error, selection bias, information bias, etc.)?
- What did the authors conclude from their analysis?
- Can the results be generalized beyond the study population?

Summary
- How strong is the case for causality? What are the implications of the results?

APPENDIX 2 | Standards for Reporting the Results of Epidemiologic and Health-Related Studies

STUDY DESIGN	REPORTING STANDARD
Observational studies	
✓ Case reports	CARE—Consensus-based Clinical Case Report Guidelines[1]
✓ Cohort, case control and cross sectional studies	STROBE—Strengthening the Reporting of Observational Studies in Epidemiology[2]
✓ Systematic review of observational studies	MOOSE—Meta-analysis of Observational Studies in Epidemiology[3]
Experimental studies	
✓ Non-randomized trials	TREND—Transparent Reporting of Evaluations with Non-randomized Designs[4]
✓ Randomized trials	CONSORT—Consolidated Standards of Reporting Trials[5,6]
✓ Systematic review of controlled trials	PRISMA—Preferred Reporting Items for Systematic Reviews and Meta-Analyses[7]
Other	
✓ Diagnostic accuracy studies	STARD—Standards for the Reporting of Diagnostic Accuracy Studies[8,9]
✓ Health care studies	SQUIRE—Standards for Quality Improvement Reporting Excellence[10,11]
✓ Health economic studies	CHEERS—Consolidated Health Economic Evaluation Reporting Standards[12,13]
✓ Qualitative studies	COREQ—Consolidated Criteria for Reporting Qualitative Research[14]

STUDY DESIGN	REPORTING STANDARD
✓ Systematic review of qualitative studies	ENTREQ—Enhancing Transparency in Reporting of Qualitative Research[15]
✓ Statistical methods	SAMPL—Statistical Analyses and Methods in the Published Literature[16]

SOURCES:

1. Case Reports: The CARE guidelines, available at http://www.care-statement.org/

2. STROBE Statement: "Strengthening the reporting of observational studies in epidemiology," available at http://www.strobe-statement.org/index.php?id = available-checklists.

3. D. F. Stroup et al., Meta-analysis Of Observational Studies in Epidemiology (MOOSE) group, "Meta-analysis of observational studies in epidemiology: a proposal for reporting," *Journal of the American Medical Association* 283 (15): (2000): 2008–2012.

4. CDC, "Transparent Reporting of Evaluations with Nonrandomized Designs (TREND)," 2014. http://www.cdc.gov/trendstatement/.

5. K. F. Schulz, D. G. Altman, and D. Moher, "CONSORT 2010 statement: updated guidelines for reporting parallel group randomised trials," *British Medical Journal.* 340 (2010): c332.

6. Consort: Transparent Reporting of Trials, available at http://www.consort-statement.org/consort-statement/.

7. PRISMA: Transparent Reporting of Systematic Reviews and Meta-analyses, available at http://www.prisma-statement.org/.

8. The STARD statement, available at http://www.stard-statement.org/

9. P. M. Bossuyt and J. B. Reitsma, "The STARD Initiative," *Lancet* 361, no. 9351 (2003): 71.

10. F. Davidoff and P. Batalden, "Toward stronger evidence on quality improvement. Draft publication guidelines: the beginning of a consensus project," *Quality and Safety in Health Care.* 2005; 14, no. 5 (2005): 319–325.

11. SQUIRE: Standards for Quality Improvement Reporting Excellence, available at http://www.squire-statement.org/.

12. D. Husereau et al., "Consolidated health economic evaluation reporting standards (CHEERS) statement," *BMC Medicine* 11, no. 1 (2013): 80.

13. International Society for Pharmacoeconomics and Outcomes Research, "Health economic evaluation publication guidelines—CHEERS: Good reporting practices," available at http://www.ispor.org/taskforces/economicpubguidelines.asp

14. A. Tong, P. Sainsbury, and J. Craig. "Consolidated criteria for reporting qualitative research (COREQ): a 32-item checklist for interviews and focus groups," *International Journal of Quality in Health Care* 19, no. 6 (2007): 349–357.

15. A. Tong et al., "Enhancing transparency in reporting the synthesis of qualitative research: ENTREQ," BMC Medical Research Methodology 12 (2012): 181.

16. T. A. Lang and D. G. Altman, "Basic Statistical Reporting for Articles Published in Biomedical Journals: The Statistical Analyses and Methods in the Published Literature or The SAMPL Guidelines," *Science Editors' Handbook*, European Association of Science Editors, 2013.

APPENDIX 3 | Answers to Problem Sets

Chapter 1

1. The crude attack rate equals the total number of persons ill divided by the total number of persons exposed. Overall, 58 recruits presented to the clinic with the same symptoms out of 535 that attended the special breakfast, or (58/535) × 100 = 11 percent of persons attending the event presented to the clinic with the same illness.

2. The food-specific attack rate equals the number of persons who ate the food and became ill divided by the total number of persons who ate the food. Example: In total, (204 + 47) or 251 recruits consumed tomato juice. Of those who consumed it, 47 became ill. The food-specific attack rate for consuming tomato juice is (47/251) × 100 = 19 percent, or 19 percent of recruits who consumed tomato juice at the special breakfast became ill.

FOOD	CONSUMED FOOD			DID NOT CONSUME FOOD		
	NUMBER WELL	NUMBER ILL	ATTACK RATE (%)	NUMBER WELL	NUMBER ILL	ATTACK RATE (%)
Tomato juice	204	47	19	263	21	7
Cantaloupe	290	53	15	177	15	8
Creamed chipped beef	147	60	29	320	8	2
Potatoes	161	44	21	306	24	7
Eggs	169	39	19	298	29	9
Pastry	204	34	14	263	34	11
Toast	238	46	16	229	22	9
Milk	301	50	14	166	18	10

3. The rate ratio for each food item equals the attack rate for those who ate the food and became ill divided by the attack rate for those who did not eat the food and still became ill. For tomato juice, RR = 19/7 or 2.7, or those who consumed tomato juice at the special breakfast were 2.7 times as likely to have become ill compared to those who did not consume it.

FOOD	ATTACK RATE (%)		RATE RATIO
	CONSUMED FOOD	DID NOT CONSUME FOOD	
Tomato juice	19	7	2.7
Cantaloupe	15	8	1.9
Creamed chipped beef	29	2	14.5
Potatoes	21	7	3.0
Eggs	19	9	2.1
Pastry	14	11	1.3
Toast	16	9	1.8
Milk	14	10	1.4

4. The likely cause of this outbreak is the creamed chipped beef. This food item produced the largest rate ratio (RR = 14.5) demonstrating that those who ate the creamed chipped beef were 14.5 times as likely to have become ill relative to those who did not eat it.

5. It is possible that not all of the batches of the creamed chipped beef were contaminated and that only the recruits who ate the contaminated batch became ill. It is also possible that some foods were cross-contaminated in the kitchen or during serving, or that recruits did not accurately remember their exposures.

6. Microbiological testing could be done to isolate and identify potential pathogens from leftover food items, stool samples (victims and food handlers), skin lesions or other potential sources of infection demonstrated by the food handlers. An investigation of food storage and sanitary practices in the kitchen and serving areas might also uncover pathogens or toxic agents that might have caused the outbreak. Careful follow-up is required to determine whether the source of contamination was local or whether it might be from a different source in the food supply chain—such as at the point of production or distribution before the item was delivered to the training center.

7. Foodborne outbreaks can be prevented through the education and training of culinary staff in proper food preparation, handling, and service. Regular sanitary inspections of kitchens and food storage areas should reinforce proper cleansing of food preparation areas, safe food storage, and the heating (cooking) and cooling (refrigeration) of prepared foods.

Chapter 3

1. a. The epidemic curve:

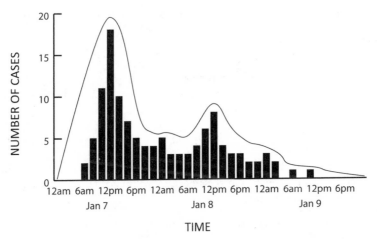

NUMBER OF CASES

20

15

10

5

0

12am 6am 12pm 6pm 12am 6am 12pm 6pm 12am 6am 12pm 6pm

Jan 7   Jan 8   Jan 9

TIME

b. The epidemic curve suggests a common vehicle outbreak. The epidemic curve is skewed to the right, with a sharp initial rise and a gradual tapering. As the time period is relatively short, the epidemic curve suggests a single exposure.

c. The bimodality of an epidemic curve suggesting a common vehicle outbreak may be the result of secondary cases contracting the agent from primary cases (serial transfer).

d. The health officer knows the distribution of times of onset of illness. The specific disease (identified as salmonella) is also known. Knowing these two factors, the health officer can estimate time of exposure.

e. Knowing the estimated time of exposure allows the health officer to seek commonalities among the cases (where they were, what they ate or drank, who they were in contact with during that time). When the commonalities are identified, the health officer may be able to locate the source of the epidemic and prevent future outbreaks of this type.

2. *Infectivity* = (*Number infected/Number exposed*) × 100

There were 4,000 susceptible persons (5,000–1,000) who were exposed to *B. pertussis* in Sunnyside Up, and 600 of them became infected. Infectivity of *B. pertussis* in Sunnyside Up is (600/4,000) × 100, or 15 infections per 100 susceptible persons exposed (15% of susceptibles were infected).

Pathogenicity = (*Number of clinically overt cases / Number infected*) × 100

There were 300 clinically overt cases of *B. pertussis* among 600 cases of infection in the most recent outbreak in Sunnyside Up. Pathogenicity of *B. pertussis* in Sunnyside Up is (300/600) × 100, or 50 clinical cases per 100 infections (50% of those infected became clinically overt cases).

Virulence = (*Number of deaths / Number of clinical cases*) × 100

There were 60 deaths from *B. pertussis* among 300 clinical cases of the disease in the most recent outbreak in Sunnyside Up. Virulence of *B. pertussis* in

Sunnyside Up is (60/300) x 100, or 20 deaths per 100 clinical cases (20% of the clinical cases died from the disease).

3. $Infectivity = (Number\ infected/Number\ exposed) \times 100$

There were 1,000 susceptible Scrambled residents exposed to the agent, and 40 had become infected. Infectivity of *B. pertussis* in Scrambled is (40/1,000) × 100, or 4 infections per 100 susceptible persons exposed.

$Pathogenicity = (Number\ of\ clinically\ overt\ cases\ /\ Number\ infected) \times 100$

There were 20 clinically overt cases among 40 cases of infection in Scrambled. Pathogenicity of *B. pertussis* in Scrambled is (20/40) × 100, or 50 clinical cases per 100 infections.

$Virulence = (Number\ of\ deaths\ /\ Number\ of\ clinical\ cases) \times 100$

There were 5 deaths among 20 clinical cases of pertussis in Scrambled. Virulence of *B. pertussis* in Scrambled is (5/20) × 100, or 25 deaths per 100 clinical cases.

4. The residents of Sunnyside Up experienced far greater infectivity with *B. pertussis* than did those from Scrambled; pathogenicity did not differ, nor did virulence differ much. The difference in infectivity suggests that the agent in the Scrambled outbreak differed from that in the Sunnyside Up outbreak, perhaps reflecting attenuation of the agent between the two episodes, or perhaps the agents came from two different sources. In any case, Dr. Over-Easy was right to be skeptical, and Mayor Poached should not charge Sunnyside Up with causing the outbreak.

CHARACTERISTICS OF THE CAUSATIVE AGENT	SUNNYSIDE UP	SCRAMBLED
Infectivity	15 cases per 100 susceptible persons exposed	4 cases per 100 susceptible persons exposed
Pathogenicity	50 clinical cases per 100 infections	50 clinical cases per 100 infections.
Virulence	20 deaths per 100 clinical cases	25 deaths per 100 clinical cases

5. The number of students who need to be immuned to forestall a measles epidemic at Pancake Row College is 2,500 (the size of the college population) × 0.90 (the desired level of herd immunity to protect the remaining unvaccinated students) =2,250 students.

   If 40 percent of the 2,500 students were previously immunized, then 1,000 students have already been vaccinated (= 0.4 × 2,500). The number of students needing to be vaccinated is therefore 1,250 (= 2,250–1,000).

Chapter 5

1. The crude death rate is the number of deaths per unit time/number of persons in the population during that same time period × 100,000.

All Knowing Senior = (20,400/1,900,000) × 100,000, or 1,074 deaths per 100,000 persons per year.

Ignorant Freshman = (22,100 deaths/2,170,000) × 100,000, or 1,018 deaths per 100,000 persons per year.

The need appears to be greater in All Knowing Senior than in Ignorant Freshman.

2. Example: The annual cause-specific mortality rate is deaths from a particular cause/population at risk × 100,000. For infectious diseases in All Knowing Senior it is (2,500/1,900,000) × 100,000 = 132 per 100,000 persons.

Note: The crude death rate is the total of the cause-specific rates.

CAUSE	ALL KNOWING SENIOR			IGNORANT FRESHMAN		
	DEATHS	POPULATION	CAUSE-SPECIFIC RATE PER 100,000 PERSONS	DEATHS	POPULATION	CAUSE-SPECIFIC RATE PER 100,000 PERSONS
Infectious diseases	2,500	1,900,000	132	3,010	2,170,000	139
Cancers	2,700	1,900,000	142	2,900	2,170,000	134
All other	15,200	1,900,000	800	16,190	2,170,000	746
Totals	20,400	1,900,000	1074	22,100	2,170,000	1,018

3. Example: The annual age-specific mortality rate for persons less than 5 years of age for infectious diseases per 100,000 persons in All Knowing Senior is (20/90,000) × 100,000 = 22.

	CITY					
	ALL KNOWING SENIOR			IGNORANT FRESHMAN		
AGE (YEARS)	DEATHS	POPULATION	ANNUAL AGE-SPECIFIC MORTALITY RATE FOR INFECTIOUS DISEASES PER 100,000 PERSONS	DEATHS	POPULATION	ANNUAL AGE-SPECIFIC MORTALITY RATE FOR INFECTIOUS DISEASES PER 100,000 PERSONS
<5	20	90,000	22	120	140,000	86
5–24	180	300,000	60	910	650,000	140
25–44	650	450,000	144	1,130	670,000	169
45–64	950	650,000	146	650	520,000	125
65 +	700	410,000	171	200	190,000	105
Totals	2,500	1,900,000		3,010	2,170,000	

4. The expected number of deaths in the standard population is the size of the standard population in each stratum × the age-specific mortality rate in the study population. Example: For the <5 years age group in All Knowing Senior, the expected number of deaths in the standard population given the infectious disease mortality rate in that city is $3,000 \times (22/100,000) = 0.7$.

   The age-adjusted rate is the sum of the expected deaths in the standard population divided by the size of the standard population and then multiplied by the unit in which the rate will be expressed.

   For All Knowing Senior this would be $(0.7 + 10.8 + 57.6 + 39.4 + 20.5)/100,000 \times 100,000 = 129$ per 100,000 persons.

   For Ignorant Freshman it would be $(2.6 + 25.2 + 67.6 + 33.8 + 12.6)/100,000 \times 100,000 = 142$ per 100,000 persons.

		CITY			
		ALL KNOWING SENIOR		IGNORANT FRESHMAN	
	STANDARD				
AGE (YEARS)	POPULATION (FROM A DATABOOK)	AGE-SPECIFIC MORTALITY RATES FOR INFECTIOUS DISEASES PER 100,000 PERSONS	EXPECTED DEATHS	AGE-SPECIFIC MORTALITY RATES FOR INFECTIOUS DISEASES PER 100,000 PERSONS	EXPECTED DEATHS
<5	3,000	22	0.7	86	2.6
5–24	18,000	60	10.8	140	25.2
25–44	40,000	144	57.6	169	67.6
45–64	27,000	146	39.4	125	33.8
65 +	12,000	171	20.5	105	12.6
Total	100,000		129		142
Age-adjusted Rate		129 per 100,000		142 per 100,000	

5. Example: The case fatality rate per 100 cases for those less than 5 years of age living in All Knowing Senior during the most recent year is $(20/40) \times 100 = 50$ deaths per 100 cases of infectious disease. The total case fatality rate for All Knowing Senior is $(2,500/9,940) \times 100 = 25$ deaths per 100 cases of infectious disease.

	CITY					
	ALL KNOWING SENIOR			IGNORANT FRESHMAN		
AGE (YEARS)	DEATHS	NUMBER OF CASES OF INFECTIOUS DISEASE LAST YEAR	CASE FATALITY RATE PER 100 CASES OF INFECTIOUS DISEASE LAST YEAR	DEATHS	NUMBER OF CASES OF INFECTIOUS DISEASE LAST YEAR	CASE FATALITY RATE PER 100 CASES OF INFECTIOUS DISEASE LAST YEAR
<5	20	40	50	120	240	50
5–24	180	400	45	910	2,275	40
25–44	650	1,900	34	1,130	2,800	40
45–64	950	3,600	26	650	1,625	40
65 +	700	4,000	18	200	2,000	10
Total	2,500	9,940	25	3,010	8,940	34

6. The expected number of deaths in Ignorant Freshman for those less than 5 years of age is $(86/100,000) \times 90,000 = 77$. The total number of expected deaths in All Knowing Senior is $(77 + 420 + 761 + 813 + 431) = 2,502$. The SMR (Observed/Expected) $= 2,502/2,500 \approx 1.0$. This indicates that the infectious disease mortality experience of the two cities was about the same.

AGE (YEARS)	STANDARD RATE (INFECTIOUS DISEASE MORTALITY RATES PER 100,000 PERSONS IN IGNORANT FRESHMAN)	STUDY POPULATION (ALL KNOWING SENIOR)	EXPECTED NUMBER OF DEATHS IN THE STUDY POPULATION
<5	86	90,000	77
5–24	140	300,000	420
25–44	169	450,000	761
45–64	125	650,000	813
65 +	105	410,000	431
Total		1,900,000	2,502

7. Years of potential life lost = (Average life expectancy—Ages at death)

AGE (YEARS)	LIFE EXPECTANCY-AVERAGE AGE AT DEATH (YEARS)	DEATHS FROM MEASLES	YPPL
<1	$75 - 0.5 = 74.5$	94	7,003
2	$75 - 1.5 = 73.5$	75	5,513
3	$75 - 2.5 = 72.5$	67	4,858
4	$75 - 3.5 = 71.5$	69	4,934
5	$75 - 4.5 = 70.5$	201	14,171
Total		506	36,479

The YPLL rate is equal to the sum of the YPLL divided by the size of the population contributing to the YPPL × 100,000. For Ignorant Freshman, this would be 36,479/140,000 × 100,000 or 26,056 per 100,000 population.

Years of potential life lost is a measure of premature mortality. The loss of 506 children less than six years of age in Ignorant Freshman due to the measles epidemic equals 36,479 years of potential life (and productivity) lost to that community. Stated as a rate for comparison with other localities, the community suffered a 26,056 years of potential life lost per 100,000 population.

Chapter 7

1. The incidence rate per 1,000 standard poodles less than two months old during 2000–2004 is (10/230) × 1,000 = 43.5. However, this rate covers a five-year time period. To get the average annual incidence rate per 1,000 standard poodles, the overall rate of 43.5 per 1,000 must be divided by five years. Thus, the average annual incidence rate is 43.5/5 = 8.7 per 1,000 standard poodles per year.

AGE (MONTHS)	AVERAGE ANNUAL INCIDENCE PER 1,000 STANDARD POODLES		
	2000–2004	2005–2009	2010–2014
<2	8.7	8.9	8.8
2–11.9	3.6	3.7	3.7
12–23.9	2.2	2.2	4.0
24+	2.6	1.5	5.3

Overall, puppies less than two months old have the highest rates, but these have not increased over time. In contrast, the rates for older dogs have increased, about doubling among dogs in their second year and showing even markedly higher increases after two years of age. Indeed, the rates among the oldest dogs appear to be rapidly approaching the rates for the youngest puppies.

2. Incidence density calculation

Half of the 1,600 dogs (n = 800) lived in the county only half of each year (0.5 years). Therefore, the dogs 2 + years of age or older during the period 2010–2014 contributed 400 years of exposure (or risk). The remaining 800 dogs each contributed one year at risk. Therefore, there are 400 + 800 (= 1,200) dog-years at risk. The number of new cases observed didn't change (i.e., 42 dogs). The incidence density is then (42/1,200) × 1,000 = 35.0 for the 5-year period, or 7.0 on an average annual basis. This figure represents a more than 32 percent increase from the average annual age-specific incidence rate of 5.3 per 1,000 standard poodles.

3. Prevalence = Incidence Rate × Duration

For the dogs 2+ years of age, the incidence rate for 2010–2014 was 5.3/1,000 standard poodles per year and the average duration was 1.5 years. The annual average prevalence of the disease is therefore 5.3 × 1.5 = 8.0 cases/1,000 standard poodles per year.

For dogs less than two years of age, we cannot simply average the incidence rates as each stratum carries a different weight (number of dogs). Instead, we calculate the annual average incidence as ((11 + 13 + 28)/(250 + 700 + 1,400)) × 1,000 = (52/2,350) × 1,000 = 22.1 per 1,000 standard poodles per year. The average duration is 0.5 years. The annual average prevalence of the disease is therefore 22.1 × 0.5 = 11.1 cases/1,000 standard poodles per year.

4. a. 2015: A, B, D, E
        2016: A, B, C, D, E
    b. First six months of 2015: A, B, D
        Last six months of 2016: A, B, C, D
    c. 1 January 2015: A, B
        1 January 2016: A, B, D, E
        1 January 2017: A, C, D

5. a. Sensitivity: 36/(36 + 4) = 90 percent
        Specificity: 251/(9 + 251) = 97 percent
    b. Positive Predictive Value: 36/45 = 80 percent
        Negative Predictive Value: 251/255 = 98 percent
    c. Accuracy: (36 + 251)/(36 + 4 + 9 + 251) = 96 percent

6. Mean age of cases (c) = midpoint of age group of cases (a).
    Mean survival time if untreated (d) was reported in problem 3 as 0.5 years (6 months) for dogs less than 2 years (24 months) of age; 1.5 years (18 months) for those two years (24 months) of age or older.
    Expected age at death if untreated (e) = mean age of cases (c) plus mean survival time if untreated (d).
    Years of companionship lost (f) = average life expectancy of a standard poodle (12 years or 144 months) minus expected age at death if untreated (e) times the number of cases (b) divided by 12 months.
    The owners of standard poodles with untreated hypothyroidism in Dr. Run's country lost 737 years of companionship (YPLL) with their animals due to the disease.

A	B	C	D	E	F
			MEAN	EXPECTED	
			SURVIVAL	AGE AT	YEARS OF
AGE GROUP		MEAN AGE	TIME IF	DEATH IF	COMPANION-
OF CASES	NUMBER	OF CASES	UNTREATED	UNTREATED	SHIP LOST
(MONTHS)	OF CASES	(MONTHS)	(MONTHS)	(MONTHS)	(YPLL)
<2	11	1	6	7	126
2–11.9	13	7	6	13	142
12–23.9	28	18	6	24	280
24+	42	72	18	90	189
Total	94				737

DALY = YPLL + YLD

YLD (Years of life with disability) = (disability weight) × (number of cases) × (average duration in years).

We have to calculate YLD in two steps because of the differences in average duration of disease depending on age.

For poodles two years of age or older:

YLD = (0.6) × (42) × (1.5) = 37.8

For poodles less than two years of age:

YLD = (0.6) × (11 + 13 + 28) × (0.5) = 16.6

The total YLD is therefore the sum of the YLD for each of these two age groups,

Total YLD = 37.8 + 15.6 = 53.4

DALY = 737 (YPPL) + 53.4 (YLD) = 790.4 years (adjusted for disability and premature death lost to untreated hypothyroidism in dogs in Dr. Run's county during the most recent time period).

Chapter 9

1. a. High stress: (9/34,400) × 10,000 = 2.6 suicides per 10,000 students
   Low stress: (2/58,980) × 10,000 = 0.3 suicides per 10,000 students
   b. Relative Risk = Incidence rate among those with high stress/Incidence rate among those with low stress = 2.6/0.3 = 8.7.

      Interpretation: Students reporting high stress are 8.7 times as likely to commit suicide compared to those who report low stress.

      The magnitude of the relative risk suggests that the association is a strong one (i.e., greater than 3.0).
   c. The risk of suicide attributable to high stress = the incidence in the exposed group minus the incidence in the less exposed group = 2.6–0.3 = 2.3 suicides per 10,000 students per month.

      Interpretation: High stress accounts for 2.3 teen suicides per 10,000 students each month in the East Eagle's Neck School District.

2. a. The risk of suicide attributable to social isolation is 3.4–0.8 suicides per 10,000 students = 2.6 suicides per 10,000 students.
   b. The attributable fraction = attributable risk/incidence in the exposed group = 2.6/3.4 = 76 percent.
   c. The formula for the population attributable fraction is:

$$PAF = \frac{P(I_e - I_n)}{I_p}$$

P = proportion of the total population exposed to social isolation. This can be determined using the overall incidence of 1.1 suicides per 10,000 students per month; 0.8 among those not socially isolated, and 3.4 among those who are socially isolated:

$$(P \times 3.4) + ((1-P) \times 0.8) = 1.1$$

Solving for P, we find $P = 0.12$, or 12% of the total student population is socially isolated.

$I_e - I_n$ = incidence of suicide in those socially isolated minus incidence of suicide in those not socially isolated $(3.4 - 0.8) = 2.6$

(Also known as the risk attributable to the exposure)

I_p = incidence of suicide in the total population $= 1.1$

$$PAF = \frac{P(I_e - I_n)}{I_p} = \frac{.12(2.6)}{1.1} \times 100 = 28 \, percent$$

An alternative formula is:

$$PAF = \frac{P(RR-1)}{P(RR-1)+1} = \frac{.12(4.3-1)}{.12(4.3-1)+1} = \frac{0.4}{1.4} \times 100 = 29 \, percent$$

The difference between the two calculations of the PAF is due to rounding error.

d. Interpretation: Addressing social isolation issues in the total school population would reduce the suicide rate by 28–29 percent; it would reduce the rate of suicide among the students who are socially isolated by 77 percent.

Chapter 10

1. a. Odds Ratios
   For baseball pitchers compared with those having no school athletic activity:

   $$OR = (13 \times 70)/(7 \times 23) = 5.7$$

   For non-pitching baseball players compared with those having no school athletic activity:

   $$OR = (17 \times 70)/(13 \times 23) = 4.0$$

   For other school athletic activity:4
   $$OR = (22 \times 70)/(23 \times 40) = 1.7$$

   b. Since the control group is a random sample of the male adolescent population, the proportions of the total populations exposed to each activity are:

   Baseball pitchers $(Bp) = 7/130 = 0.05$
   Non-pitching Baseball Players $(Npbp)$: $13/130 = 0.1$

   Other School Athletic Activity (Osa): $40/130 = 0.3$

   The odds ratios are used as a proxy for the relative risk in the PAF equation.

   $$PAF_{Bp} = \frac{P(RR-1)}{P(RR-1)+1} = \frac{0.05(5.7-1)}{0.05(5.7-1)+1} = \frac{0.24}{1.24} \times 100 = 19 \, percent$$

   $$PAF_{Npbp} = \frac{P(RR-1)}{P(RR-1)+1} = \frac{0.1(4.0-1)}{0.1(4.0-1)+1} = \frac{0.3}{1.3} \times 100 = 23 \, percent$$

$$PAF_{Osa} = \frac{P(RR-1)}{P(RR-1)+1} = \frac{0.3(1.7-1)}{0.3(1.7-1)+1} = \frac{0.21}{1.21} \times 100 = 17 \ percent$$

Interpretation: Elimination of baseball athletics (or changes in how baseball was played to eliminate whatever in the game was causing these injuries) would reduce the occurrence of knee injuries by 42 percent (19 + 23 percent), even though only 15 percent (20/130) of the adolescent male population play baseball at school.

INDEX

Page numbers in *italics* indicate figures and tables.

American Association for Cancer Research, 34
American Cancer Society Hammond-Horn study, 36
American Statistical Association, 33
Amish, 161
Amniocentesis, 255
Analysis, cohort studies and, 187–188
Analytic studies, 15, 167–168. *See also* Experimental epidemiology; Observational epidemiology
Anecdotal case reports, 289
Animalcula, 23
Ankylosing spondylitis, 53
Anonymous data sets, 135
Antagonistic causal effects, 66
Antecedent causes of death, 75
Anthrax terrorist episode, 123, 125, 273
Applied epidemiology. *See* Field epidemiology
AREDS. *See* Age-Related Eye Disease Study
Arms of studies, 216
ART. *See* Assisted reproductive technologies
Artifacts, 59–60, 101–105, *102*, 106
Asbestos exposure, 4–5, 22, 67–68
ASDR. *See* Agency for Toxic Substances and Disease Registry
Aspirin, 215
Assessment stage, 272
Assisted reproductive technologies (ART), 113–114
Atomic Bomb Casualty Commission (ABCC) Studies, 173
Attack rates, 12–14, *14*. *See also* Incidence proportion
Attributable fraction, 179–181
Attributable proportion. *See* Attributable fraction
Attributable risk, 178–179
Attributable risk percent. *See* Attributable fraction
Australian Bureau of Statistics, 128
Australian Health Survey, 157
Autopsy rate, 76–77

Average life expectancy, 87
Avian virus (H7H9), 279–280

Babington, Benjamin G., 28
Bacillus anthracis, 273
Background rate of disease. *See* Endemic rate of disease
Barriers, 46
Bartlett, Elisha, 33
Baseline information, 234, 236
Bassi, Agosino, 23
Bath Breakfast Project, 225
Behavioral factors, 4, 48
Behavioral Risk Factor Surveillance Survey (BRFSS), 157
Belmont Report (1978), 222
Beneficence, 221
Benzene, 183
Berkson, Joseph, 199
Berkson's bias/fallacy, 199
Bernoulli, Daniel, 26
β-Error, 219–220
Beta-carotene, 215
Bias
    case-control studies and, 198–201
    cohort studies and, 184–186
    community and cluster randomized trials and, 234
    disease screening and, 251–255
    information, 185–186, 199–200
    interviewer, 199–200
    lead time, 252, *253*, 254
    length, *252*, 252, 254
    observer, 185
    overdiagnosis, 253
    publication, 226–227, 291, 294
    randomized controlled trials and, 226–227
    recall, 200
    selection, 184–185, 199, 234
    surveillance, 185–186
    in systematic reviews, 294
Bills of Mortality, 25
Biological factors, 4
Biological samples, 13
Biometrika, 33

Bioterrorism, 123, 125
Birth cohorts, 112–113, *113*
Birth data, 113
Birth outcomes, 112–113
Birth rates, 7
Births. *See* Natality
Birth to 20 Study, 170, *173*
Birth weight, 89, 160
Blinding, 200, 222
Block randomization, 222
Blood clots, 7
Bloodletting, 26
Bogalusa Heart Study, *172*
Bovine spongiform encephalopathy
    (BSE), 159
Bowditch, Henry I., 33
Bradford Hill criteria, 61
Breast cancer, 201–202
Bretonneau, Pierre-Fidèle, 23
BRFSS. *See* Behavioral Risk Factor
    Surveillance Survey
Bright, Richard, 28
Brill's disease, 153–154, *154*
British Birth Cohort Studies, *172*
British Doctors' Cohort Study, *172*
British Doctors Study, 36, 178–180, 184
British Medical Journal, 287
BSE. *See* Bovine spongiform
    encephalopathy
Budd, William, 30–31
Buffer zones, 46

C2. *See* Campbell Collaboration
Campbell, Donald, 289
Campbell Collaboration (C2), 289
Campbell Systematic Reviews, 289
Campylobacter spp., 15, 196
Canada Health Survey, 157
Canadian National Breast Cancer
    Screening Studies, 252
Cancer, 34. *See also Specific forms*
Cancer registry, 34
Cannibalism, 159
Cardano, Girolamo, 22
CARE. *See* Consensus-based Clinical
    Case Report Guidelines

Carriers, 44
Case-based registries, 121
Case-cohort design, 206
Case-control studies
    additional analyses for, 201–204
    bias and, 198–201
    confounding and, 205–206
    designing, 201
    design variations, 206–207
    Farr on, 29
    in hierarchy of evidence, 288
    measuring association in, 194–196
    misclassification and, 204–205
    overview of, 167–168, 193–194,
        207–208
    population attributable fraction
        and, 196
Case-fatality rates, 79, 273
Case-finding screening programs,
    120–121
Case series, 193, 289
Case tracing, 270
Causal association, 60
Causal criteria frameworks, 60–63
Causal factors. *See* Etiologic factors
Causal inference
    confounding and effect modification
        and, 63–66, *65, 66*
    legal and policy implications
        of, 67–68
    overview of, 59–63, *62*, 68–69
Causal pies, 62
Causal risk difference. *See*
    Attributable risk
Causation, correlation vs., 36
Causative agents, 269, 270
Causes of death, 25
Cause-specific death rates, 78–79
Cavities, 5–6, *6*, 9
CBPR. *See* Community-based
    participatory research
CDC. *See* Centers for Disease Control
    and Prevention; Communicable
    Disease Center
CDC WONDER, 75, 81
Censoring. *See* Data censoring

Decision trees, 257, *258*
De-identifying. *See* Recoding
Delafield, Francis, 33
Delta, 218, 220
Dementia, 159–160
Demographic and Health Survey (DHS)
    Program, 126
Demographic factors, 4
Demographic studies. *See* Descriptive
    studies
Dental caries, 5–6, *6*, 9
Descriptive studies, 10, 15, 71–72, 289.
    See also Vital statistics
Deterministic models, 63
DHS program. *See* Demographic and
    Health Survey Program
Diabetes mellitus, 8, 214
Diabetic retinopathy, 214
Diet, Cancer, and Health cohort study,
    187–188
Differential misclassification, 205
Diminished causal effects. *See*
    Antagonistic causal effects
Diphtheria, 23
Directly observed therapy (DOT), 224
Direct standardization. *See*
    Age-adjusted rates
Disability, morbidity statistics and,
    162–163
Disability-adjusted life years (DALYs),
    139–142, 162–163, 259
Disability programs, 119–120
Disasters, 273–274
Discordant pairs, 202
Disease etiology, theories of, 21–24
Disease registries. *See* Registries
Disease screening, 251–255
Disease surveillance programs, 7
Disinfectants, 32
Disparities, 1
DMC. *See* Data Monitoring Committees
Doctors without Borders, 270
Doll, Richard, 4–5, 35–36
Donabedian model, 259–260
Dopamine, 213–214
Dosage, 50

Dose-response effect, 29, 156
Dose-response relationships, 61, 177, 184
DOT. *See* Directly observed therapy
Double-blinded studies, 223
Down's Syndrome, 158
Drinking water, 5–6, *6*, 9
Drug abuse, 162
Duration, Farr on, 29
Dutch Famine Birth Cohort
    Studies, 173
Dynamics of spread, 45, *47*

Ears of the hippopotamus, 45
Ebola hemorrhagic fever, 270–271, *271*
EBP. *See* Evidence-based practices
EBPH. *See* Evidence-based public health
ECDC. *See* European Centre for
    Disease Prevention and Control
Ecological data, overview of, 10–11
Ecological fallacies, 11, 167
Economic status, 111–112, 182
Effect modification, 66
EHR. *See* Electronic health records
EIS. *See* Epidemic Intelligence Service
Electronic health records (EHR),
    125, 261
Embase, 291
Endemic rate of disease, 12, 152
Endemic typhus, 153–154, *154*
Endogenous factors, overview of, 39
English Privy Council, 268
Enhanced causal effects. *See* Synergistic
    causal effects
Enhanced surveillance. *See* Syndromic
    surveillance
Enhancing Transparency in Reporting of
    Qualitative Research (ENTREQ), 302
Environment
    in epidemiologic triad, 39–41, *40*,
        54, 297
    genetic factors and, 157
    population effects vs., 107
Epi-Aids, 268
EPIC Study, *173*
Epidemic curves, 12–13, 50–54, *51*,
    54–55, 270

Epidemic Intelligence Service (EIS), 268
Epidemics, 11, 24
Epidemiologic triad, 39–41, *40*, 54, 297
EPIET. *See* European Programme
    for Intervention Epidemiology
    Training
Epi Info, 275
Epstein-Barr virus, 43, 206–207
EQ-5D. *See* EuroQol Instrument
Equipoise, 223
Errors, data validity and, 129
Estonian Study of Chernobyl Cleanup
    Workers, 183
Ethnicity and race, 110–111, 159–161
Etiological studies, evaluating, 4–6
Etiologic factors, 4
Etiologic fraction. *See* Attributable
    fraction
Etiology, 1, 4
European Centre for Disease
    Prevention and Control
    (ECDC), 268
European Programme for Intervention
    Epidemiology Training
    (EPIET), 268
European Prospective Investigation
    into Cancer and Nutrition (EPIC
    Study), *173*
EuroQoL Group, 141, *263*
EuroQol Instrument (EQ-5D), *263*
Eurostat, 128
Evidence, Expertise, Exchange (3e)
    Initiative, 289–290
Evidence-based medicine (EBM),
    287–294
Evidence-based practices (EBP),
    250, 285
Evidence-based public health (EBPH),
    286–287
Examination data, validity of, 129
Examiner and Compiler of
    Abstracts, 74
Excess risk. *See* Attributable risk
Exclusion criteria, 218, 224
Exogenous factors, overview of, 39
Experiment, causal association and, 61

Experimental epidemiology, 9–10,
    301. *See also* Community and
    cluster randomized trials;
    Randomized controlled trials
Exposure assessment, 184
Exposure status, 183–184
External sources. *See* Exogenous factors
External validity, 182
Extremely low birth weight, 89
Extrinsic sources. *See* Exogenous
    factors

FACT-B. *See* Functional Assessment of
    Cancer Therapy, Breast
Factorial trials, 216–217
Fallacies, 11, 167
False negatives, *129*, 129
False positives, *129*, 130, 255
Familial clusters, 157
Familial hypercholesterolemia, 39
Family of International Classifications
    (FIC), 134
Farr, William, 28, *29*, 48, 74, 105, 112
Feasibility determinations, 272
Feline leukemia virus, 155
Fetal deaths, 88, 91, 112–113
FIC. *See* Family of International
    Classifications
Field epidemiology
    clusters and, 271–272
    disasters and, 273–274
    investigation process, 268–271, *269*
    overview of, 250, 267, 280
    rise of, 268
    surveillance and, 277–280
    terrorism and, 272–273
    tools of, 275–280
Field trials. *See* Community trials
Finland, 49
Finnish Cancer Registry, 252
Finnish Diabetes Prevention
    Study, 214
First National Cancer Survey
    (FNCS), 34
Fisher, Ronald A., 35, 36
Fixed effects model, 292

Healthy migrant effect, 105
Healthy worker cohorts, 124
Healthy worker effect, 183
Henle, Jacob, 23, 60
Henle-Koch postulates, 60, 69
Hepatitis, 182
Herd immunity, 1, 29, 48–50, 54,
    155, 158
HIE. *See* Health information exchanges
Hierarchy of evidence, *288*, 288
Hill, A. Bradford, 34, 35–36, 61
Hill's postulates, 61
HIPAA. *See* Health Insurance
    Portability and Accountability Act
Hippocrates, 21
Hiroshima, 52–53, 156, 182
Historical design. *See* Retrospective
    cohort design
History of epidemiology
    continued developments in, 33–34
    disease etiology theories in, 21–24
    early American efforts, 33
    London Epidemiological Society
        and, 28–31
    method development, 24–28
    modern, 34–36
    other European efforts, 31–32
    overview of, 21, 36
HIV (Human Immunodeficiency
    Virus), 43, 62, 159, 162, 254–255
Holmes, Oliver Wendell Sr., 33
Homogeneity, 294
Honest brokers, 135
Hospital-based disease registries,
    121, *122*
Hospital epidemiology. *See* Field
    epidemiology
Hosts, in epidemiologic triad, 39–41,
    40, 54, 297
Hot spots, 275
HPV. *See* Human papillomavirus
HRQoL questionnaires, 217, 261,
    262–263
HUI. *See* Health Utilities Index
Human immunodeficiency virus.
    See HIV

Human papillomavirus (HPV), 7, 161
Human spongiform
    encephalopathy, 159
Hygienic Laboratory, 34. *See also*
    National Institutes of Health
Hypercholesterolemia, 244
Hypocenter, 52
Hypothesis testing, 175

Iatrogenic illness, 260
ICD. *See* International Classification of
    Diseases
Iceberg phenomenon, 45
ICF. *See* International Classification
    of Functioning, Disability,
    and Health
ICHI. *See* International Classification
    of Health Interventions
ICMJE. *See* International Committee of
    Medical Journal Editors
ID. *See* Incidence density
ILSA. *See* Italian Longitudinal Study
    of Aging
Immunity, herd. *See* Herd immunity
Inapparent infections, 44
Incidence, 29, 135–138, 139
Incidence density (ID), 137, 176
Incidence proportion, 136, 139
Incidence rates, 136–137
Incidence studies. *See* Cohort studies
Incident rate. *See* Incidence density
Inclusion criteria, 218
Incubation periods, 50, 51, 54, 151
IND. *See* Investigational new drugs
Independent variables, 66
Index cases, 270
Indian Ocean Tsunami, 276
Individual factors, overview of, 10
Individual matching, 198
Individuals, descriptive studies and, 71
Induction period, 42, 44, 54
Inductive science, 61
Infant mortality rate, 91, 113
Infants, 89
Infectious period, 44, 54
Infectivity, 42

Inference of causality, 61, 67
Influenza, 39, 152–153, *153*
Information bias, 185–186, 199–200
Informed consent, 220–222
Infoveillance, 279
Initial contact and response, 272
Institutional Review Boards (IRB),
    75, 221
Institut National de la Santé et de la
    Recherche Médicale, 34
Intent to treat (ITT) population, 225
Interaction. *See* Effect modification
Internal sources. *See* Endogenous
    factors
International Classification of Diseases
    (ICD), 75, 103–104, *104*, 134
International Classification of
    Functioning, Disability, and
    Health (ICF), 134
International Classification of Health
    Interventions (ICHI), 134
International Committee of Medical
    Journal Editors (ICMJE), 216
International Standard Randomised
    Controlled Trial Number
    (ISRCTN) Register, 216
Inter-observer variability, 133
Interval incidence density. *See*
    Incidence density
Interventional trials, 213
Intervention epidemiology. *See* Field
    epidemiology
Interviewer bias, 199–200
Interviews, 184
Intra-observer variability, 133
Intrauterine devices, 175–176, 202
Intrinsic sources. *See* Endogenous
    factors
Investigational new drugs
    (IND), 215
IRB. *See* Institutional Review Boards
ISRCTN Register, 216
Italian Longitudinal Study of Aging
    (ILSA), 128
ITT population. *See* Intent to treat
    population

JAMA. *See Journal of the American
    Medical Association*
Japan, 49, 76
Jarvis, Edward, 33
Joint Policy Committee of the Societies
    of Epidemiology (JCP-SE), 67
*Journal of the American Medical
    Association* (JAMA), 287
JUPITER study, 214
Justice, 221
Justification for the Use of Statins
    in Prevention: an Intervention
    Trial Evaluating Rosuvastatin
    (JUPITER) study, 214
Justinian (Byzantine Emperor), 22

Kaplan-Meier approach, 226
Kappa (κ) statistic, 133–134
Kircher, Athanasius, 22
Koch, Robert, 23, 60
Koch's postulates, 60, 69
Kuru, 159

Laboratory investigations, 13
Langmuir, Alex, 268
Large-simple trials (LST), 227–228, 288
Latency period, 43, 44, 54, 186
Laws of epidemics, 24
Laws of mortality, 24, 25
Lead poisoning, 39
Lead time bias, 252, *253*, 254
Legal implications of causal
    associations, 67–68
Length bias, *252*, 252, 254
Leprosy, 22, 42
Leukemia, 52–53, 155, 183, 218
Level of significance (α), 219
Levin, Morton L., 36
Liability, causal association and, 67
Life Span Study, 182, 186
Lifestyle intervention trials. *See*
    Community trials
Life tables, *25*, 177
Lifetime prevalence. *See* Period
    prevalence
Likert-type scales, 133

Protocols, 217–218, 234

PsycINFO, 291

Publication bias, 226–227, 291, 294

Public Health Service Reye Syndrome Study, 194, *195*

Public health services, basis for, 7–8

Public Participatory GIS (PPGIS), 276–277

Publishing results of systematic reviews, 293–294

PubMed, 291

Pubmed Central, 291

Puerperal fever, 31–32

PulseNet International, 277

Purposes of epidemiologic inquiries, overview of, 4–8

P-Values, 175

QALYs. *See* Quality-adjusted life years

Quality-adjusted life years (QALYs), 139, 140–142, 162–163, 259

Quality Initiative in Rectal Cancer Trial, 243

Quality of care, 259–260

Quality of Reporting of Meta-analyses (QUORUM) Statement, 293

Quality of Well-Being (QWB) Scale, *263*

Quarantine laws, 22

Questionnaires, 184, 217

Quick and dirty surveys, 274

QUORUM Statement, 293

QWB Scale, *263*

Rabies virus, 43

Race and ethnicity, 110–111, 159–161

Radiation exposure, 52–53, 155–156

Radon, 188

Random effects model, 292

Randomization, 222

Randomized controlled trials
  clinical trials, 215–216
  conducting, 217–227
  crossover trials, 217
  evidence-based practices and, 286
  factorial trials, 216–217
  in hierarchy of evidence, 288

history of, 34–35

informed consent and, 220–222

limitations of, 227–228

overview of, 168, 213–215, 228–229

randomization and, 222

Randomized trials. *See* Community and cluster randomized trials; Randomized controlled trials

Rate and degree of immune response, 50

Rate ratios, 13. *See also* Relative risks

RCC. *See* Renal cell carcinoma

Reading epidemiologic literature, 285, 299–300

Reasoning, sequence of, 10–11

Recall bias, 200

Recoding, 135

Record linkage, 134

Recruitment, 218, 235–236

Rectal cancer, 243

Reference population, 218. *See also* Control groups

Refractory disease, 218

Registrational trials, 216. *See also* Phase III trials

Registries, 34, 121–123, *122*, 216

Relative risks, 66, 174–176, *175*, 193, 292

Reliability, 128, 132–134, 224–225

Religion, 161

Remote sensing, 276

Renal cell carcinoma (RCC), 217

Reporting results, 285, 301–302

Reproducibility, 128. *See also* Reliability

Research Ethics Committees, 221

Reservoirs, 46, *47*, 153–154, 270

Respect for persons, 221

Responsiveness of epidemiology, 297–298

Restriction, confounding and, 64

Results, cohort studies and, 187–188

Retrospective cohort design, 169–170, *170*, *173*, 183

Reye's syndrome, 193–196, *195*

Rheumatic fever, 154

Ring-vaccination technique, smallpox and, 48

Risk, defined, 178
Risk difference, 292
Risk estimates, 91–92
Risk ratio. *See* Relative risks
Roswell Park Memorial Institute, 36, 200
Royal Society of Medicine, 36
Royal Statistical Society, 28
Rumors, 279–280
Rush, Benjamin, 23

Salicylate, 193–196, *195*
Salk vaccine, 7
Salmonella spp., 15, 44, 46, 52
SAMPL. *See* Statistical Analyses and Methods in the Published Literature
Sample size, 218–220
SARS. *See* Severe acute respiratory syndrome
Satellite imagery data, 276
Scarlet fever, 23
Schizophrenia, 228
Scope of epidemiology, Farr on, 29
Screening programs, morbidity statistics and, 120–121
Scrutinium Pestis (Kircher), 22
Scurvy, 26
Seasonal distributions, *152*, 152, 157
Secondary attack rate, 139
Secondary cases, 270
Secular trends, 101–106, *102*, *104*
"Seeds of contagion," 22
SEER registry, 124, 156
Selection bias, 184–185, 199, 234
Selective factors, 107
Self-reporting, 128–129, 132–133
Sellafield cluster, 155–156
Semmelweis, Ignaz, 31–32
Sensitivity, 129, 130, 156, 255
Sensitivity analyses, 225
Sentinel health events, 124
Sentinel surveillance, 123, 124, *126*, 277
September 11, 2011 terror attacks, 123, 125, 274
Sequence of epidemiologic reasoning, overview of, 10–11

SES. *See* Socioeconomic status
Severe acute respiratory syndrome (SARS), 48, 125, 278
Seveso Women's Health Study, *173*
Sexual behaviors, 162
Sexually transmitted infections, 162. *See also Specific infections*
SF-36. *See* Short Form Health Survey
Shapefiles, 275
Shattuck, George C. Jr., 33
Shattuck, Lemuel, 33
Shiga toxin-producing *E. coli* (STEC), 15
Shigella spp., 15, 277
Shoe leather epidemiology. *See* Field epidemiology
Short Form Health Survey (SF-36), *141*, 261, *262*
Sicily conference, 287
Sickness Impact Profile (SIP), *262*
Sickweather.com, 278–279
Silkworms, 23
Simon, John, 28, 268
Single-blinded studies, 222
SIP. *See* Sickness Impact Profile
Skew,of the epidemic curve 50
Skoda, Joseph, 31
Slone Epidemiology Center, 200
Smallpox vaccination, 23, 26
Smallpox virus, 42, 46
Smith, Stephen, 33
Smoking, 5, 8–9, 35–36, 62, 157, 174, 178–180. *See also* Tobacco
SMR. *See* Standardized mortality ratio
SNOMED CT, 103–104
Snow, John, 28–30
Social class. *See* Socioeconomic status
Social contagions, 48
Social epidemiology, 112
Social media, 278–279
Socioeconomic status (SES), 4, 111–112, 182
Sojourn period, 42, 44, 54, 252
South Korea, 253–254
Space, 155–157
Special populations, 181–182
Specific death rates, 78–79, 156

Weighted odds ratios, 202
Wennberg study, 260
West Nile virus, 277
Whitehall Study I and II, *172*, 182
WHO. *See* World Health
    Organization
WHO-FIC. *See* World Health
    Organization Family of
    International Classifications
WONDER website, 75, 81
World Health Organization (WHO), 75,
    88–92, 134, 216, 240
World Health Organization Family
    of International Classifications
    (WHO-FIC), 134
World Population Standard for
    2000-2025, 85
World Standard Population, 85
World War II, 221
Wynder, Ernst, 36

Xerophthalmia, 241
X-ray exposure, 53

Yaws, 46
Years of life with disability (YLD),
    140, *141*
Years of potential life lost (YPLL),
    87–88, 140
Yellow fever, 23, 46
Yelp, 279
Yersinia spp., 15
Yield. *See* Positive predictive value
YLD. *See* Years of life with disability
YPLL. *See* Years of potential life lost

Zaire ebolavirus, 270
Zero time shift bias. *See* Lead time bias
Ziprasidone Observational Study of
    Cardiac Outcomes (ZODIAC), 228
Zoonotic diseases, 270